D1256193

WITHDRAWN

Contemporary American Leaders in Nursing

AN ORAL HISTORY

GWENDOLYN SAFIER, Ph.D.

McGRAW-HILL BOOK COMPANY
A Blakiston Publication

New York St. Louis San Francisco Auckland
Bogotá Düsseldorf Johannesburg London
Madrid Mexico Montreal New Delhi Panama Paris
São Paulo Singapore Sydney Tokyo Toronto

*This book is dedicated to
the memory of my father,*
JOSEPH W. STYRVOKY . . .
a man of great courage and generosity.

*Contemporary American Leaders in Nursing:
An Oral History*

1 2 3 4 5 6 7 8 9 0 KPKP 7 8 3 2 1 0 9 8 7

This book was set in Helvetica Light by National ShareGraphics, Inc.
The editors were Orville W. Haberman, Jr. and Elysbeth H. Wyckoff;
the designer was Nicholas Krenitsky;
the production supervisor was Angela Kardovich.
Kingsport Press, Inc., was printer and binder.

Library of Congress Cataloging in Publication Data

Safier, Gwendolyn.
    Contemporary American leaders in nursing.

    "A Blakiston publication."
    1. Nursing—United States—History. 2. Nurses—United States—Interviews. I. Title
[DNLM: 1. History of nursing—United States. 2. Nurses—United States—Biography. 3.
Leadership. WY11 AA1 S2c]
RT4.S23   610.73′092′2   [B]   76-46352
ISBN 0-07-054412-3

Contents

Preface

Contemporary American Leaders in Nursing: An Oral History is intended to supplement courses in nursing history, women's history, and studies of leadership in general. The book presents a number of American nursing leaders who were selected by their peers and who, through the medium of oral history, give accounts of their careers.

This book was written for several reasons. At the present time there is a paucity of books available on the recent history of American nursing. Although nursing as a profession has undergone profound changes since World War II, neither the changes themselves nor those persons instrumental in bringing them about have received sufficient public recognition or scholarly attention. Many of the changes resulted from the new directions taken by nursing leaders. This book is based on interviews with seventeen wartime and postwar nursing leaders.

The interviews illuminate some of the principal areas of change and showcase the specific contributions, along with brief biographical sketches, of these notable leaders.

Oral history is defined here as interviews with knowledgeable people, recorded on tape. It seems to be an ideal tool of inquiry, since it gives each leader an opportunity to relate her experience within the context of the profession's development. The author is a trained nurse and has had previous interviewing experience in a psychiatric clinic. In addition, her doctoral dissertation in sociology employed the tool of oral history to present the work of one eminent woman sociologist. Furthermore, she has had the privilege of knowing some of the outstanding nursing leaders who were getting on in years, and it seemed a meaningful venture to document in their own words their thoughts and feelings about their leadership roles and their opinions on sometimes controversial issues.

Contemporary American Leaders in Nursing: An Oral History fills a need in history-of-nursing courses and leadership courses at both undergraduate and graduate levels. Increasingly, history-of-nursing courses are being developed and introduced into curricula. Nurses are becoming more interested in their history, perhaps because of such factors as the "youth" of the nursing profession, the growing popularity of historical research, and the recent emphasis on feminist studies. History of nursing is rapidly becoming a popular area of research, and an increasing number of articles and books relating to the subject will probably be published within the next few years.

This book is different in three essential ways from other history-of-nursing texts: (1) The approach is that of oral history. (2) The primary focus is the living individual leader and her contribution; that is, the trends and issues are discussed only as they relate to the particular leader. (3) The time covered is limited to the last few decades in the United States. This book is in no sense presented as an exclusive historical source. It is meant as a corroborative guide and is, therefore, a beginning. The purpose is to provide discussion and to further an interest not only in nursing history but in women's history in general. It is hoped that what is presented here will give present nurses and nurses of the future a sense of heritage as well as knowledge and pleasure. Examples of leadership and leadership technique will have significance for women's studies and for anyone concerned with leadership in general. In addition, this book will have relevance to anyone who is interested in examples of the struggles of women to achieve and to contribute in a male-dominated world.

ACKNOWLEDGMENTS

I wish to thank the following individuals who have given me much support and encouragement: Fred Safier, Ph.D., a relative and dear friend; Mrs. Willa K. Baum, Director of the Regional Oral History Office, University of California, Berkeley, for her wise counsel; Lucile F. Newman, Ph.D., Brown University, Rhode Island, for her insight and delightful chats; Marie C. Behm, M.D., a friend of over twenty years; to my editors, Cathy Dilworth Somer, who is much more than an editor, and to Betsy H. Wyckoff; to my typists, Mary Ann Holstein and Mrs. Joan Kapsimalis; and to the nursing leaders who participated. I also want to thank the individuals who took the time to read the various chapters and who gave helpful, critical comments. Special thanks is given to Jessie M. Scott, Assistant Surgeon General, Director, Division of Nursing, Public Health Service, Department of Health, Education, and Welfare, who read the chapter on Leone, to Marion Sheehan Bailey, the chapter on Freeman, and to Anna M. Fillmore, the chapter on Nahm. Several of the leaders portrayed in this book appeared originally in shorter form in *The Oral History Review, 1975.* I am grateful to that publication for permission to reprint portions of the material. I am grateful to the American Nurses' Foundation for a grant which enabled me to travel to different geographical places in the United States to meet with the nursing leaders and to the University of California, San Francisco, for granting me one quarter's sabbatical leave and several research grants which helped me conduct my work.

I want to thank my son, David, who was burdened with excessive responsibilities for his years and who with "good cheer" put up with my many trips away from home.

Gwendolyn Safier

Introduction

Historical Background

World War I provided the necessity to expand the supply of nurses in the United States and led to the organization of the Army School of Nursing in 1918.[1]

Feminism surged in the 1920s; women finally won the right to vote, and they sought emancipation from restrictive modes of conduct and morality. They were beginning to enter some professions but not in any large numbers. The societal expectations were that a woman's ultimate goal should be marriage. Teaching and nursing were accepted women's occupations but were looked upon only as a stopgap until marriage and a family, or as "security" if a woman's husband died or if she did not get married at all and had to earn her livelihood at something respectable.

World War II produced a crisis situation and the responsibility of recruiting and training a massive work force of nurses. The U.S. Cadet Nurse Corps was launched in 1943 with the passage of the Bolton Act, in response to the urgent need for more and better-trained nurses to meet the wartime emergency. Under the terms of the Bolton Act, the Corps was granted a $60-million appropriation to subsidize scholarships and subsistence grants to attract prospective cadets. Lucile Petry Leone designed and directed the Corps. It was a landmark in the development of American nursing, for it marked the first time federal money was allocated for nursing education.

---

[1] The Army School of Nursing was designed as a wartime measure. Because the war might last a long time, it was thought that nurses ought to be prepared to supplement the civil nurses who were available to enter military service. There were 10,000 applicants for the Army School of Nursing, and 2000 were accepted. There were 500 in the first graduating class in 1921, the largest class of nurses graduating at one time in the world's history. Although designed for wartime, the school continued into the postwar period and was discontinued in 1932 for economic reasons. For a brief overview of the school, see Josephine A. Dolan, *Nursing in Society*, W. B. Saunders Company, Philadelphia, 1973, p. 268.

1

According to one account, between 1944 and 1946 the Corps over-saw the education of some 170,000 cadets, who constituted 90 percent of the total enrollment in nursing programs for those years and nearly doubled the number of nursing students previously enrolled. Indeed, as the study explains, "This was a remarkable achievement, considering the competing appeals for women war workers at this time and the difficulties met in expanding the teaching, clinical housing, and other facilities needed for these enlarged quotas."[2]

Many forces operating in society created changes that influenced nursing. There had been the passage of the Social Security Act in 1935 (amended in subsequent years), which influenced the expansion of health programs and services.

One major event in nursing was the unification in 1952 of several nursing associations into the National League for Nursing (N.L.N.). Men started to enter nursing. There was an influential study of basic nursing programs, commissioned by the National Nursing Council and conducted and written by Dr. Esther Lucile Brown, a nonnurse anthro-pologist.[3] She recommended that if society's future nursing needs were to be met, the profession would have to prepare two types of nurses: professional and vocational. This recommendation, along with the en-tire report, provoked a spirited controversy within nursing circles, but ultimately the National Committee for the Improvement of Nursing Serv-ices (N.C.I.N.S.) was established to implement the Brown plan. The committee agreed that improvements in nursing services could not re-sult without a noticeable upgrading in nursing education. The Brown study had been based on visits to fifty representative schools, and the committee broadened the inquiry to encompass all state-approved schools of nursing in the United States. Questionnaires were mailed to these institutions, and the data collected were subjected to statistical analysis. Schools were ranked according to certain agreed-upon crite-ria relating to curricula, faculty preparation, student welfare, finances. The highest 25 percent were classified as Group I schools, the middle 50 percent as Group II schools, and the lowest 25 percent as Group III schools. Lists of the schools in Groups I and II were then published in the *American Journal of Nursing (A.J.N.)*.

In 1949 the National Nursing Accrediting Service (N.N.A.S.) was in-stituted, and Dr. Helen Nahm was appointed its first director. "For the first time in history the nursing organizations [the N.C.I.N.S. was re-

[2] Isabel M. Stewart and Anne L. Austin, *A History of Nursing*, G. P. Putnam's Sons, New York, 1962, p. 221.

[3] Esther Lucile Brown, *Nursing for the Future*, Russell Sage Foundation, New York, 1948.

sponsible to the joint board of directors of six national nursing organizations] had had the courage and the strength to make public their knowledge about the status of nursing education programs in the United States."[4]

Different types of nursing programs were being initiated, for example, the two-year junior college program. There still were a number of three-year hospital diploma programs, but professional nursing education was moving into the colleges and universities. In fact, the American Nurses' Association (A.N.A.) in 1965 took the position against opposition that to turn out a professional nurse, nursing education should be housed in institutions of higher learning.[5]

Methodology

Oral history is a relatively new phenomenon in American historiography, and a note about its development, purpose, and procedures may serve to put this book in perspective.[6]

Oral history is defined as a technique of collecting information on recent events by interviewing knowledgeable people, recording the data on magnetic tape, and keeping it available for the use of researchers. The interviews are structured in question (interviewer) and answer (interviewee) form from preplanned interview guides.

There has been oral history for centuries, but it was in 1948 that the term "oral history" was used by Professor Allan Nevins, a historian at Columbia University, to refer to his systematically conducted interviews. Professor Nevins is considered the pioneer in advocating this tool. The interviews should gather material that not only will meet the immediate needs but will be broad enough in scope so that the edited transcript will be of value to researchers in the future.

As Benison points out, *oral history is in an important sense misnamed* because, although the oral historian gathers oral memoirs, "it is equally true that such an account is based on a written record."[7]

[4] Dr. Helen Nahm to author, Feb. 19, 1974. For a judicious treatment of the entire question of accreditation, see William K. Selden, *Accreditation: A Struggle over Standards in Higher Education,* Harper & Brothers, New York, 1960.

[5] A.N.A. Position Paper, 1965. For the current status of programs, consult the National League for Nursing, Division of Nursing Education, 10 Columbus Circle, New York, N.Y.

[6] There is a growing oral history movement in the United States, which started about 1948 with Professor Nevins's work and is expanding rapidly nationally and internationally. In 1967 the Oral History Association, a national association, was organized at Columbia University. The present membership is over one thousand. For a succinct account of oral history, see Gwendolyn Safier, "Answer to What Is Oral History?" *Nursing Research* (in press). See also Gwendolyn Safier, "'I Sensed the Challenges': Leaders among Contemporary U.S. Nurses," *The Oral History Review,* 1975, pp. 30–58.

[7] Saul Benison, *Tom Rivers: Reflections on a Life in Medicine and Science,* The M.I.T. Press, Cambridge, Mass., 1967.

The interviewer has to plan the interview guide from primary and secondary sources. The final transcript that results from the taped interviews may have to be edited and reedited many times until it says what the subject wants it to say.

There is the advantage of the *interaction* between the interviewer and the interviewee, so that in-depth probing may be done.

The oral history material can be used to "improve upon the record"[8] for future scholars. Also, by getting a subject to talk in his or her own words, the interviewer hopes to capture to some extent the personality and conversational style of the person. It is the position here that even the best oral history interview cannot serve as a substitute for traditional reading and archival research. Both the interviewer and the interviewee should be well prepared.

Oral history has its limitations. One is that the interviewee material may be too subjective. The assumption is that the subject is giving honest answers, but the issue of confidentiality is raised and must be respected.

Oral history is an extremely time-consuming tool, and it is expensive in terms of money and energy. The interviewer frequently has to travel long distances to meet with the subject, and the interviews may range in length from a few hours to several hours over a period of days. The cost of transcribing the tapes is not negligible.

The sample of nursing leaders was selected during the summer and fall of 1973 by the reputation method. This method permitted other nurses to determine who is a leader and why. First, a letter outlining the project's research objectives was sent to all deans and directors of accredited nursing education programs and to presidents, executive directors, and chairpersons of professional nursing organizations and national commissions; their cooperation was requested. Specifically, they were instructed to list the names of thirty living American nursing leaders at present in or near retirement, and to indicate the reasons governing their selections. Respondents were asked to keep all areas of nursing—administration, research, education, and practice—in mind. To encourage candor, they were assured confidentiality for their choices.

The rationale for choosing the leaders by reputation was that it seemed to provide more appropriate evidence than a listing drawn from

[8] *Ibid.*, p. ix.

Who's Who, a reference work that excludes many nursing leaders, or one compiled from professional publications, since quality of research alone does not determine a leader's qualitative contributions to the development of the profession. A strength of the method was that it allowed respondents to indicate why they chose the individuals rather than imposing a strict set of criteria for their selections. A possible shortcoming of this approach was that respondents may have had a conscious or unconscious tendency to compromise their professional judgment by displaying inordinate consideration for friends.

Out of 432 letters sent, 345 responses were received. The thirty names most frequently cited were then compiled into an alphabetical list, which was subsequently sent to sixty nurses picked at random from the original list of 432. Each respondent was asked to rank the top sixteen, a number chosen to accommodate time and funding limitations.

After the sixteen leaders were determined,[9] each one received a letter in which the author identified herself, informed the leader that she had been selected for a study, asked if she could be interviewed in depth, and requested that she forward her photograph and curriculum vitae to help prepare specific interview questions.

General questions of a biographical nature were designed for all interviewees: What is your family background? What early childhood experiences were influential in your life and career? What type of education did you receive? Why did you enter nursing? How was your education financed? Did you ever desire to leave nursing and take up something else? Did you ever want to switch from nursing to medicine? What do you consider your unique contributions to nursing? What do you consider your failures? What obstacles, frustrations, and disappointments did you encounter? What help did you get along the way? What do you consider the most critical decisions you have made? What impact did these have? What social and personal conflicts did you have? How did you resolve them? What are your work habits? What is your life-style? What do you consider the biggest changes in nursing? Where do you think nursing is going? What, if anything, would you now do differently in your life if you had the opportunity? What was your first

[9] Before commencing any interviews, the author was required to submit fifteen copies of her entire research protocol and procedure for approval to the University of California, San Francisco, Committee on Human Subjects and Experimentation. The committee recommended that a provision be included whereby if any subject became tired and desired to discontinue her participation in the project, she could. Upon inclusion of this provision, the research plan was approved Sept. 12, 1973.

leadership position? How did you get it? Did you ever feel discriminated against? By whom? Why did you stay (or, if you left, leave)? If married, did you ever feel that your home life was neglected because of your career? If unmarried, did you ever want to get married and have a family? Did you ever feel that you had to make a choice between marriage and a career?

Next, a list of specific questions was prepared relative to each leader's career. These were formulated after the author scrutinized the leader's curriculum vitae, did preparatory reading about her and her activities, and engaged in informal conversations with people who had worked with her or who knew her well. A list of general and specific questions was forwarded prior to the actual interview. Each interviewee was told the interviews would be taped and the interview time would run approximately one-half hour to two hours. All were assured that interview material would be kept strictly confidential and that each interviewee would be sent a copy of the transcript. Should the leader desire, she could select one other person familiar with her career to read and comment upon the edited transcription.

Fourteen of the sixteen leaders[10] agreed to be interviewed. Of these, one became too ill to participate and another later decided to discontinue her involvement in the project. There was then space to add two more leaders. The next *three* names on the list were chosen because all lived in the same geographic region of the country (the East) and only one trip would be necessary. Therefore, the total number is seventeen.

The definition of who was a leader emerged from the respondents: a nurse whose ideas and activity had produced a major impact upon the course of nursing.

Each leader has only one category after her name, although many of the early nursing leaders by necessity had multiple roles, such as administrator, educator, and clinician, either simultaneously or sequentially. Each one was asked how she would categorize herself with only one label in one area. Her selection always correlated with the reason the respondents had chosen her.

The length of the interviews varied in accordance with the two primary factors: (1) the extent and variety of the individual's activities and (2) how well prepared and organized the individual was for the interview.

A word about what this book is *not*. It is not meant in any way to be

---

[10] While the sample selection was in process, two nursing leaders, Margaret Arnstein and Katherine Dolan, died. Both were included by many respondents.

exclusive or inclusive. There are *seventeen* leaders represented; therefore the length of each chapter is limited. Several leaders by nature of their stature and accomplishments could warrant a biography each. A few selected aspects of major events in American society and nursing are touched upon briefly to place the leaders in perspective. The focus is a number of American nursing leaders whose strong leadership helped to shape nursing into what it is today. By no means did they operate in a vacuum.

Let the leaders speak for themselves.

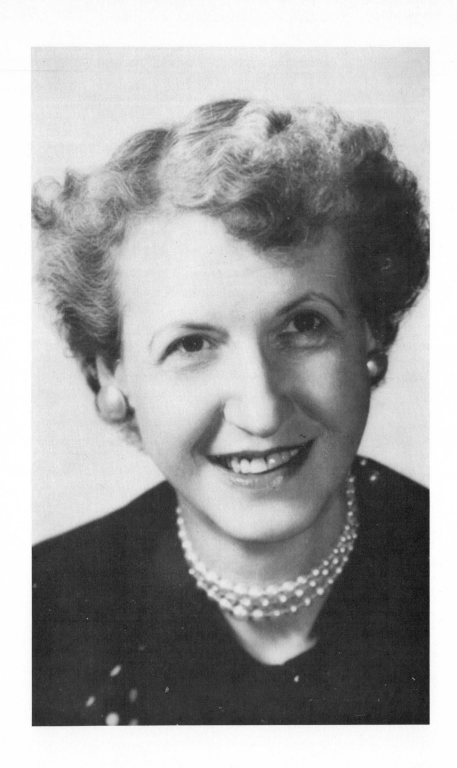

1

. . . For outstanding leadership and
contributions to the nursing care of children
through creative nursing, inspirational
teaching, distinguished clinical research and
excellence in professional writing.[1]

[1]Award from the American Nurses' Association, Division of
Maternal-Child Nursing Practice, June 1974.

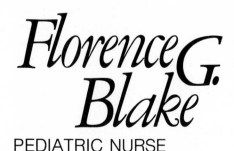

Florence G. Blake

PEDIATRIC NURSE

*F*lorence Blake is a tall, distinguished-appearing woman who devoted her life to improving the nursing of children. She was a pioneer in teaching the importance of understanding children, parents, and co-workers when providing care for children.

Florence G. Blake was born November 30, 1907, in Stevens Point, Wisconsin. Her background was middle-class. Her father was a Baptist minister who had been educated as an Episcopalian minister in England, and her mother was a talented musician who taught music and played the pipe organ in church. Florence Blake was the younger of two girls, and she looks back upon a "pretty happy" and "very active" childhood. She grew up always knowing that she would be a nurse. When she graduated from high school, she went to the Michael Reese Hospital School of Nursing in Chicago because it was considered to provide the best clinical experience. She graduated and received her registered nurse diploma in 1928. Following graduation she worked as an instructor and head nurse at the hospital, where she later became a supervisor of pediatric nursing. She stated that in all her earliest experience in the care of children, she felt inadequate and in need of more education; she perceived that the behavior of sick children was complicated and was undoubtedly a response not only to illness and treatment but also to their relationships with their parents and hospital caretakers. Today there is a sophisticated stance regarding the psychological development of children, but at the time Florence Blake was a student and a young, inexperienced supervisor, a psychological orientation to the care of sick children was nonexistent. Florence Blake knew intuitively that a hospital for children should provide an understanding and nurturing environment. The only way she knew to achieve this was to quickly develop rapport and happy relationships with the children, the parents, and the professional staff.

To prepare herself, she obtained a B.S. in teaching at Teachers College, Columbia University. In 1942 she received an M.A. in child development from the University of Michigan. Some of the credits for the degree were earned at the Merrill-Palmer School in Detroit. Later she was invited to be part of the first group of lay people to study at the Institute for Psychoanalysis, where, in 1951, she received a diploma in psychoanalytic child care.

In addition to her positions at Michael Reese Hospital, she was on the faculty of the School of Nursing at the Peiping Union Medical College and at the University of Michigan, Yale University, and the University of Chicago. In 1963 she established a graduate program in pediatric nursing at the University of Wisconsin, Madison, and after retirement in 1970 she became a professor emeritus.

Florence Blake has served on many panels relating to child care and, in addition to being a consultant, has presented papers at professional meetings. Her textbooks in pediatric nursing[2] were among the first to appear in this field.

Into Nursing

GS: What made you decide to go into nursing?

FB: My first memory of a wish to be a nurse came after my father had an operation to remove gallstones. I can picture myself at about six years of age changing the abdominal wound dressing. I am not sure whether this is fantasy or an actual memory, but I surmise that it had an impact on the development of my interest in hospitals and nurses. Being a minister, my father visited sick people in the hospital and I often accompanied him on these trips. My uncle was a surgeon in a nearby town, and in both my own and his home I heard much about medicine and nursing. There was never any doubt in my mind that both my father and my uncle thought that nursing was a great profession, with preparation that every woman should have.

My sister attended the hometown normal school to prepare herself for teaching. Neither teaching nor a hometown school intrigued me; I wanted to get into a hospital as quickly as I could, take care of people, and travel as my father had done extensively before coming to America. I felt certain my father wanted me to study nursing. He had accompanied me to Chicago to be interviewed by several directors of nursing, and was interested in all details of my preparation for nursing school.

GS: How did the Great Depression affect you, if at all?

FB: It didn't affect me at all. I was in my first position as a graduate nurse and earning $100 a month with room, board, and laundry. I had so much more money than I had ever had before; I felt rich and able to save money so that I could go on to school.

GS: Did you like nurses' training? Were you ever ambivalent about it?

---

[2] *The Child, His Parents and the Nurse*, J. B. Lippincott Company, Philadelphia, 1954; with Philip C. Jeans and W. Rand, *Essentials of Pediatrics*, 4th ed., J. B. Lippincott Company, Philadelphia, 1946; with Philip C. Jeans and F. Howell Wright, *Essentials of Pediatric Nursing*, 7th ed., J. B. Lippincott Company, Philadelphia, 1963; with F. H. Wright and E. Waechter, *Nursing Care of Children*, 7th ed., J. B. Lippincott Company, Philadelphia, 1970.

FB: At one point I was terribly discouraged. Student nurses carried heavy assignments of patients, and I was nearly ready to quit. Mother suggested I change schools and go to a Baptist school of nursing in Minneapolis. My father came to visit me in Chicago and took me out to dinner, and my fatigue and anger vanished. I stayed, and especially enjoyed my senior year. No, I'd say I liked every service but pediatrics. My dislike of that service was due to the supervisor, not to the children. She was deprecating, critical, and completely insensitive to our problems in dealing with sick children and their parents. I had always liked children and babysat with them often, and remember vividly my enjoyment of play when I was a child. I collected dolls and every kind of prop I needed for house play.

GS: What was it, then, that brought you back to your active interest in children?

FB: After my first year of study at Teachers College, I was supervisor of a private pavilion for adults. I was twenty-one then, and wonder now how I ever thought I could cope with that much responsibility. Because I had disliked pediatric nursing so much when a student, I never dreamed of supervising the care of sick children; but when the pediatricians asked to have me replace the supervisor I'd had when a student nurse in pediatric nursing, I decided to do it, after much deliberation and assurance of support from the Director of Nursing. During the first year of supervision in pediatric nursing I learned to enjoy the experience but felt a great need for more education, clinical practice, and work with healthy children.

GS: And yet, here you are, considered to be one of the leading contributors in the area of pediatric nursing. Did you stay with it, then, from that time on?

FB: Yes, I never wanted to do anything else. The more education I got, the greater the challenge became.

Major Contribution

GS: What do you see as your major contribution to nursing?

FB: I think probably it was helping students to discover the value of ongoing study of children and parents in the planning and evaluation of nursing care.

GS: Will you elaborate on that?

FB: While at Yale University School of Nursing I served as chairman of a National League of Nursing Education (N.L.N.E.) committee to plan an advanced course in pediatric nursing then in 1946 I went to the University of Chicago to establish one of its first two advanced clinical courses in nursing. Having been on the N.L.N.E. committee was indeed helpful to me in meeting my responsibilities in Chicago, but I soon discovered that teaching graduate students required more preparation than I had had. I knew they needed depth of knowledge and exposure to new kinds of clinical experiences. They also needed other kinds of supervision than I had had. When I was invited to enroll in a program of study which was being developed for persons outside the medical profession at the Institute for Psychoanalysis, I seized the opportunity with enthusiasm, even though I knew all classes would be held in the late afternoon and evening. Before going to Yale in 1942 I had had experience in teaching children in nursery schools, and felt that it had increased my understanding of children and improved my skill in nursing. Therefore I felt that study of psychoanalytic child care would give me more insight into patients' behavior and provide the kind of experiences I had been searching for in the schools I had already attended.

The three-year program of study at the Institute was exceedingly valuable. My concept of nursing broadened, and my respect for the role that nurses could play in the prevention of ill health as well as in the care of sick people increased considerably. I had an opportunity to study with members of several professions, and being the only nurse in the group, I had many opportunities to present case material from observation in the wards and clinics and to get help in understanding the behavior of the children and parents with whom my students and I were working. Discovering how interested my classmates and teachers were in nursing was, of course, satisfying. That was one of the factors which prompted reevaluation of the role that nurses were playing in the area of family health. I remember vividly the first time I was asked to discuss nursing with my classmates. Because I thought case material would enrich and enliven my presentation, I observed a toddler ambulating about a ward for an hour and a half, without interacting with her. This experience brought life to my presentation and more importantly, it opened my eyes to what could be learned from observation of children and parents in both in- and outpatient services of the medical center. At the end of ninety minutes the toddler I was studying was in anguish. She was so desperately in need of help, I had to intervene. The experience was a revelation to me! This child sought help from every adult in the ward and made contact with some of them several times; yet none of them responded in a way which changed the behavior I had interpreted to be the outgrowth of loneliness, fear, and helplessness. This experience saddened me and told me again how much more we nurses needed to learn to fulfill more adequately the needs of sick children. It also stimulated the development of a plan for the study of patients and for involvement of my students in nursing activities they had never experienced before. The initial plan was revised many times, as was the curriculum for presentation of theory and direction of clinical study. Questions from clinical experiences motivated my students and me to identify elements of nursing care which we could test in our attempt to reduce children's distress from illness and from treatment and care in the hospital. A method which evolved from clinical experiences of this kind is illustrated in the study of Suzie, which I did while at the University of Chicago.[3]

One of the most exciting parts of the program for students at the Institute was the study of patients to whom we were assigned. In individual weekly conferences, the student's study and plan of therapy for each patient were closely supervised by faculty members—Helen Ross, Dr. Emmy Sylvester, Dr. Irene Josselyn, and Dr. Adrian Van der Veer. I had all of these people as supervisors during the three years. They were outstanding teachers and stimulated me to expand continually the content for advanced courses in pediatric nursing. It wasn't long before I became convinced that study of patient-nurse and nurse–child patient relationships could increase the quality of nursing care and also become a tool which nurses could use to enhance their personal and professional growth.

GS: When you say children, what age are you referring to?

FB: The whole age range from earliest infancy through adolescence.

GS: Within that age range, did you have any preference?

FB: I think I really enjoyed most working with toddlers and preschoolers; and yet, when I studied school-agers and adolescents, I found them mighty challenging and enjoyable too.

GS: Why do you suppose you preferred toddlers and preschoolers?

FB: Probably because they seemed most in need of care. Outwardly they certainly appeared to need more help from nurses than did most older children. Young children in the hospital taught me so much about responses to separation and identified so clearly their needs for care when they were ill and confronted by fearsome new experiences. From

---

[3] *Open Heart Surgery in Children: A Study in Nursing Care*, U.S. Maternal and Child Health Service, Rockville, Md., 1964.

observation of the nursing care of many young children, I felt sure that continuity of nursing care given by their own mothers, as by nurses the children came to identify as their own, was the most important factor in minimizing anxiety from illness and hospitalization. After revising the section on nursing care of adolescents for the seventh edition of *Essentials of Pediatric Nursing*, I had greater awareness of the problems confronting adolescents when they are chronically ill, subjected to periods of life in a hospital, or both. I decided that they needed nearly as much help in the hospital as younger children do to protect their potentials for optimal character development.

GS: Did you notice in your work with children whether or not there were differences between those children who came for operations and those who were in the hospital because of an acute or chronic illness? Were there differences in their reactions to the hospital experience?

FB: That would be difficult to say because there are so many variations in the way children react to each part of a new situation. So many factors influence the way children perceive and react to both new and familiar parts of any experience: age, physical and psychological resources, past experiences at home and in the hospital, type of treatment measures used, parental response to their children and their own current life situation, degree of illness, type of preparation before admission, and, not of least importance by any means, the quality of physical and emotional support available to children and the degree to which they can make use of it. Experience leads me to believe that all hospitalized children live with some degree of fear, anger, disappointment, and guilt. Too often they never know what is going to happen next. Even when they've been prepared for treatments, and so on, the experiences they are subjected to often turn out to be quite different from what the children had imagined they would be like. Or the nurses the children expected to be with them weren't available when needed the most. In such instances trust is easily lost, and children can quickly become disappointed in, and furious with, their caretakers. Young children just don't have the inner resources needed to cope with separation and other frightening experiences unless they have continuity of care from their own mothers or from trusted nurses who have become of significant importance to them.

GS: Would you say that your major contributions in the area of child care have dealt with identification of problems that children confront in the hospital and of those elements of nursing care which supported their struggle to cope with them? Would you hold workshops to teach the hospital staff?

FB: Yes, I participated in many institutes which were held in various parts of the country. My greatest interest was in finding ways to prevent children from being traumatized in the hospital. My goal was to help students to use their eyes, ears, head, and heart to provide nursing care which would make illness and hospitalization a growth-producing experience for children rather than one which left them with residual feelings of fury, fear, guilt, and anxiety. Psychoanalytic theories of child development and guidance increased my insight into behavior and the needs of both healthy and sick children. Classwork at the Institute also heightened my interest in studying parents of handicapped and chronically ill children. Study of expectant parents and of parents of young infants also became a challenge. My interest in maternity nursing was kindled while studying at the Institute and at Lying-In Hospital, Chicago, and I perceived tremendous potential in it for the prevention of health problems. But before we could intervene effectively, we had to identify the problems people had during the maternity cycle and to discover the elements of nursing care which promoted growth in preparation for parenthood and enjoyment of parental roles after the delivery. We didn't call pregnancy and delivery "crises" in those days, but study of couples during the maternity cycle made us aware of the fact that they weren't as happy as we expected them to be. I was always aware of suffering in pediatric units, and I wanted to become more helpful to both children and parents. When in school before, I was always searching for courses which would help me to become a better nurse and develop content for the courses I was teaching. The more I observed the outcome of the nursing care my students provided, the more convinced I became of the importance of skillful nursing during the kinds of crises met by nurses in the field of maternal and child health nursing. My purpose in writing was to share what I had learned with nurses so they could lighten the burden not only of sick children but of other family members as well.

GS: *Did any of your work at that time consist of preplanning—getting together with the family before a child's hospitalization for elective surgery, for instance, or for special medical treatment which was planned far ahead of time?*

FB: At the University of Wisconsin, Madison, we often did this. Students worked with selected chronically ill and handicapped children and then their parents for a long time, sometimes throughout the entire period students were in school. Students knew when another period of hospitalization or a clinic visit was scheduled, and it was planned for with child and parent. Usually students met new patients in the lobby and assisted parent and child in coping with the clinic visit or in adjusting to an initial or another period of hospital life.

GS: How would you get your ideas across, and how did you approach administration to get the nursing and medical staff to cooperate with you? Wouldn't they sometimes say to you, "Well, that's fine, but you're not working here. You don't know how busy we are; go mind your own business."

FB: Yes, I've heard similar statements on quite a few occasions. If such comments weren't made directly to me, I surmised that such thoughts were in the minds of the staff from observing their behavior in response to my suggestions or activity with parents and children in the ward or clinic.

Yes, I had many problems—far more at the University of Chicago than at the University of Wisconsin, Madison. At both of these universities, graduate programs in pediatric nursing were the first to be established. That in and of itself made for many of the problems I had. When I went to the University of Chicago in 1946, there was only one other graduate program in pediatric nursing in the country, and the Children's Hospital at the University of Chicago had never been used for students of nursing at either the baccalaureate or the graduate level. Yes, problems were knotty and painful. Yesterday, while anticipating your visit, I recalled many experiences associated with establishment of graduate programs. I wondered how I had ever lived through them.

GS: Could you give a specific example of how difficult it was?

FB: The staff at the University of Chicago couldn't understand why students were assigned to only one child at a time and for the entire period of the child's hospitalization. Head nurses thought assignments of patients should be changed daily so the children wouldn't become attached to students. They also thought assignment to five or six children would increase the students' knowledge and skill and certainly heighten the level of their efficiency. But I knew from experience it would be difficult, if not impossible, to learn to study children and to use observational data to plan and evaluate nursing care if field work was planned as assignments were being made for staff nurses. Some doctors thought students should be assigned to a ward and be placed under the direction and supervision of the head nurse, who would make patient assignments, teach, and evaluate student performances. This, however, wasn't the opinion of doctors and nurses at the University of Wisconsin, Madison. In fact, the situation was totally different from what I found it to be in Chicago. There, the doctors often requested that a specific child and family be assigned to a graduate student. After conferences with the students, this was usually done because it provided rich experience in expanding skill in collaborative activity, not only with the doctor but with other team members as well. None of the pediatricians at the University of Wisconsin, that I know of, ever criticized the size of student assignments or suggested that parents not be made a part of the team providing care for their children. Yes, we had problems at Wisconsin, but most of them resulted because there were students from several disciplines working with the families that came to the medical center for in- and outpatient care. Teams were large, and coordinating activities of all types of personnel and establishing common goals was indeed a difficult and time-consuming process. There were other reasons why problems were fewer and more easily resolved at the University of Wisconsin. In the first place, I didn't make the same mistakes I had made in my first experience with graduate students. For example, infinitely more planning was done with the medical and nursing staffs in my second experience than in my first. In Chicago I was unsure of myself. I didn't know what the content of graduate education in clinical nursing should be. I was feeling my way at the University of Chicago. I was attempting to increase my understanding of the families which used the university health services and to determine how and in what ways the nurse's role could be expanded. I was also trying to identify the kinds of educational experiences graduate students needed to play a more significant role in the prevention of disease and in strengthening physical and psychosocial resources during family crises associated with child health problems, hospitalization, and the maternity cycle. As a consequence, plans and goals weren't as easily defined when I was teaching at the University of Chicago as they were while I was teaching in Wisconsin.

GS: Was your formal role at that time as an instructor?

FB: Yes. I had no administrative responsibility or authority to make changes except while teaching at the Peiping Union Medical College and Yale University. At the University of Michigan and the University of Chicago there was no direct route for problem solving with nursing service personnel either. Until I received my master's degree from Merrill-Palmer School, Detroit, and the University of Michigan, I had been a supervisor (administrator) as well as an instructor of pediatric nursing. Then, while at the University of Michigan School of Nursing, I was given only teaching responsibilities. I never had such a miserable, frustrating year. That was the year Dean Rhoda Reddig began to separate teaching and administrative responsibilities. All administrative responsibilities were delegated to the head nurses in the pediatric department, and their power with doctors and nursing service personnel increased.

Upon arrival I took over the responsibility of assignment, teaching, and evaluation of student nurse performances. I did this without first learning how the teaching program had been carried out in the past, from other faculty members or from the head nurses. Little wonder the head nurses were critical of my educational methods, and perhaps also envious of the teacher-student relationships which were established. Now I can see why head nurse–instructor relationships were so disharmonious. We were all deprived of satisfactions we'd enjoyed previously. I was deprived of the pleasures I'd had as an administrator and instructor in Peiping. While there I'd had doctors, nursing service personnel, and students looking to me for help in difficult clinical situations. Nursing service personnel wanted and needed my approval as much as the students did. They were dependent upon me for recommendations and promotions, and I presume this heightened their motivation to learn from me. No such experiences were forthcoming at Michigan. I was stripped of a title which had previously given me duties I'd enjoyed. Previous to my arrival at Michigan, head nurses had assumed major responsibilities for the students' clinical experience. They made assignments, taught them how they wanted procedures and routines carried out, and evaluated their performance as it related to the nursing staff's need for speed and efficiency. This no doubt gave them security, feelings of competence, and also prestige in the eyes of students and doctors. In retrospect the dynamics of the situation seem simple to me now. Had I perceived them then, perhaps I could have worked out plans with the head nurses which would have protected the students' needs for sound educational experiences and promoted our professional growth as well. I feel sure the care of the children would have been greatly improved too.

GS: Would you say you had a great deal of what is called "role conflict"?

FB: My, yes. I never heard that term in those days. If I had I probably wouldn't have understood it anyway. Even if I had understood the term, I'm not sure that I was mature enough then to make replanning a growth-producing experience for us. Dr. McQuarrie, whom I worked with in Peiping, became Professor of Pediatrics before my arrival at the University of Michigan. One of the reasons I took the position at Michigan was because I had enjoyed working with him in Peiping. He too had trouble with the staff nurses in Michigan. Their loyalty was to the previous Professor of Pediatrics, who continued to have a place on the faculty and medical staff. Everyone was under strain and on edge most of the time, so it was a year of minimal productivity as far as I was concerned.

GS: How did you resolve some of your problems?

FB: None of the above problems got resolved. I took flight at the end of a year and went to Yale University as Supervisor and Assistant Professor of Pediatric Nursing.

GS: Did someone invite you to Yale?

FB: I think I made application there, but I'm not sure of this. Being at Yale was as different from being at the University of Michigan as night is from day. All of the students at Yale had degrees, many of them master's degrees; others had Ph.D.'s. It was a superb experience. I never worked harder nor enjoyed teaching as much. Head nurses in the pediatric wards needed help when I arrived. There was an epidemic of diarrhea in the premature population, and I was able to make needed changes at once. There was little resistance to change; medical and nursing staff wanted it. Dr. Grover Powers was Professor of Pediatrics. They didn't come any better than he. Dr. Edith Jackson, a child analyst, was there, too, to plan the rooming-in unit for the maternity department as well as to do therapy with children. She was of great support to me as I set up meal, rest, and play programs on the wards, which were similar to those in the nursery schools where I'd been a practice teacher. This was done not only to improve the care of the children but also to give the students an opportunity to observe and interact with groups of children having experiences which were specially planned for them. Students observed in the Gesell nursery school and also functioned in the ward activity program. They thoroughly enjoyed the experience, and the program did a great deal to make the hospital environment more appropriate for the learning of children, students, and nursing services personnel. Parents appreciated it, too, and often functioned as teachers, as did the students. I did not fully comprehend the value of play for hospitalized children at that point in time. Intuitively I knew that play preparation for new experiences, the case method of assignments, group meal periods, and so on, would make life more comfortable and productive for the children, but I didn't have any theories or research findings to back up my convictions. I acquired those later, when studying at the Institute in Chicago. Both Dr. Powers and Dr. Jackson supported me in what we were doing, and the students seemed infinitely more comfortable with the children after they'd had experience in the hospital activity program. Head nurses resisted this addition to the educational program when it was first introduced in 1943, but it wasn't long before they and the staff nurses began to participate in and learn from it.

After four satisfying years at Yale I was invited to the University of

Chicago to establish advanced courses in my specialty. Again I had no administrative responsibilities, and the situation with nursing service personnel was similar to what I'd lived through at Michigan. I could see similarities in the two situations; yet I could see differences, too. The head nurses and the supervisor of pediatric nursing in Chicago had not worked with students at either the baccalaureate or the graduate level. Their first exposure to students was to those with degrees, and this was perhaps a threat to them. Only when one of our graduates became supervisor did conflict end. She knew the goals of the advanced clinical courses, she had profited greatly from study of patient care, and she wanted to participate in the teaching of graduate students. Head nurses who were interested to learn soon replaced those who had "run" the pediatric department since it opened in 1929–1930. When the pediatricians learned that I had been invited to be a member of the first class in psychoanalytic child care, I noticed a marked change in their relationship with me.

GS: *Would you say you had more resistance from the nurses or from the physicians at the University of Chicago?*

FB: It's hard to say. Before one of our graduates became the supervisor of pediatric nursing, doctors and nurses seemed allied in their criticism of our activities. I think head nurses went to the pediatricians with criticism rather than expressing it directly to me. Staff nurses didn't believe that nursing care included observation of children, preparation for treatments, support during potentially traumatizing experiences, interviewing parents, or the institution of self-regulatory schedules of feeding for babies. Provision of continuity of nursing care during the maternity cycle was designated as a "frill," and rooming-in for mothers and newborns was considered to be completely unnecessary to prepare parents for greater enjoyment of their infants at home.

Early in my experience at the University of Chicago (1946–1947) we used an orthopedic unit for field study. In this instance I feel certain that it was the head nurse who prompted the Professor of Orthopedics to tell me that I couldn't use his ward unless I assigned students to the head nurse and let her make their activities similar to those carried out by staff nurses.

GS: *How did you cope with this?*

FB: I could see no other solution but to remove students from the unit. I wasn't going to have patient assignments changed every day. Nor could I approve of assignments to large groups of children, making it impossible for students to improve their ability to sustain relationships with children and parents. The students at the University of Chicago were mostly from hospital schools. They had had wards of children assigned to them for evening and night duty; they had been "medicine" and "treatment room" nurses, and so on, and needed a different kind of clinical experience than they'd had previously. My focus was on study of children and their families, with opportunity to test methods of intervention to reduce fear and anxiety and to support constructive problem solving. Observation in the medical center had proved to me that purposefully planned nursing care could make a difference in the kind of experiences children had while they were ill or in the hospital for correction of a physical handicap.

GS: Since you received so much opposition in working situations, did you ever feel at times like giving up?

FB: Heavens, yes!

GS: What kept you in Chicago?

FB: Probably Dr. F. Howell Wright, the Professor of Pediatrics with whom I revised a textbook of pediatric nursing several times. We got to know each other in these collaborative experiences. We discovered what we each believed in. We learned the concept we had of each other's professional roles and discussed values, treatment measures, hospital policies, and resistance to change in persons working in obstetrics and pediatrics. Having a graduate of our program of study as Supervisor of the Children's Hospital made a great difference in all relationships throughout the department. Then I discovered that staff nurses wanted help, too, and also exposure to some of the experiences the students were having. I hadn't surmised this from their behavior, but if I'd been more astute, I'm sure I would have tried more methods of reaching them than I did. It wasn't until one of the staff nurses had the courage to share her thoughts with me that light began to dawn. She said, "We're jealous of your students' having all the supervision they have from you." Then, of course, I began to focus more attention on them, and changes in the behavior of staff nurses began to appear. As a consequence I was infinitely better prepared to understand the needs of staff nurses at the University of Wisconsin, Madison, than I was of those in Chicago.

GS: In working with students and nursing service personnel, are you saying that in the beginning of your career in teaching graduate students you were trying to increase awareness of children's and parents' problems, feelings, strengths, and needs, and then later you were trying to motivate students and staff to participate in the changing of policy routines, and methods of providing care?

FB: Exactly. At first students and I were so engrossed in the study of patients' behavior, to determine their problems and needs, and of our own feelings, thoughts, and responses to the persons with whom we worked, that we couldn't see the forest for the trees. Later I began to suggest to students that they share what they were learning about patients and their families with nursing service personnel and other members of the team. When students also began to share the purposes of their nursing care with others, the staff began to perceive the rationale for studying patients, and participated more actively in planning nursing care than they had previously.

GS: Would that be an appraisal, then, of your major contributions in child care?

FB: Yes, the clinical experience (field study) which took place in homes, clinic, and medical center had many objectives, another of which was to provide opportunities for students to increase their skill in collaborating with others. Quickly the students learned from experience that collaboration was worth the time and effort it took. They couldn't help but see improvement in the quality of care that their families received.

GS: You mentioned that your students used play materials in giving nursing care so their patients could have more opportunities to deal constructively with the feelings that were aroused by illness and care in the hospital or clinic. Would you comment more about this?

FB: Yes, providing time for play with hospital equipment, dolls, raw materials such as clay, paste, and paint, and other appropriate toys, as selected by the student, was considered to be an essential part of each child's plan of care unless there was an acute illness which depleted the child of energy for play.

GS: Was a personal psychoanalysis a prerequisite for admission to the program of study at the Chicago Institute?

FB: Yes, for the first group of students invited to register for the program. I didn't have a complete analysis, but I had psychoanalytically oriented therapy, which was very helpful to me.

At the Institute we studied theories of play and had the help of our supervisors in interpreting the play of the children we had in therapy. I had a three-year-old boy and a nine-year-old girl assigned to me soon after the program began. Later a mother was assigned to me when her child was being treated by a classmate.

GS: *Where did you get these children?*

FB: They were assigned to us at the Institute and we provided therapy hours for them there.

After studying the theories of play and observing the use children made of them in their hours of therapy at the Institute, I could see many ways that nurses could use play materials in the provision of nursing care. While in the children's ward of the Peiping Union Medical College, I learned a great deal about play from the children who could be out of bed. They spent hours playing hospital with dolls and cribs used in the care of premature infants. They begged to use hospital equipment like syringes, catheters, emesis basins, tongue blades, ether masks, and so on. I watched their play with great interest, never dreaming they were providing themselves with self-directed play therapy. Yet their absorption in it told me it was mighty important to them. Had I been able to understand Chinese better, I probably would have learned more about the purposes it was serving for them. However, having already observed Chinese children at play in the hospital, I could see sense in an analytical theory of play. Thereafter, opportunities for self-directed play became a regular part of the students' plans for nursing care.

GS: For example, if a child were coming into the hospital for an operation, how would you use play in the provision of nursing care?

FB: Each student had a skate case, which was equipped with a family of dolls, hypodermic syringe, needles, medicine cups, Band-Aids, sponges, cotton balls, tongue blades, paper, paste, scissors, bandage, ether mask, and stethoscope. When the student learned that other equipment would be used in the care of the child, it was added to the supply of equipment used for play.

GS: What are skate cases?

FB: They are inexpensive, gaily colored suitcases used to transport skates. Students didn't have to scramble about to get appropriate items for their patients to play with; they had them easily available to use. They took the case of toys to the bedside each day so the children could learn that their nurses understood their play, and to take steps in solving their problems. When an operation was scheduled, the student learned what preparation the parents had provided for admission to the hospital and for surgical treatment. Then the child was introduced to the use of the toy case in a way which encouraged freedom to use its equipment in a self-directed way.

When the student learned that further preparation was needed for preoperative medication or for anesthesia or for what the child would see, feel, and be subjected to postoperatively, bits of information were introduced as the child was able to listen and make use of the preparation that was provided. Unless the operation was an emergency, there was usually time to gauge the speed of preparation to the child's ability to make use of it in play in mobilizing the child's resources to cope with fearful events. Dolls were made of sponge rubber, so giving them hypodermic injections was simple. Hypodermic syringes and needles were used by the children more often than any other equipment, and it was remarkable how much the children had learned from observation of their caretakers' activities.

GS: So the purpose of this was to familiarize the child with unfamiliar equipment and details of the situation that would be confronted in the future. Is this correct?

FB: Yes, and to give children the opportunity to ask questions and talk about the preparation and treatment they already had, if they were able to use this method of reducing their worry and fear of oncoming events. At this time the students also made an effort to assure children and parents that they would be there when the children got their medicine, so they wouldn't feel it when, for example, the child's heart was being fixed. Teaching children ways in which they could help themselves before and after an operation was also a part of the preparation. We learned, too, that most children needed assurance that this nurse would be with them when they awakened from anesthesia. Periods of self-directed play were also provided postoperatively to assist children in assimilating the events which had taken place. At the University of Wisconsin we also had a playroom where students could take their patients to play. They scheduled time for its use so as many children as possible could use it. There was a telephone there, and calls to the home were often made, which kept the children in closer touch with their family when parents had to be away from Madison.

GS: Is there anything you want to add about your major contributions?

FB: Provision of weekly supervisory conferences with students, relating to problems they were having learning to plan and provide supportive nursing care during crises, was a learning experience for all of us. Soon after the establishment of advanced clinical courses at the University of Chicago, process recordings became a part of student experiences with families. Supervisory conferences and recordings of therapeutic sessions with patients were important learning experiences for me at the Institute. With some variation, they became useful to students of nursing as well. Courses in supervision given by Charlotte Towle in the School of Social Work guided me in providing supervision for nursing students, as did conferences I had with an unusually well trained supervisor of social work students. With this help I was more able to provide helpful educational experiences for students when they were struggling with problems in interpersonal relationships with children, parents, or other members of the health team.

At the University of Chicago some of my colleagues thought limitation of admission to six students per year was a mistake, but personnel in the Children's Bureau understood what I was trying to do and knew that large classes would make it impossible to meet the students' or my objectives.

GS: It sounds to me as if you had stimulation and encouragement from many highly qualified, outstanding people.

FB: That is so very true. I was indeed fortunate to be invited to study with the first group admitted for study of psychoanalytic child care. They were unusually well-prepared classmates who contributed much to my learning. As I said before, the faculty at the Institute was an inspiring group of people who were mighty interested in the progress of their first group of students. In each university where I taught, there were people who were generous with their time and interest and supportive of our efforts to provide advanced preparation for nurses. Faculty associated with nursery and laboratory schools cooperated enthusiastically when we expressed the need of our students for observation and practice-teaching experience with healthy children. Personnel in selected community agencies also assisted wholeheartedly in providing advanced preparation for students of nursing.

GS: As a result of your insight into the need of nurses for understanding of human development and behavior in health and during crises associated with disease and disability, have there been other schools of nursing which used nursery schools for student experience?

FB: I hope I influenced curriculum change so nurses receive better preparation for doing preventive work than they used to get. So many people have had an impact on the curriculum changes which are being introduced today. In 1933 my adviser at Teachers College couldn't understand why a nurse would want courses in child development and practice teaching in nursery schools. However, Grace Langdon, Professor of Early Childhood Education, understood and supplemented my education further by giving me experience in a home where two healthy preschoolers needed care while their mother taught for short periods in a nursery school. That was a great experience—one I wouldn't have wanted to miss.

University of Wisconsin

GS: *Were you invited to come to the University of Wisconsin, Madison?*

FB: Yes. One of the many reasons I chose to teach there was because the pediatricians were assembled to greet me when I arrived for interviews. They shared with me their special interests in research and establishment of a graduate program in pediatric nursing, and they assured me of their readiness to teach in Wisconsin's first graduate program for nurses. I found them to be as helpful and enthusiastic with the productivity of graduate students as I had expected them to be. I rectified the mistakes I'd made in Chicago. Or perhaps it would be more correct to say that the design of the program at Wisconsin evolved from study of past experiences and the educational needs of graduate students. During the years 1946–1958, students came to the graduate program with infinitely more knowledge of disease and pathophysiology than of the behavioral sciences. Content for teaching advanced courses in maternal and child health nursing was limited. As a consequence the students and I were absorbed in the study of human growth, development, and behavior and in determining ways in which the study could be used to expand our role in the delivery of primary and secondary health services for families. I didn't negate the importance of physical care and knowing the scientific principles upon which it is based, but there was a limit to what could be accomplished in a program as short as the one at Chicago. Before going to Wisconsin, I was aware that our graduate program needed more emphasis on the ways in which disease affects the bodies of children at different age levels, and on preparation to increase skill in appraising the responses of the body to disease and in providing the particular kinds of support the body needs in its fight against disease. The faculty in Madison was agreeable to a broader program of study than we'd had in Chicago. Most of the students came to the graduate program in Wisconsin from baccalaureate programs, with greater depth of knowledge in both the biological and the behavioral sciences. When graduate courses in these sciences were provided, we could discern student progress in fulfilling an extended role in the delivery of health services for families. This was especially observable in the work of those students who chose to take the practicum in the clinical-specialist role during the last two months of the two-year program.

Inclusion of advanced content in the biological sciences threatened me at first. I wanted very much to master the knowledge the students were acquiring, but I had neither the foundation nor the time needed to absorb it. Anxiety vanished when I realized how much I wanted nurses to get the knowledge they needed to gain expertise in carrying out an extended role in the delivery of health services. I certainly did not want to do anything which would prevent our students from going beyond what their teachers of nursing had already accomplished. In designing the curriculum, we hoped some of our graduates would be able to assume a leadership role in designing new and more effective kinds of health services for families.

Teaching at the University of Wisconsin was a joy, but it would have been more satisfying if I had not been director of the graduate program as well as the developer of the graduate courses in nursing. At first I enjoyed this amount of responsibility, but when enrollment and the number of committee meetings increased, there was little time left for the supervision of practice in the field. Patient population in the University Medical Center differed markedly from the population in the University of Chicago hospitals. In the University of Wisconsin hospitals there were few acutely ill children. Most of them were chronically ill, handicapped, or both. They were in the hospital for long periods, and family situations were often complex and complicated. Students needed a great deal of supervisory help in planning care for them in the hospital and at home. Frustration mounted when clinical supervision and time with nursing service personnel had to be reduced to the barest minimum. Those were the experiences from which my stimulation for continued learning and the challenge of teaching came. Without contact with the clinical field, frustration increased and motivation for teaching became less and less. I was glad when retirement time arrived. I felt sure I'd find plenty to do and become as deeply involved in other activities as I had been in nursing.

Major Publications

GS: *What are some of your major publications, and what impact did they have?*

FB: I think the first book I did alone contributed the most. That was *The Child, His Parents and the Nurse.* I had revised *Essentials of Pediatrics* with Dr. Jeans, of Iowa, twice before writing it. Dr. Jeans didn't want so much growth and development in his book, nor was he enthusiastic about inclusion of content relating to emotionally supportive nursing care. When he suggested I cut content in prenatal care to three paragraphs, I decided to do a book of my own so I could control its content. When Dr. Jeans died, I chose F. Howell Wright, M.D., to work with me on revisions. I think it has influenced nursing care. I certainly hope it has. Perhaps *Open Heart Surgery in Children: A Study in Nursing Care* contributed more toward helping others perceive what is meant by nursing process and the value of the case method of assignment for children and their families and for nurses, too. I enjoy most writing about the children and parents with whom I've worked. They have taught me so much and have been the source of much of my inspiration and motivation to learn and to change policies and procedures in hospitals and clinics for the care of mothers, fathers, and children.

Major Issues

GS: *What would you say have been the major issues in nursing during your career, and what has been your role and your own particular relation to them?*

FB: The issues which were most important to me in my role as teacher of nursing grew out of these questions: Should parents be permitted to visit daily? Should hours for visiting be extended for children? Should experience with families during the maternity cycle be a part of graduate programs in pediatric nursing? Should fathers be allowed in delivery rooms and be permitted to have close contact with their wives and newborns? Should mothers room in with their newborns and their sick children? Should all schools of nursing be a part of a college or university? Should the case method of assignment to patients be instituted?

Should research or acquisition of increased knowledge of clinical nursing receive priority in graduate programs? Should children's nurses be allowed to be with them while being anesthetized and in the recovery room with them thereafter? Should teachers have any administrative authority in clinical units? How should clinical supervision be provided for students of nursing at the baccalaureate and graduate levels? Should all faculty be required to do pure research for promotion?

The issue I have discussed most was the pros and cons of empirical versus experimental research. In Chicago and also in Madison, the case method of research wasn't valued as highly as I thought it should have been. My students and I were always searching to verify the description of development and the interpretation of behaviors we read about. Theories and methods of child guidance and counseling didn't mean much to me until I had tried them out and learned from repeated experience that they had usefulness in the provision of nursing care. However, if I had my life to live over again, I'd take courses in research. I'd also get involved with persons who could help me design and carry out studies to provide evidence to demonstrate a need for changes which I believe should have been made long ago.

GS: *It seems to me that you've been very involved with improvement of patient care. That is applied research. Why did you want to study pure research?*

FB: Because ideas take root more quickly when statistically proven findings are available to support hypotheses relating to change.

GS: *But you had the ideas—and that's the important thing—but not the research tools.*

FB: Right. I didn't have the tools I needed to do pure research. I have a tremendous amount of observational data which will never be used because it wasn't collected in a systematic way under controlled conditions.

GS: *Would you classify that as a current issue in nursing?*

FB: Yes. So many persons believe that all faculty should be involved in pure research. Personally I can't believe that productivity grows from coercion or constant reminders that research is necessary for promotion. I'm glad I wasn't exposed to that until I came to Wisconsin, or I might never have written anything. I recall the energy expended in gripe sessions after faculty meetings which were weighted with pressure to do research. I used to hypothesize that more research would be done if the energy dissipated in coercion would be diverted into study of how time could be made available to faculty members who had already identified problems worthy of, and appropriate for, controlled research. Faculty who are interested in doing research should have support in doing it, but I can't see why every faculty member must be cast into the same mold. Is this really the best use of the varied, unique talents observable in faculty members? Other activities might contribute more to safeguarding family health than do some research studies. Shouldn't this be studied too? I would like to see some of our best-prepared faculty become more involved in nursing service than they are today. Maybe then some of the stumbling blocks to our professional growth might vanish. I wouldn't want to see the faculty of the school assuming the same administrative responsibilities supervisors carried in the past. That would be inappropriate use of nurses with advanced degrees. Teachers and nursing service personnel have a great deal to share with one another, and I think progress could be made faster if we could all learn to work together.

I'm convinced that graduate students need tools and motivation for continued learning; but I trust that their programs of study don't get so heavily weighted with research methodology that there is no time or energy left to acquire the competence, self-respect, and confidence which seem to me to be necessary ingredients of effective collaboration with colleagues in all professions. Isn't it also important for researchers? Now that pure clinical courses are being offered at the baccalaureate level, it seems even more important to make room for intensive clinical study at the graduate level. I just hope the felt needs and goals of graduate students aren't being overlooked when changes are made in program designs.

GS: What is your view of those who presently advocate such concepts as nurse-practitioner and physician's assistant?

FB: I wish there weren't so many different categories of nurses. It's confusing, especially to lay people and others on health teams. I can't quite see why settings should determine the titles provided for nurses. I think educational experiences to help nurses learn to make thorough physical assessments of patients are great. Nurses need data derived from physical assessments of the persons with whom they're working, regardless of their physical status. Nursing diagnosis and plans for care or for continued health supervision require it. We've glossed over the area of preparation for planning patient care in the recent past, and I'm delighted to learn that more thorough preparation for making total health assessment is being provided. I just hope nurse-practitioners are doing nursing and not just doing those procedures and routines delegated to them by doctors. I don't see why physicians' assistants should be a threat to nurses. I'd much rather see them meeting physicians' needs for help than for nurses to do it. I say this because I know there are many people in our society who need the kind of help that well-prepared nurses can provide.

GS: Do you think it's a sellout to nursing to get someone to go and hang up a sign "Nurse-Practitioner?"

FB: No, I don't think so. There's no doubt in my mind that nurses have always been able to do more than they've done in the past, and they can learn to do much more nursing than they're doing now. They'll succeed, too, if they are smart enough to know their limitations, to use consultation freely to help people get what they need, to respect their strengths, and to make honest evaluations of their work a continuing process.

GS: Do you think physicians and nurses are becoming more competitive than they were previously?

FB: Yes, I think so. Certainly nurses and doctors need to become better acquainted with one another's values, role definitions, goals, and methods used to reach them, and with each professional's unique contribution in the delivery of health services. Conflict and competition in doctor-nurse relationships consume so much energy which should be invested in effective collaboration to achieve optimal care of people. I think there's a great deal of anxiety in doctors about where nursing is trying to go.

GS: Where would you like to see it go?

FB: I'd like to see nurses expand their role to the limits of their capacity. They can do a great deal more in the prevention of all types of disease than they have in the past. There is plenty for all professional workers to do which isn't being done well enough now. Nurses can play a significant role in rehabilitation and in helping people learn how to protect themselves from disease and from further disability if they already have a chronic disease. People need so much more knowledge about their disabilities and the purposes of the treatment prescribed than doctors are giving them. If they got it, they would be much better prepared to help themselves and would value themselves more highly as a consequence. I don't think young married couples are getting the help they need today, when problems of all kinds seem to have multiplied. So much time is being devoted to the care of aging citizens in the community. Heaven knows they need it and should have it, but young families in the throes of child rearing also need much more help than they're getting. Raising children today is a tremendously difficult task, and parents are reaching out for the kind of help nurses can become prepared to give them.

Frustrations

GS: I discern two frustrations in your career: one, not being able to influence to a greater degree the care of newborns and children in hospitals through direct educational experiences with staff nurses, and, two, not having research tools to get evidence to support hypotheses made from the participant-observation studies you and your students were doing. Is that right?

FB: Yes.

GS: What were some other frustrations, disappointments, or blocks along the way in your career?

FB: I've mentioned the major ones.

GS: What strategy did you use to get your ideas across?

FB: When I was a supervisor and a teacher, effecting change was infinitely easier than when I had no administrative authority. First I shared my suggestion and the purpose for change with all personnel who would be affected by it. Then I became active in helping the nurses to make the change. I thought that helping the staff make the change was an important supervisory activity. I worked to help others see that the change had value for patients, families, and themselves too. When the staff found they derived pleasure from the change, then I could focus my energy on finding solutions to other problems.

In Madison I got professionals in other disciplines and in nursing service involved with us when the first graduate program in nursing was being designed and implemented. I had learned by that time that resistance to change is reduced when the persons affected by it can participate in planning for it. I don't believe we ever introduced an innovation without first discussing it with nursing service personnel and also with the pediatricians. I can't remember ever suggesting a change in the program without a positive response which later became expressed in cooperation. I think because they helped to plan the program, they also wanted to see it succeed. In Chicago I just barged ahead, doing what I thought needed to be done for patients or parents or to further the education of students. When I did this without conferring with all the people who expected or wanted to be consulted, tension mounted and little progress was made.

High Points in Life

GS: You mentioned earlier, when you were talking informally, that you thought two of the highest points in your life, in terms of growth and development in nursing, were your experiences at Yale and in Peiping. You mentioned Yale a little bit, and if you care to add anything about that, fine; if not, we can talk about your experiences in China.

FB: At Yale doctors and nurses worked together closely, with splendid cooperation from social workers too. Teams weren't nearly as large as they were at the University of Wisconsin. At Yale I had as much support from nursing service as from the Dean of the School of Nursing. I've often looked back on my experiences at Yale and in Peiping and wondered if my contributions to nursing education weren't greater there than in other universities. In those two schools I carried dual responsibilities (teaching and supervision) and thereby was more able to influence the kind of nursing care provided and the milieu in which students, staff, and children learned. Staff nurses gave superior care, and, as a consequence, the students had excellent models from which to fashion themselves. Energy wasn't dissipated in dissension, resistance, and bucking the system; it was channeled into constructive activity.

GS: How did you go to China? What took you there?

FB: I had always wanted to work in a foreign country, but while in training I dismissed this from my mind. Only when I went to Teachers College in New York City the second time did the interest become revived. I lived at International House and became well acquainted with several nurses from the faculty of the Peiping Union Medical College. A book I read on nursing in Japan also kindled my wish to go to the Orient. The Chinese students suggested that I make application to the Rockefeller Foundation. I did this, and, soon after, I was offered a position teaching nursing arts. By that time, however, I was engrossed in pediatric nursing and wasn't about to change my area of specialization again. Two years later I went by boat to China as Supervisor and Instructor of Pediatric Nursing. I made the trip with Gertrude Hodgeman, Dean of the School of Nursing and one of the greatest leaders in nursing I've ever known. The years I spent there were three of the very best years of my life, professionally as well as socially.

GS: What years were you there?

FB: 1936 to 1939. It was a collegiate school of nursing. Gertrude Hodgeman achieved that. The students were the most avid students I ever had, and I've never seen any better nursing care given anywhere in the world than was given in that entire medical center.

GS: What else would you say you learned from your experiences in Peiping?

FB: I saw children with many kinds of disease I'd never seen before, and I learned much about the importance of physical nursing care and the potent emotional components associated with it. Most of the children were desperately ill upon arrival, and without intensive, meticulous care around the clock, the mortality rate would have been higher than it was. The Chinese nurses were warm, loving people. Intuitively they knew the children needed more than physical care, and they saw to it that they were well cared for and loved. I think one of the reasons why doctors and nurses worked so well together there was because orders were always carefully carried out. When the doctors discovered that nursing care entailed a dimension over and above what they had prescribed for the children's care, they became interested in learning our goals and then did much to help us reach them. What the Chinese nurses gave of themselves wasn't termed "emotional support" in those days. Nor could I put into words then the purposes it served for the children, but I know that the caring and commitment that grew out of the case method of assignment, when it was instituted, made a difference in the children's physical and behavioral responses to disease and to the rigorous, frightening medical care that they had to endure to survive.

Living conditions in Peiping were excellent. It was great having no shopping or housework to do. Two of us shared a luxurious house, and together we had seven servants. Entertaining was simple for us, and the social life was satisfying. Shopping for the exquisite art of China was a marvelous pastime, and there was much to see and do in the beautiful city of Peiping. There were also unusual opportunities for travel while on holiday. En route home I spent a month in a small mission hospital in the south of India, where I knew the director of nursing. The contrast in the care given in that hospital with the nursing provided for patients in Peiping was striking and sad to see. We had children with cholera, typhoid, and dysentery; and 30 miles from where I was, an epidemic of plague had broken out. Needless to say, I was frightened and wished for the supplies that were needed for adequate treatment measures and for isolation precautions. After seeing pictures of children in a hospital, which a friend of mine took while working in Pakistan recently, I wondered if any progress had been made in the care of children since I was in India in 1939. The friend I had been traveling with, until she left me to visit friends in Burma, joined me again in Calcutta. We traveled across India, and then met up with the friends I'd visited in the mission hospital near Madras, and shared a houseboat moored on a river in the Vale of Kashmir. I've never seen any sight more beautiful than the snow-covered Himalaya Mountains looming on high as we walked through the flower-filled Shalimar Gardens on Easter Sunday.

Significant Others

GS: Who are the persons who have influenced your thinking the most?

FB: Fortunate I was to have had the influence of Mary Marvin Whalen at Teachers College (1928–1929) so early in my career. She believed in clinical study of patient care. What I learned in that first year at Teachers College gave me an excellent foundation on which to build. I had no unlearning to do, as many of my graduate students at the University of Chicago did. Gertrude Hodgeman, Dean of the School of Nursing at the Peiping Union Medical College, Effie Taylor, Dean of the School of Nursing at Yale, and Helen Bunge, of Wisconsin, were stimulating colleagues. I already mentioned the teachers I found most helpful at the Institute for Psychoanalysis, Chicago. I also mentioned the professor of pediatrics whom I admired and greatly respected. At the University of Wisconsin Dr. Mark Hansen and Charles Lobeck were wonderful helpers in developing the graduate program. Dr. Hansen was interested in nursing, and I valued highly the many opportunities I had to share ideas with him. Students, children, and parents were invaluable teachers too. They really should head the list of ''significant others'' because I believe they contributed the most to my education and were the source of my motivation for learning, teaching, and writing.

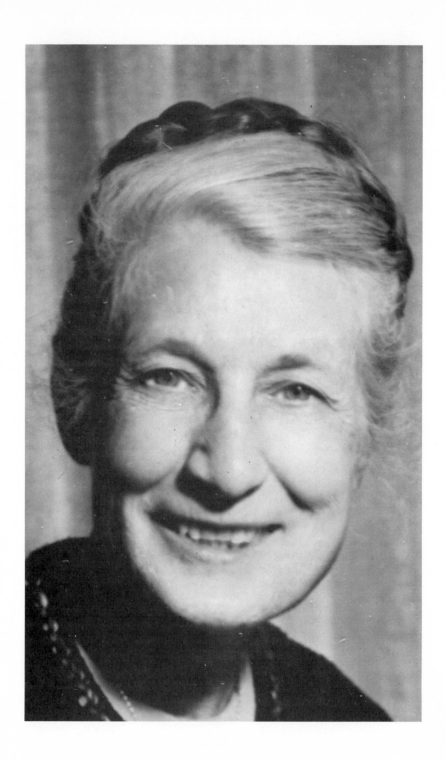

2

Nurse, educator, author, administrator, leader and innovator, first Director of the program in public health nursing at the University of Colorado from 1943 to 1957, first Dean of the School of Nursing at the University of Arizona from 1964 to 1967, and now Professor and Dean Emeritus, former President of both the Colorado Nurses' Association and the Colorado League for Nursing, one of the founders of the Western Council on Higher Education for Nursing, widely honored for outstanding professional leadership, admired and loved by students and colleagues.

For your keen and challenging approach to nursing education, and for the profound influence you have exerted for thirty years on nursing and nursing care in the United States and the West . . . [1]

[1]From Doctor of Science, honoris causa, University of Colorado, 1970.

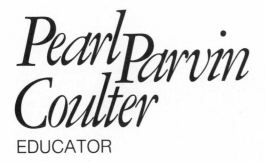

Pearl Parvin Coulter

EDUCATOR

*P*earl Parvin Coulter[2] was born August 19, 1902, in Almyra, Arkansas. She was the second oldest in a family of five children. Her father was a Methodist minister whose parents were committed to the Union cause in the Civil War. Her mother, a housewife, had deep roots in an early German settlement in Pennsylvania. Her father's profession required the family to move around considerably, but Pearl Coulter lived most of her life and childhood in little towns around Colorado.

She attended the University of Denver, where she majored in biological science and psychology and earned her B.A. in 1926. In 1927 she received her M.S. from the same institution. She attended the University of Colorado School of Nursing and was granted a diploma in nursing in 1935. She then went to the George Peabody College for Teachers in Nashville, Tennessee, where she received her certificate in public health nursing (1936). Further study was at the Yale School of Public Health, 1946–1947.

Pearl Coulter started out as a rural schoolteacher in Idaho (1922) and taught elementary and high school in Colorado. Her first nursing position was over ten years later as a staff nurse with the Visiting Nurse Association in Colorado Springs, Colorado, from 1935 to 1936.

After serving on the faculty at the University of Colorado, the George Peabody College for Teachers, and the University of Wisconsin, she started the baccalaureate program in nursing at the University of Arizona in 1957 and later became its first Dean.[3]

Pearl Coulter was a member of the Committee of Seven, appointed by the Director of the Western Interstate Commission for Higher Education (W.I.C.H.E.), 1956–1961.[4] She has authored many publications.[5]

---

[2] In 1928 Pearl Parvin married her teacher and was happily married until 1931, when her husband was killed in a tragic accident.

[3] She retired from the deanship in 1967 and remained as a Professor of Nursing until her retirement in 1970 as Professor Emeritus.

[4] First meeting March 1956 in Denver.

[5] *The Nurse in the Public Health Program,* G. P. Putnam's Sons, New York, 1954; with V. A. Christopherson and M. O. Wolanin, *Rehabilitation Nursing Perspectives and Applications,* McGraw-Hill Book Company, New York, 1974; "Winds of Change," *A Progress Report of Regional Cooperation in Collegiate Nursing Education in the West, 1956–1961,* Western Interstate Commission for Higher Education, 1963; with Hannah Erickson, "New Patterns for Field Instruction in Public Health Nursing," *Nursing Outlook,* February 1956.

*D*ecision to Take up Nursing and Special Interest in Public Health Nursing

GS: What made you decide to take up nursing?

PC: My father must have believed in women's liberation. He wanted his daughters to prepare for a profession such as medicine, dentistry, or law. He considered working for a salary distasteful. While there was no question that I would progress from high school to university, I must have lacked initiative. I didn't know how to break into the masculine professions, and there were very few choices for young women in those days. I drifted into teaching.

I married my major professor, head of the botany department at the University of Denver. His death, after a happy but brief marriage, left me to consider my future from a more mature posture. I might have chosen nursing earlier, had an opportunity to combine it with higher education presented itself. I liked science and had acquired a good background in biology. During the time I was married I took graduate courses in anthropology at the University of Denver and in bacteriology at the University of Colorado Medical School. In addition to the sophomore medical students, a School of Nursing faculty member, Ruth Colestock, was in the class, which she usually attended in uniform. I was impressed with her competence when patients were brought to class.

After my husband's death a friend of his, a professor from the University of Pittsburgh, visited me. He said he could help me obtain a scholarship in Pillsbury if I wanted to work toward a Ph.D. in microbiology. I went to my teacher at the University of Colorado Medical School for advice. It was his opinion that while I had competed well with medical students, it would be a different matter if I tried to be competitive in a work setting. Those were Depression days, and nobody was looking for a woman scientist. The experience in the medical school and my glimpse into the hospital rekindled my interest in nursing, and I made inquiry about entering that field. The Director of the School of Nursing at the University of Colorado suggested that my background, far from being an asset, would militate against becoming a happy, well-adjusted student nurse.

GS: Why was that?

PC: I am not sure, but I can guess. Even though located in the University Medical Center, it was really a hospital school, possibly one in transition. I was older than the usual student, had been married, and had a better education than any of the nursing faculty, though I was not aware of their meager preparation at the time. These factors were never verbalized. The Depression had created a paucity of demand for nurses; many were unemployed. I was warned that even after three years in the school, there might not be any employment opportunities. Since I had a little income and it would be some time before I would be looking for work, I persisted in saying that I would enter the school if acceptable. It would have been easy to avert me by telling me of the two graduate programs in basic nursing, Yale University and Western Reserve University, but they were not mentioned. Perhaps the Director was not aware of them or did not think them suitable. She was an austere woman, and she finally said, "Very well. You know nothing about nursing. We will assume that you have come here to learn. We will teach you."

GS: What made you decide to pursue studies in public health?

PC: My curriculum included an "affiliation" with the Denver Visiting Nurse Service. I loved every minute of it. One of the supervisors there, Margaret Blee, who later went to Chapel Hill to teach in the School of Public Health, was interested in me. She was the only teacher during the three years who let me know that my unusual background might be useful. One day she asked, "Why don't you go to Peabody and study public health nursing?" I had never heard of George Peabody College for Teachers, nor did I know that there were special programs for the preparation of public health nurses. I learned that the program was in Tennessee and initiated correspondence with its Director, Aurelia B. Potts. I thought I might like to do school nursing, since I had taught in a public school system; so I applied in the Denver schools, knowing that a position there would enable me to return to my little house and continue to live in Denver. It was disappointing to learn that I did not qualify. I was told that I would need a certificate in public health nursing from an approved program. My first public health nursing position was in Colorado Springs. I replaced Ms. Brown, who had just retired, and along with her position I inherited her winter coat. She must have been about 8 inches shorter than I. The winter was cold, the work not very challenging, and the coat a misfit. A letter from Aurelia Potts, saying that I had been accepted for admission, urged me to begin study in the winter quarter. She also encouraged me to believe that by using transfer credit I might be able to complete the certificate requirements in two quarters. At the beginning of the spring quarter I was given an opportu-nity to teach two courses in health education for freshman and sopho-more students who were preparing themselves as elementary teachers. I did receive the certificate in public health nursing at the end of the spring quarter, and was offered the option of remaining for another quarter to take two required graduate courses in education, which would yield a master of science degree with a major in public health nursing. It seemed to me that there was something wrong, almost dis-honest, with a system that permitted one student to earn a master's degree with essentially the same curriculum that supported the bacca-laureate degree or the certificate. Since I already had a master of sci-ence degree, I saw no advantage in accumulating another. Such was the status of graduate work in nursing at that time! Failure to qualify for a nursing degree proved to be a mistake. Some years later a master's degree in nursing became a useful credential, regardless of its content.

By summer I was back at the University of Colorado School of Nurs-ing. The Director, of whom I was still in awe, had written me that a plan was under way to move nursing into a baccalaureate program which would include public health. Integration was the word in those days, and since I had met the requirements, I was to be the integrator. During the summer there were no students. With two other faculty members I was to revise and update the hospital nursing manual and plan the new curriculum. In the fall, my assignment would be teaching nursing arts. By some strange alchemy the "public health point of view" was expect-ed to ooze into all of the courses. The new curriculum would lead to a bachelor of nursing degree, a route chosen because it would permit recruitment of students with disparate backgrounds, comprise two years of college, and relieve the school of complying with demands of the arts and science degree. Nurses had been dictated to long enough! There seemed to be no expectation that the nursing curriculum would have a foundation in arts and science courses, or that students with that background had greater potential than those with a miscellany of credits. It took seven or eight years for the folly of this decision to be fully realized. Then a new Director was appointed, a massive curriculum revision was undertaken, and unit credit was assigned to nursing cours-es for the first time. Early in this new atmosphere I was to be on hand again, which I shall explain later.

My tenure in nursing arts lasted fourteen months. I was invited to return to Peabody College with the rank of instructor. New federal sti-pends had greatly expanded the enrollment. For four quarters of teaching my salary was to be $2000. I wanted to become more closely identified with public health nursing, so I agreed to return with the proviso that I be given assignments including practice. I was keenly aware of my lack of experience. I taught school nursing theory and practice, which included direction of the health programs in the demonstration and nursery schools. These two facilities were available for the field teaching of graduate nurses registered in the certificate or degree program. After two years my assignment was changed to teaching Principles of Public Health Nursing and supervising students' fieldwork at the Nashville Health Department. I was also responsible for public health nursing practice for students from the Hubbard School of Nursing, associated with Fisk University.

From reading professional journals and attending national meetings, I had begun to realize that the future of public health nursing education was in the baccalaureate schools of nursing, while the program for registered nurses was an expedient that had served its purpose and was destined to disappear. During the five years at Peabody College I had progressed to the rank of associate professor, and my annual salary was still $2000. I had learned a great deal about the southern region, and was impressed with the cooperative spirit of planning and sharing that was pervasive. I had come to know a great many nurses from that region, some of whom had been my students. The decision to leave was not easy. However, in September 1941 I went to the University of Wisconsin, where a baccalaureate program in nursing was administered by the medical school and the university hospital, with the College of Letters and Sciences conferring the degree. Its public health nursing program had just been accredited by the National Organization for Public Health Nursing (N.O.P.H.N.). I taught theory courses and arranged for student field experience in rural areas, the educational integrity of which I questioned. Shortly after I arrived in Madison, the Japanese bombed Pearl Harbor, and from then on war was in the air. Toward the end of my second year I was told that an administrative decision had been made to eliminate all frills from the nursing curriculum so the students could help win the war by working more hours in the hospital. To my dismay I learned that public health nursing had been designated as one of the frills. I was asked to stay. My salary would be paid, and an effort would be made to find something useful for me to do for the duration of the war, at the end of which the teaching of public health nursing would be resumed. If I preferred, a leave of absence would be arranged for me and I could go elsewhere until the war was over. I resigned with no expectation of returning.

About this time a letter from the University of Colorado announced that the B.N. degree had been found wanting and would be replaced by a B.S. degree supported by a totally revised curriculum and better-qualified faculty. I was invited to teach public health nursing. Nothing could have pleased me more than returning to my alma mater. In September 1943 I was in Boulder and entirely immersed in the excitement of the new program. I stayed there until February 1957, when I came to Arizona to start the baccalaureate program in nursing at the University of Arizona. I was ready to leave the University of Colorado despite my love for the institution. Increasingly I realized that I had given and gained all I could at that time and place, and, because of continuing differences between me and the administrator of the School of Nursing it seemed best to leave. The situation in Arizona was challenging. It was the last of the then forty-eight states to support a baccalaureate nursing program. Such an opportunity might never present itself again.

GS: What do you consider your major contributions to nursing?

PC: I would like to mention three, though others will have to judge how major they are:

1 Teaching and influencing a large number of public health nursing students.

2 Work with the Western Council on Higher Education for Nursing (W.C.H.E.N) of W.I.C.H.E.

3 Initiating and administering a baccalaureate program in nursing under pioneer conditions.

TEACHING

During and immediately following World War II, nursing education moved substantially forward toward professional quality. Teaching in a specific clinical area became a specialty, and a great deal was done to separate the goals of service from those of education. Student nursing practice was regarded as a laboratory experience with the right to learn under the direction of skilled teachers. Only public health nursing differed from this pattern. The practice of relying on the public health agency for teaching persisted. Each student was assigned to a staff nurse, and the school abdicated its responsibility for teaching. A large percentage of staff nurses were graduates of diploma programs with only work experience to give them competence in community nursing. Some of the agencies welcomed students because of a genuine interest in helping them acquire insight into public health nursing, while others welcomed them because their services added to the production of the staff. Still other agencies saw the student as a liability and demanded reimbursement for the time the staff invested in her. Some nursing faculty members believed that they could accomplish their educational objectives more effectively by omitting the community nursing experience altogether, replacing it with a curriculum enriched as much as possible with community-based experiences under faculty direction.

When the University of Colorado School of Nursing proposed to the public health agencies the placement of faculty in the field with students, the response was negative and in some cases hostile. The agency nurses felt that it was belittling, though they were aware that they did not qualify as faculty members. The general consensus was that we could continue with fieldwork on their terms or not at all. They were assured that if they could provide space and case materials for students, their policies would be learned and followed, and the welfare of the community they served would be safeguarded while the faculty took responsibility for student teaching. When Bernice diSessa became State Director of Public Health Nursing in Colorado, she listened to complaints voiced against the student program. She pointed out that the state needed a continuing supply of qualified public health nurses, more federal funds were becoming available, and more more positions remained unfilled. She suggested that they listen more carefully to the university's suggestion. Eventually, written agreements were signed by agency and university officials, and public health nursing was established as a course with a well-developed teaching plan and adequate faculty.

When this new pattern had been operative long enough to test its effectiveness, it was described in *Nursing Outlook*.[6] Experiences shared in a generous spirit are not always received with joy. The magazine was besieged with reactions to the article, mostly negative and some quite abrasive. They suggested that we were trying to sabotage the cordial relationship that had for years been enjoyed between edu-

---

[6] Pearl Parvin Coulter and Hannah Erickson, "New Patterns for Field Instruction in Public Health Nursing," *Nursing Outlook*, February 1956.

cational institutions and public health agencies. Probably as a result of the consternation generated by the article, the National League for Nursing (N.L.N.) convened a conference on public health nursing field instruction at Gull Lake, the W. K. Kellogg home, which was then owned and maintained by the state of Michigan. I was invited to attend and to explain the Colorado pattern and participate in a subsequent question-and-answer session. Neither the N.L.N. nor the University of Colorado had any funds for travel, so I went at my own expense. I was received with noticeable coolness by some of my public health nursing colleagues. I overheard one of them remark, "I can hardly wait for that session on field instruction tomorrow morning. I have feelings about it."

The presentation went well, and as I talked, some attitudes appeared to change. One of my friends whispered to me, "You must feel like a rattlesnake stripped of its venom." The chief concern now was how to get budget for salaries for the additional public health nursing field teachers. Unlike laboratory work in some of the sciences, where graduate assistants are utilized for laboratory teaching under the direction of a more senior faculty member, it was felt that the public health nursing field teacher should have preparation comparable with that of other faculty.

The following summer the University of Colorado School of Nursing conducted a conference on field instruction in public health nursing. Nurses came from all over the country, not only public health nursing faculty and agency nurses but also their deans or directors. Gradually skepticism was replaced by acceptance, and long before the N.L.N. adopted the pattern as standard, many educational institutions and public agencies had already implemented it.

REGIONAL PLANNING FOR NURSING

When western nurse leaders learned of the potential for nursing held by W.I.C.H.E., they eagerly sought an alliance with this regional organization. They were aware of hopes for utilizing a few centers for medical education in the Western states. Students from states with a small population could be sent to well-established medical schools in neighboring states. This "exchange arrangement" meant expansion for some medical schools with fixed quotas for enrollment in order to accommodate nonresident students whose out-of-state fees would be absorbed by the sending state. The plan brought added revenue to the state operating the school and probably reduced its unit cost. It provided professionally trained personnel for the sending state while relieving it of the enormous cost of operating a professional school for a few students, and it created a sense of community sharing within the region. Nursing groups assumed that every western state would eventually support a baccalaureate nursing program but that the smaller states would not have the clinical richness, the synergistic momentum of graduate students in allied disciplines, or the financial resources to develop and maintain graduate programs in nursing. It was further assumed that the existing graduate programs in nursing might develop specialties in areas of their greatest resources and that students would choose the school that provided the specialty in which they were interested. It did not seem likely that every school would have clinical resources or prepared faculty to offer all majors.

Looking back, the exchange system for the preparation of professional personnel seems to have worked in the western region, though in the intervening years more medical schools and graduate programs in nursing have developed than were anticipated in the 1950s. Because of the availability of federal funds, nursing did not ask states to pay non resident fees for nurses wishing to study in another state.

Probably the nursing leaders who did the most in the initial stages to promote W.C.H.E.N. were Lulu Hassenplug, Henrietta Loughran, and Katherine Hoffman. Their activity started about the time that preparation was under way to move the W.I.C.H.E. headquarters to the campus of the University of Colorado in Boulder. Following a survey of western nursing education by Helen Nahm, then on the staff of the N.L.N., and a subsequent conference attended by western nurses in Berkeley, Harold Enarson, W.I.C.H.E.'s Executive Director, appointed the Committee of Seven.[7] The purpose of the ad hoc committee was to implement the Berkeley conference recommendations.

GS: *What criteria did he use?*

PC: Economy was a factor; the committee had to be small. Representation from each school, or even from each state, was not possible, but an effort was made to get representation from each type of program. Action was given high priority; the committee had to produce with very

---

[7] The seven members of the committee were Lulu Hassenplug, chairman, Pearl Coulter, James Enoch, Katherine Hoffman, Amelia Leino, Annette Lefkowitz, and Kathryn Smith. For more information see "Winds of Change."

little time at its disposal. I do not know why I was chosen. Possibly it was because I could represent both the University of Colorado and public health nursing, and had served as chairman of the Continuing Education Committee at the Berkeley conference. Dr. Enarson made no commitment beyond convening and funding this committee. The future of western nursing was in its hands. It was charged with producing plans for action and financing within a maximum time period of five days. It had available the Nahm survey; the proceedings and recommendations of the Berkeley conference; and a group of able consultants from organized nursing, from the U.S. Public Health Service (U.S. P.H.S.), and from some of the schools of nursing. I believe that each member felt a terrible sense of urgency, an almost overwhelming burden of responsibility, and much enthusiasm for the potential which lay hidden in the week ahead.

The first morning we received our respective assignments. Mine was to chair the Continuing Education Committee. The three of us, Kathryn Smith, Margaret Taylor, and I, seemed to be working in a vacuum. At that time continuing education was not particularly popular in any field, and in nursing it was almost nonexistent. We reviewed the Berkeley conference report and tried to assess the need for continuing education and its present status. We talked about the inadequate initial training of most nurses; the poverty of any mechanism to help them update their practice; the established license renewal system, which required no continuing proof of competence; the difficulty nurses experienced in getting away to study because they could not be replaced at work and because many of them had home responsibilities, including the care of young children. It was thought that many nurses did not feel the need for further education and that some were too old for extended periods of study to be practical. We had to refine the work of the previous group and to focus on a feasible program that would be a positive force in improving patient care and health services. We kept coming back to the question of financing, somewhat despairingly. We did not believe that nurses could afford to finance even short terms of study; we knew that the educational institutions which we represented would not be warm toward making such a contribution; and we had the message loud and clear that W.I.C.H.E. would be unable to undertake such a project. So our work became twofold: what type of program could be developed in such a way that it would touch most employed nurses so effectively that they would become better practitioners, and how it could be funded? We finally realized that the first step was to produce an irresistible plan, a plan so practical, so attractive, and so full of promise that some "angel" would see that it was implemented.

Tabling the financial problem momentarily, though it always lurked near us, freed us to focus on a plan that proved to be both pragmatic and innovative. This was probably the first time that continuing education for nurses had been planned on a regional basis with objectives carefully considered. Essentially, the format was:

1   Each agency wishing to participate in a continuing education conference series would be asked to send two nurses. They would support and reinforce each other in their work setting when they tried to share their newfound knowledge with their coworkers.

2   Continuing education would be offered in a series of short exposures, for example, one to two weeks each quarter over a period of five years. The participants might reach the saturation point during this short, intensive learning experience. Intervals of learning interspersed with periods of work not only would help nurses accept their need for updating, but would culminate in a conviction that continuing education was a way of life for all professions based on scientific knowledge. The short release period would also be more acceptable to employers as contrasted with a quarter or a semester of sustained study.

3   Faculty would have to learn how to package content material in small, concentrated units. They would have to devise ways of finding out what their students already knew in order that only relevant content would be included. They would have to learn to identify new information that would be translated into practice and to help students learn how to extract information independently from the literature. Attitudes had to be changed from "I was well trained and will always be a good practitioner" to "Nursing is a science-based discipline and therefore subject to continual change. I must keep on learning in order to keep my practice current."

4   The first conference series, two weeks per session, would be conducted over a five-year period by three institutions well established and strategically located for convenience of travel—the two California universities working in cooperation, the University of Colorado, and the University of Washington. The recruits would be top leadership personnel in nursing service and nursing education because the leaders were in the best position to influence change.

The serial pattern persisted, but experience showed that two weeks and five years was too long, so it became more standard to utilize five days and two years. On Thursday of the week the Committee of Seven met, each subcommittee chairman was expected to be ready with a report. The continuing education plan, after undergoing rigorous editing, was eventually taken to the W. K. Kellogg Foundation by Lulu Hassenplug and Harold Enarson, with an appeal for funding.

GS: Did the entire package get funded by the W. K. Kellogg Foundation, or just continuing education?

PC: To some extent the entire package was funded, first for five years, and parts of it for some years longer. The Foundation had a special interest in continuing education at the time, but its administrators were persuaded that the purposes of W.C.H.E.N were broader than continuing education. It would require a director and a skeleton structure, including the graduate and baccalaureate seminars, in order for any program to be effective. It is my impression that without the continuing education component, the Foundation would not have funded W.C.H.E.N. When federal funds became available, W.C.H.E.N. applied at intervals for grants to maintain and expand the continuing education program.

The western regional plan was well publicized through reports at national meetings and in the literature.[8] In subsequent years more continuing education centers were developed, which were visited by observers from throughout the United States and some foreign countries, and the pattern was replicated many times. Gradually, as leadership personnel had the continuing education experience, they asked for opportunities for their staff; and, in time, conference series were available for head nurses, team leaders, and staff nurses. Apprehension about continued attendance soon disappeared. A high percentage of nurses who came to the first conference of a series were present for the final one. Institutions reluctant to send two nurses to the first series were now asking for space for five, ten, or twenty. There was consensus among the group who had completed one or more series that the nurses who had experienced continuing education were able to translate their new knowledge into improved service. As they came under the influence of university faculty and better understood the baccalaureate and graduate programs, their attitude became more charitable toward modern trends in nursing education.

W.C.H.E.N. was the first W.I.C.H.E. council, and some of the commissioners expressed pride in its activities.

[8] Pearl Parvin Coulter, "Continuing Education Program for Nurses in the West," *Nursing Outlook,* February 1962.

As soon as funds were available, the search for a director started. A number of prospects were interviewed, but the position was not filled.

GS: Was the salary too low?

PC: No, but nurses with the desired qualifications were in short supply, and the new venture into regional leadership may have seemed a bit too challenging. They were oriented toward positions in universities. Eventually Faye Abdullah came on loan from the U.S.P.H.S. to get the program started. Jo Eleanor Elliott was finally persuaded to abandon her doctoral program at the University of Chicago, at least temporarily, and she seemed to bring the right mixture of leadership and diplomacy that was needed in this pioneering effort. My greatest involvement with W.C.H.E.N. was with developing the continuing education plan in the early days and later in the baccalaureate seminar, at which I represented the University of Arizona.

AT THE UNIVERSITY OF ARIZONA

Perhaps I made a substantial contribution to nursing education in the West by becoming the first director of the baccalaureate program in nursing at the University of Arizona. At that time, February 1957, there were forty-eight states in the Union, and Arizona was the only one without a baccalaureate program in nursing. For obvious reasons Nevada, Wyoming, and New Mexico had also been laggards, but they all had programs prior to Arizona's. The U.S.P.H.S. had undertaken the survey of nursing resources in each state, following the war, and Margaret Arnstein did the survey and prepared the report for Arizona. It revealed lack of qualified faculty in the five existing diploma schools. Very few nurses in Arizona held baccalaureate degrees, and most of those who did had earned liberal arts degrees superimposed on a diploma in nursing. Since the dearth of appropriate education among the leadership nurses was made apparent, many of the nurses who read the Arnstein report concluded that Arizona needed a graduate program.

GS: By graduate you mean master's?

PC: Yes. Nobody was thinking beyond a master's in nursing at that time. It took a great deal of explaining to help them understand that a backlog of nurses with baccalaureate degrees in nursing would have to accumulate before a master's curriculum could be supported. For some, the master's program still remained the ultimate goal. The leadership nurses in Arizona had for years been hoping to move nursing education into the institutions of higher learning. I was invited to come from the University of Colorado and teach a course for registered nurses. Nurses seemed eager for help, and it was hoped that the Governor, who was an ex officio member of the Board of Regents of the University of Arizona and the state colleges, might realize Arizona's problem in importing a teacher from another state.

So I commuted to Arizona during the fall quarter of 1951 and taught a class in Tucson on Friday evening and repeated it in Phoenix on Saturday morning. I believe there were about seventy-five in the combined group. Governor Pyle came to the final class in Phoenix and said that he would not be averse to starting a baccalaureate program in nursing at one of the state institutions, but he was very much opposed to a medical school because it would be too expensive. During the sessions in Tucson I had had several conferences with Vice President Nugent at the University of Arizona. He told me that they had taken Margaret Arnstein's report seriously and had invited Margaret Bridgeman from the N.L.N. for a consultative visit. She had expressed some doubts about the quality and amount of clinical material in either Phoenix or Tucson to satisfy the needs of a baccalaureate program, but she thought the state was in great need of the graduates from such a school. President Harvill at the University of Arizona had prepared a report for the Board of Regents with a proposal for a degree in nursing. This raised questions about the best location for such a program, and since there was no inclination to start one in each of the three contending institutions, the debate was resolved by not approving any.

One of the school administrators believed he already had a baccalaureate program in nursing because he had agreed to accept a diploma graduate and grant two years of credit for her training, upon which two additional years of liberal arts courses were superimposed. The nurse graduated with essentially no upper-division major, but her transcript indicated "a concentration in nursing." A number of the nurses who availed themselves of this opportunity believed that they had a major in nursing.

Eventually the Regents were persuaded to authorize two programs in nursing, one at the University of Arizona in Tucson and the other at Arizona State College in Tempe. After this action of the regents in the fall of 1956, I was invited to the University of Arizona for a consultation visit and was then asked to assume the director's position. My Dean at the University of Colorado had been consulted, and she arranged to release me for the spring semester. By April I was expected to resign from the University of Colorado or replace myself at the University of Arizona.

After attending the W.C.H.E.N. meeting in San Francisco as the University of Arizona's representative, I arrived in Tucson early in February to face perhaps the biggest challenge of my life. I had a few months to decide whether or not I would remain permanently on that faculty and eight months to develop a curriculum, to learn about the resources and internal workings of the University of Arizona, and to recruit students and faculty to start the academic year.

I felt it was important to become acquainted with the nurses in the state and especially in the Tucson area. For the most part their attitude was friendly but skeptical. No doubt some of them felt threatened by the approaching change in nursing education, though the threat was mixed with pride because at long last something good for nursing was happening in Arizona.

I also had to acquaint myself with the clinical facilities in the community and to negotiate agreements with them for student experience. It was evident that some unique cultural experiences might be developed. Tucson has a large Mexican-American Spanish-speaking population; many live in discrete communities and preserve their native customs. Some of our students and eventually a faculty member were drawn from this group, and students encountered many of them as patients. Tucson is only about 60 miles from the Mexican border. There is also a large Indian population in Arizona, composed of several different tribes. Some of these Indians live in Tucson. In addition, the Papago Indian Reservation's border is only 6 miles from the campus. One of our challenges was to learn to make use of these rich resources in such a way that students would understand cultural influences on health practice. In this effort we were helped immeasurably by the department of anthropology.

The more conventional facilities also had some unique features. St. Mary's, the oldest hospital in Arizona giving continuous service, had developed from a twelve-bed unit started during territorial days. It was conducting its own diploma program and had a large and vocal alumnae group. I was told that when the summer rains came, the roof leaked and patients' beds had to be moved from place to place to avoid the drips. The administrators of this program were friendly and indicated that any resources not needed for their own students could be available to the university. Tucson Medical Center occupied a number of cottages scattered about the desert. Due to pressures of population growth, it had developed from an abandoned sanitorium for the study of chest conditions. It was not uncommon to see patients directly from the operating room wheeled along a desert path to a room in one of the cottages, exposed to the blazing sun, wind, and blowing dust or to a spring shower. The night supervisor told me that snakes often crept into patients' rooms to escape the desert chill. They were harmless bull snakes, but still disconcerting when at large in a sickroom. She said that if prodded, they would curl themselves around a broom handle and could then be carried outdoors. They were not easily persuaded to abandon the broom, so she learned to leave the snake-entwined broom on the ground, and usually when she returned on her next rounds, the snake would be gone and she could recover her broom for future use. Each patient's room opened directly to the outdoors, and the nurse carrying medications from room to room went outside between patients. During storms it was difficult to answer signal lights, but most of the time the weather was mild. The county hospital was also housed in a series of cottages, most of which were in poor repair. The Veterans Administration Hospital was also an old structure; it serviced tuberculosis patients only, and I was told frankly by the chief nurse that they did not have anything to offer students. A trip to Washington to confer with the Veterans Administration's Chief Nurse revealed that it had not been visited by nursing service for many years and had been practically written off as hopeless. However, I left with a promise that she would see what could be done. While there was no dearth of patients, the existing facilities did not look promising.

Perhaps due to a variety of converging forces, things did begin to work out. Tucson Medical Center gave up a patient room in order to provide students with a classroom. Both its nurses and its doctors were supportive in every way possible. Over the ensuing years it developed into a large, modern hospital. New buildings sprang up and the old cottages were rehabilitated beyond recognition. St. Mary's Hospital eventually discontinued its school, went through a modernization period, and built a new, modern hospital on the east side of town, which the same order of nuns maintained. Some useful outpatient clinics developed at the county hospital, the Veterans Administration gave general services and underwent modernization, and influences from Washington brought more adequate nursing staff to replace or expand the old. A working agreement was negotiated with the Papago Tribal Council, the new private psychiatric hospital, and the new mental health clinic. As our enrollment and needs increased, miraculously resources became available. It would be hard to estimate the impact of the W.C.H.E. N. continuing education program on patient care. A total of ten or twelve nurses represented Arizona in the first conference series. Five of them were from Tucson; some from Phoenix were from state agencies such as the State Mental Hospital and the State Board of Nursing.

I was appointed to serve two consecutive five-year terms on the Arizona State Board of Nursing. This was a dedicated group, which had a great deal of influence on upgrading nursing education and nursing service in Arizona. It gave me insight into problems on a state level and made it possible for me to share my knowledge of baccalaureate nursing education with other members of the Board, whose experience had been long and rich but different.

We were convinced that the University of Arizona's responsibility for helping the current practitioner of nursing was almost as great as that of developing an excellent baccalaureate program. Through the years, continuing education was given a great deal of emphasis. We regarded this effort as supportive rather than competitive with our other work. The University of Arizona, in cooperation with Arizona State University, became a center for W.C.H.E.N. continuing education. In addition to the three-a-year-for-two-years series under the aegis of W.C.H.E.N, we conducted a number of others each year, beginning in our first years with focus on such subjects as rehabilitation, child development, operation of nursing homes, communication, culture and nursing, and cardiac nursing that included a series on chest surgery. (One morning in Tucson, three surgeons conducted three chest surgeries simultaneously in three different hospitals in order to permit conferees to observe and learn more about the nursing care of these patients.) For leadership it was our policy to recruit one person of national prominence, known in the field to be covered, and in addition to utilize our own faculty as well as faculty from other disciplines. As a result many nurses from Arizona and from some other states had at least one exposure, and some several exposures, to continuing education. It helped create a ferment which resulted in improved nursing care, brought some nurses back for longer periods of study, and helped nurses understand the advantages of allying nursing with higher education.

The school of nursing was housed in scattered rooms in various buildings about the campus for three years; then it was moved into a section of the new home economics building. These quarters were soon outgrown, and we were never really adequately housed until we moved into the new million-dollar College of Nursing building, paid for by a federal grant with matching state funds. During the first four years we graduated two or three registered nurse students who came with transfer credit. By the end of the first four years, the original forty-two students had dwindled to ten graduates. A short time before the end of the fourth academic year, we received accreditation from the N.L.N.

When I made the recommendation for an autonomous school, the President kept his promise and honored my recommendation. The timing was right, it seemed to me. We had gained vitality and had a substantial enrollment, and a medical college had been approved which would have immediate autonomy. We had graduated a fair number of students who went on for master's degrees and a few for doctorates. In 1967, before we moved to the new building, our own master's program was accepted by the graduate college, and prior to that we had already started a nurse-scientist Ph.D. program.

During the years I directed the program at the University of Arizona, we accomplished a number of things:

1 Achieved a substantial enrollment in the baccalaureate program and attracted a number of students to the master's and nurse-scientist programs.

2 Employed a well-qualified faculty.

3 Achieved adequate housing.

4 Became an autonomous college.

5 Developed good working relationships with a number of colleges and departments on the campus and with agencies throughout the state.

6 Throughout the period we enjoyed good administrative support.

GS: *Obviously you decided to stay and not go back to Colorado.*

PC: Yes, I discovered that I was barely started in laying the foundation for a baccalaureate school of nursing, and despite my best efforts I had not been able to find anyone interested in the position.

GS: *It seems to me that in the back of your mind you kept thinking of going back to Colorado.*

PC: Yes, probably not back to Colorado but to someplace where I could get out of the heat. By this time I saw the challenge clearly: the eagerness of nurses for this long-overdue program, the lack of facilities for good nursing service and good health practices, the willingness of local institutions and agencies to cooperate in any way possible, and the always-available administrative support.

GS: *You said that recruitment of faculty was a problem.*

PC: It was not easy. We had reasonably high standards. During the first summer we had many local applicants who were shocked when told that we required the minimum of a master's degree. We could offer new faculty the opportunity to be innovative in developing a new program in an unusual setting: a warm, mild climate; a casual way of life; and colorful cultural surroundings. The chamber of commerce literature sometimes helped. The deans of nursing in the West also helped. We got faculty from the University of California at Los Angeles, from the University of Colorado, and from the University of Washington as well as some from farther east. Many of them came with experience in other baccalaureate programs. We persuaded the administration that we could not stay within the established university ratio of faculty to student. We wanted our best teachers for clinical teaching, and this required small groups of students. Since we did not make demands for expensive laboratory space or equipment, most of which was provided by the community agencies, we felt that we merited a larger budget for faculty. I'm afraid that my annual report was always accompanied by a memorandum giving examples of our clinical practice, the need to provide a learning experience for students in difficult situations, and an impassioned plea for more money for faculty salaries.

Leaves the Deanship

GS: What was your reason for relinquishing the deanship?

PC: At the time I was employed, I had been told that it was the policy for deans to retire at age sixty-five with the possibility of remaining on the faculty. I was approaching that age. Knowledge of the policy prompted me to take steps early to provide for a successor. Gladys Sorensen came from the University of Colorado at the beginning of our second year. She had been an outstanding faculty member at Colorado and had acquired some preparation toward her doctorate. Subsequently we granted her two years of leave to complete the doctorate. She was capable, well liked by the faculty, and ready to assume the responsibility when the time came. After I had made preparations for retirement, the President said he recommended that I be permitted to remain as Dean for two more years so I could reap the fruits of occupying the Dean's office suite in the new building which I had worked hard to finance. I thanked him for his generous gesture, but asked if I might instead remain on the faculty for a few more years as Professor of Nursing. I was tired of administration and wanted to be back with students in the classroom. Since this was a routine arrangement for superannuated deans, it created no problem. I told the President and the new Dean that I would be glad to help her in any way I could when she requested my advice. For two years I had a full-time teaching schedule, and the last year, 1969–1970, I asked for half time. I thought retirement might be easier if I learned to adjust gradually.

Shortly after the beginning of the academic year, the State Board of Nursing asked me to come on the staff as half-time educational consultant. This position had been vacant for some time, and if I took it on a temporary basis, it could be filled when the right candidate appeared. Two half-time positions equal a little more than one full-time, but I enjoyed that last year, half of which was spent in Phoenix at the State Board of Nursing office or traveling to visit the schools of nursing in the state. I think in this position I was able to interpret to some of the nursing leaders the educational problems in Arizona. The community college system was developing rapidly. I visited them all, talked with faculty and college administration, and tried to help them see the importance of qualified faculty—that nursing, like other disciplines, needed teachers who had preparation in the discipline taught, beyond that of the student. Most of the community college nursing faculty had baccalaureate degrees and some of them had master's degrees, but very few, if any of them, were in nursing. When I said to the administrator, "You probably would not employ a chemistry major to teach English," he got the point.

GS: How would you describe the University of Arizona College of Nursing in a few words?

PC: As it was when I was there, or as it is now? I am not sure, but I assume that it has progressed on somewhat the same lines.

GS: What comes to your mind, then, in descriptive words?

PC: We had goals which required the development of a high order of intellectual activity. The faculty had to be more innovative than the average in order to make use of unusual facilities to accomplish goals. They had to be continually evaluative of their own and their students' accomplishments. I think they had a very definite feeling of team relationship with the students; they succeeded or failed together. We had some evidence of real patient-centered attitudes on the part of students; for example, two honors seminar students chose to work a few hours in the hospital every day during a vacation period in order to apply theory to practice. The report which they wrote showed that they had made real progress. I think of faculty and student contributions to nursing literature and, in the latter half of our first decade, the development of some research sophistication. We never assumed that a faculty member published or taught or that she did research or taught. These intellectual activities were not regarded as mutually exclusive. The more gifted teachers tended also to be the ones who engaged in research and publication.

GS: *What do you like best about the things you have done?*

PC: I enjoyed teaching students and watching their careers develop. Some of my former students are now in positions of leadership and high-level responsibility in nursing. Through correspondence I hear from a number of them, and not infrequently some of them come to see me.

Developing a new baccalaureate program was interesting and challenging. It required my best efforts, and many times I was aware these were not good enough. There were aspects of administration that I found rewarding. When I was director of the program, I appreciated the counsel of the Dean of the College of Liberal Arts. He was not accustomed to women in administration, though he never gave me the impression that he wanted to take over the nursing program. I suppose in a way he was a male chauvinist, though a benevolent one. The chief difference in becoming Dean was the direct access to the President that it afforded and a place on his council, which met once a week. The university was still a man's world. I was the only woman academic Dean. Some of the men looked at me with misgivings. For the most part they were cordial, courteous, and, I think, sometimes curious about how I would react to certain issues. Unless there was a threat to losing some of their prerogatives, they tended to be supportive and even protective. I got some satisfaction from seeing an article published or hearing favorable comments about a speech I had made, though I agonized during the preparation of every one.

I enjoyed the work I did with organized nursing. It gave me an opportunity to know many leaders in nursing and often gave me insight into the direction nursing was going. I am most appreciative of the honors which came to me from nursing groups—receipt of the Pearl McIver Award, honorary recognition by the American Nurses' Association (A.N.A.) at its forty-seventh convention in May 1970, and, a few weeks later, the honorary degree from the University of Colorado. Peer approval is a source of great satisfaction.

Nursing changed tremendously during my career, and I feel privileged to have been active during that time. Nursing has always had a good supply of energetic and intelligent leaders. Since they had to live within the social structure of their time, I am filled with wonder at their accomplishments because they had educational limitations and experienced deprivation imposed by the culture.

RETIREMENT

Perhaps everyone whose career has been demanding and has yielded many satisfactions is apprehensive about retiring. I was no exception. What would I do with my time? How could I become acquainted in a strange community? How could I balance my activities to include more play but some service to others? Fortunately for me, there are a number of retired nurses in Sun City, some of them career officers from the U.S.P.H.S. whom I had known for years. This gave me an immediate nucleus of friends on whom I could depend for social activities. I have always believed that it is not necessary to go far afield to find someone who needs help. I have been able to apply this theory in this retirement community. It seems to me that Sun City is a little cul-de-sac of age, the one thing that we all have in common. Actually the residents here are quite diverse in background, and many have had unusually interesting and productive careers. Some must live frugally while others are affluent. Though not necessarily financial, there are problems relating to aging; for example, malnutrition may debilitate people who are no longer able or who lack incentive to shop and prepare their own meals. Because of this obvious problem one woman initiated a meals-on-wheels program. I was invited to join the group, and participated in some of the original planning. Special diets come from the local hospital, and a restaurant provides the regular meals. More volunteers than can be utilized are available to deliver meals. They are very glad to give their time and the use of their cars to deliver meals one day a week. The clients find them friendly, and welcome them not only because of the meals they bring but also for the brief visit that is part of the delivery service. This project has gradually grown. During 1974, the third year of operation, about 14,000 meals were delivered. The meals were paid for by the client receiving them. Some clients are blind; some are confined to wheelchairs; and some, because of such conditions as diabetes or cardiac disease, require special diets. The community has gradually learned about the service, and more doctors are now referring their patients and prescribing the diet needed. I am currently president of Meals on Wheels. Working with this program are a number of persons of professional quality. The Admissions Committee is chaired by a social worker. This committee visits each prospective client, explains the service, and determines eligibility. Some clients reach a point where receiving meals is not enough. They are faced with selling or closing their homes and planning for another type of care. If drivers observe such needs, the clients are referred to the Service Committee, which is composed of a mental health nurse and two social workers. They have been skillful in getting in touch with relatives, helping select a nursing home, or assisting with plans for other types of care.

We find that many people do not know where to turn when a resource is suddenly needed. Recognition of this need has motivated me to work with another group developing an information and referral service. An administrative board has been organized, volunteers to answer the telephone have been recruited and trained, an office has been found, and the service was recently launched. The community response has been immediate.

Since my retirement I have done a little volunteer nursing. I usually have one or two patients who are being cared for at home, where some help with nursing is needed. They have tended to be terminal cancer patients. I am far from a clinical specialist, but some of my old skills still seem to be useful. On several occasions I have taught the home nurse to give hypodermic injections to relieve pain. I have also taught them a few ways to make the patient comfortable. The other day the husband of one of my patients said, "If someone had tried, they couldn't have devised a crueler way for a person to die." I think this is true. I feel particularly sorry for the family members of terminal patients, and sometimes my help is to them rather than directly to the patient. I have read extensively about chemotherapy and some of the newer treatment modalities. One of the faculty members at the University of Arizona who knows of my interest frequently sends me duplicated copies of articles she thinks will be helpful. Occasionally I am called in the night because I let the home nurse know that I am willing to come if she is frightened or needs help. During the past few months I have been with two patients at the time of death and have, I believe, been of some help to the surviving spouse. One night a woman called me and said she was terribly sick. When I reached her home a few minutes later, she was on the floor in shock. Her husband was ill at home with terminal cancer. I called another neighbor and together we called an ambulance and got her to the hospital, where emergency surgery was performed for an obstructed, gangrenous intestine caused by adhesions. She required hospitalization for several weeks, so it was necessary to take her husband to a nursing home, where he died about six weeks later.

As long as I am able, I would like to continue nursing. Some patients have asked me to talk to their doctor for them because they have been unable to explain their problems or to understand the doctor's orders. I have stayed in the hospital while a patient is in surgery, so she will know that someone cares about her and will be there when she regains consciousness. I have stayed with women while their husbands were undergoing surgery, to give them a little support.[9] All of this keeps me busy, and though I do a substantial amount of reading every week, I have not had as much time for reading as I would like.

[9] Pearl Coulter received the Distinguished Citizen Award Nov. 7, 1974, from the University of Arizona, upon the recommendation of the College of Nursing faculty.

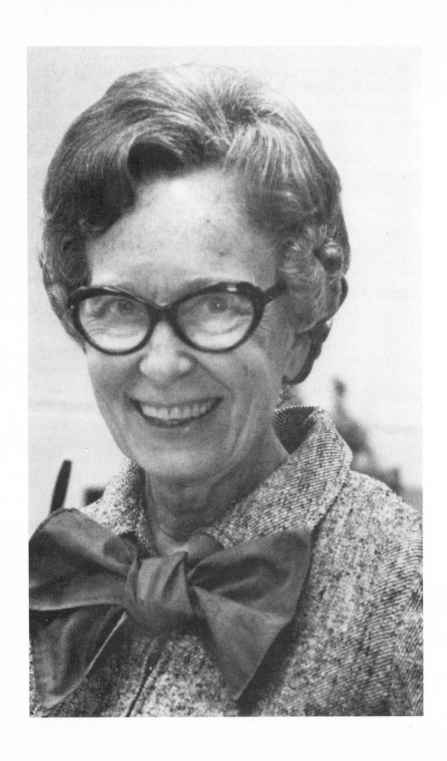

3

Ruth B. Freeman's contributions to public health have been of the highest quality and substance. Her extraordinary combination of energy, talent, and background has produced a continuous stream of significant ideas, writings, and disciples. All this productivity has taken place in a variety of settings. Dr. Freeman has been a public health nurse, a supervisor of visiting nursing, and an administrator of nursing services . . . Dozens of organizations have sought and benefited from Dr. Freeman's wisdom and leadership. They range from the United States Air Force to the World Health Organization . . . President of the National Health Council and the National League for Nursing.[1]

[1]Bronfman Prize for Public Health Achievement, American Public Health Association, 1971.

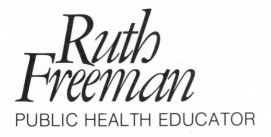

Ruth Freeman

PUBLIC HEALTH EDUCATOR

*R*uth Freeman was born in Methuen, Massachusetts, December 5, 1906. Her father earned his living as owner of a livery stable and in real estate activities. Dr. Freeman describes her family as "sort of middle-class Protestant." She was the oldest of three children; the others were boys. Her mother, to whom she felt very close, died when she was eight. Her father remarried but Dr. Freeman never felt the same close relationship with her stepmother, who soon had three children of her own. Mainly to become independent of home, she entered nurses' training at Mt. Sinai Hospital School of Nursing, where she met her future husband. She married Anselm Fisher in 1927 after receiving her registered nurse diploma. She has had a long and happy marriage and has one daughter, Nancy Ruth. Dr. Freeman worked and went to school intermittently. She received her B.S. in 1934 from Columbia University and her M.A. (1939) and Ed.D. (1951)[2] from New York University.

Ruth Freeman has made significant contributions both to nursing and to public health. She retired as Professor Emeritus in 1971 from Johns Hopkins School of Hygiene and Public Health, where she had a long and distinguished career.[3] Before that she was with the American National Red Cross (1946–1950); she was a Professor of Public Health (nursing) at the University of Minnesota School of Public Health (1941–1946) and an instructor at New York University (1937–1941); and she was with the Henry Street Settlement Visiting Nurse Service (1928–1937). During her American Red Cross appointment, she was on leave to the National Security Resources Board for a year and a half as consultant.

She has published extensively—over fifty articles in public health and nursing journals. Among the five books she has authored, her *Public Health Nursing Practice (1950)*[4] is a classic.

Dr. Freeman has been extremely active in professional organizations at local, state, national, and international levels. She has been elected and appointed to many offices. Some of these are President of the National League for Nursing (N.L.N.), 1955–1959, President of the National Health Council, 1959–1960, President of the Minnesota State

---

[2] The title of her doctoral dissertation was "Supervision in Public Health Nursing."

[3] She went to Johns Hopkins in 1950.

[4] *Community Health Nursing Practice*, W. B. Saunders Co., Philadelphia, 1970. The other books are *Techniques of Supervision in Public Health Nursing*, W. B. Saunders Company, Philadelphia, 1945; with Dr. Ramona Todd, *Health Care of the Family*, W. H. Freeman and Company, San Francisco, 1946; and, with Dr. E. M. Holmes, *Administration in Public Health Services*, W. B. Saunders Company, Philadelphia, 1960.

Nurses' Association, 1944–1946, and Vice-President of the National Organization for Public Health Nursing (N.O.P.H.N.), 1946–1950. With the American Public Health Association (A.P.H.A.) she has served at various times as a member of the Governing Council, the Executive Board, the subcommittee on Handicapped Children, the Editorial Board, the Technical Development Board, and the Awards Committee.

In addition, she has served on many governmental task forces and commissions. To cite only a few, she was consultant to the U.S. Air Force; on the Advisory Board, International Cooperation Administration; a member of the White House Conference on Children and Youth with the Children's Bureau; on the Advisory Committee for Pan-American Health Organization and World Health Organization (W.H.O.); a member of the W.H.O. Expert Advisory Panel on Nursing; director of a survey of nursing in W.H.O.; and a member of the International Council of Nurses (I.C.N.).

She has received recognition from her peers for her many accomplishments. In addition to the Bronfman Prize, she received the Pearl McIver Award, the Nursing Award from New York University, the Mary Adelaide Nutting Award, and the Award of Merit from the Pennsylvania League for Nursing.

Since her retirement, Dr. Freeman has been writing, serving as a consultant, and, "best of all," having more time to enjoy her husband and their 130-acre farm in Virginia.

Early Training

GS: Why did you go into nursing?

RF: I enjoyed working with people who were disabled and older, but didn't have any feeling that nursing was my career. It was just a way to get out of an unchallenging situation. My aunt happened to be at Mt. Sinai Hospital in New York City, working as a secretary, and she suggested I go to Mt. Sinai, which I did. Nursing was accidental, but I found it really absorbing. I was always in trouble, but I enjoyed it.

GS: When you say "always in trouble," what do you mean?

RF: I was in trouble because I talked to the social workers and the doctors and you weren't supposed to; and I was in trouble because I didn't "know my place" with respect to the doctors. I went to observe a postmortem without getting prior permission. There are all kinds of episodes of that sort.

Although I was in a typical diploma school, I found it intellectually very challenging. I spent a lot of time at the library reading; whether it was just an escape from things, I don't know, but in any event I'd read anything that I could get my hands on. So it seemed rather natural to me when I finished at the School of Nursing to go on to college, and I enrolled at Columbia. It was more that it was a thing to do that was there—and it sounded interesting—rather than because I'd planned ahead. Maybe that's kind of the story of my life. I do what's at hand and enjoy it very much. When I leave it, I go to something else. I never had a long-range career goal [or] career ambitions. That sounds sort of silly, but when something came up and my husband and I weighed it at that moment, it either seemed as though I could do it or I couldn't, and it would be exciting or it wouldn't. The decision was made then and there, so that it was all happenstance that things came along as they did. Having taught planning, that's a very damaging kind of admission to make.

Henry Street Visiting Nurse Service

Immediately after graduation from Mt. Sinai, I applied and was accepted for a staff nurse position at the Henry Street Visiting Nurse Service. My purpose was to have working hours that would allow me to attend Columbia University's part-time program for nurses seeking a degree. This experience had a profound influence on my concept of nursing and upon my commitment to it as a career. It was a sobering, joyful, sharing experience. For the first time I felt free to do what *I* wanted to do for people, and saw people as people rather than patients struggling with overwhelming problems, winning the battle of making a decent life despite depression, illness, and inadequate health resources. I remember most the rush of gratitude I felt toward families who taught me things I needed to know—that dying wasn't calamity, that "making do" was not demeaning, and that helping wasn't controlling. My immediate superior, Helene Buker, and the central office staff, Elizabeth Mackenzie, Marguerite Wales, Elizabeth Phillips, and, of course, Lillian Wald, taught me much in terms of patience and optimism, but through their example reiterated the primary place of the family in making its own decisions. It was Helene Buker who finally persuaded me that becoming a supervisor wouldn't really separate me from nursing practice. I knew that no other field of nursing could ever be as deeply satisfying.

New York University, Department of Nursing

It was Dr. Helen Mauzer, director of the nursing program at N.Y.U., who picked me out of a class she was teaching to ask whether I would like to teach. At first reluctant, I was persuaded that teaching was also a service, and we started. Classes were huge—often over one hundred—and students were largely full-time employees coming to class after a day's work. Resources were minimal, but Dr. Mauzer was a "can do" leader who believed firmly that anything could be done if it were needed, and her optimism spilled over to all of us. Coming from the "real world," students were encouraged to challenge their instructors—a healthy experience for all! It was long afterward that Dr. Vera Fry (now Maillart), who took Dr. Mauzer's place at N.Y.U., persuaded me to complete my doctoral work.

Professor at the University of Minnesota School of Public Health, 1941–1946

GS: What took you to Minnesota?

RF: Primarily because, while I enjoyed New York and felt comfortable there, I felt that there was a whole area of nursing that I didn't know, that had to do with the main part of the country, and that this was an opportunity to learn what went on in that kind of state. A second reason was that Dr. Gaylord Anderson, who was Dean of the School of Public Health at Minnesota, was an extraordinary fellow in that he believed thoroughly in nursing. I think at that point his was perhaps one of the few, if not only, schools that required physicians and others to take a course in nursing. His whole concept of public health was so broad and so fascinating that the opportunity of working with a man like that was tremendous. It's unlikely that I would have been accepted if it weren't for Marion Sheehan's recommendation, because their feeling was that people who came from Eastern schools didn't understand the rural situation at all and were not very helpful in meeting the people's needs.

The University of Minnesota was one of about ten schools of public health at that time. At Minnesota we had baccalaureate as well as graduate programs for nurses. We had relatively large numbers of students, [although] in general schools of public health had smaller enrollment than other schools. An average counseling load for a faculty member in nursing at that time was about fifty. We had a large number of part-time people, a large number working for baccalaureate degrees, and a smaller number engaged in graduate work. Looking back on it, I think we did far too little with the graduate program and more than we should, proportionally, with the undergraduate program. On the other hand, we all participated very actively in all aspects of the graduate program and with the seminars. [Nurses] were expected to carry their weight as scholars, and I think they did what was expected.

Dr. Anderson was an innovator, and he was a people lover. He wanted his staff to think. He might not like some things we did, but he never didn't like us. He would insist on certain standards; he expected us to do a good job of teaching. It was very clear if he thought we hadn't come up to his standards, without his ever making an issue of it.

There are one or two other things I want to comment on with respect to Minnesota because it was really one of the most satisfying periods in my life. We were involved with agencies and with local groups in a very responsible way. For example, I did a great deal of work in the province of Manitoba, largely in the form of consultation or surveys or workshops, and we had a good many students from Manitoba on a regular basis. When I went out as a consultant there or in Minnesota, which I did a great deal, I was held responsible for the results, not what went on or how happy people were. At one time I can remember Dr. Jackson, Deputy Director of Health and Welfare, Manitoba, saying that someone had come to summer session, and when they went back to work in a remote area in Manitoba, he didn't think they knew what to do. He felt that we had fallen down on their education. I said, "Well, what do you want us to do?" He said, "I want you to get the so-and-so up there and see what went on." I talked with Dr. Anderson about this, and we decided that was an entirely reasonable request, but we didn't have any money. So we again talked to Dr. Jackson and said, "We haven't any money to travel." He said, "Fine!" and worked out with the nursing group a consultant job in Winnipeg so I could go up to see these women. I saw what was wrong. What we had been doing was taking people who had long experience in remote areas, submitting them to a great deal of theorized knowledge, and we hadn't spent the amount of time we should have spent discussing experience. The young students could make the transfer because their basic nursing was different. With these older women what we should have had was more conferencing. As a result of that trip we changed our methods. If a graduate of any one of our programs didn't measure up, we were very likely to hear about it. People would want to know why: "Why are you teaching this?" At one point a physician in a smaller county called and said, "You were talking about nurse-physician relationships in class. Now I've come to this county and the nurse is in the office that I feel I should have, and she refuses to move out. What am I going to do?'' He had a situation in which the nurse had been the only county health worker; she was so firmly entrenched and so threatened, she said she had worn out two health officers before him and she was going to wear him down too. He finally worked his way out of that by a series of concessions, and even got the office after a year. But the point was that he was holding me responsible for not having prepared him to deal with a situation which was a very common one.

[In Minnesota] the state health department was on the same grounds as the university, and there was a terrific, supportive back-and-forthing between the school and the agency. This was based on trust and affection as well as expediency. We were expected to be as concerned about the health department as they were about the School of Public Health. I find in some places there's competitiveness among departments or between service and educational agencies, or even a downgrading of the contributions made by the nonacademics. This never would have been tolerated in Minnesota.

GS: Why did you leave Minnesota when you did?

RF: We left Minnesota primarily because it was not turning up anything useful for Al [my husband]. I think that I would have stayed merrily on if we hadn't had a second career to be concerned with.

American National Red Cross[5]

RF: The American Red Cross job needed to be done; it looked as though I could do it; and I saw it as a temporary kind of job, which it was. I was not unhappy about the move; it was administrative experience I could never duplicate. It was the most complex administrative job, I think, that could be imagined. It was working between the voluntary groups and the paid staff and the local communities: somebody was always unhappy about what you were doing. They had very traditional things going that had to be changed, and a staff that didn't want to change. It was a very challenging, interesting job, and I enjoyed every minute of it. But I was ready to leave at the time I left.

[5] Dr. Freeman went to the American National Red Cross as the administrator of its Nursing Services in 1946 and remained there until 1950. For about a year and a half preceding 1950, she served as a consultant to the National Security Resources Board.

Coordinator, Nursing Programs, Johns Hopkins School of Hygiene and Public Health, 1950–1971

GS: How did it come about that you went to Johns Hopkins?

RF: The Johns Hopkins School of Hygiene and Public Health never had a nursing program. They had had nurse lecturers, but never a nursing program. Dr. Stebbins didn't know what was needed, and he invited me to come in with an absolutely open hand to develop the program. I was asked whether I would expect to have a department of nursing. It became very apparent, as I looked around and lived at Johns Hopkins, that the departments were very compartmentalized and very competitive. I did not think that I could do what was needed if I placed nursing in a a competitive position, simply creating another little capsule, when I wanted in effect to do something that would cut across all of the departments. I thought that was the job, and, still think that is the job that needed doing.

GS: So how did you get nursing into the structure?

RF: Simply by again feeling absolutely comfortable about walking in and saying, "I hear you're talking about adding a nurse to your staff. What kind of a nurse are you looking for and can I help?" Or, if I saw something going on, I might go in and say, "You know, a good many of the things you're doing could be very much improved if you had a nurse on your faculty. How about getting one if I can find the money?" It turned out that in the long run they not only got one, but they found the money themselves. As the number of nurses employed increased, we also formed a nurse faculty council to share ideas and coordinate the nursing effort. I think Dr. Stebbins had in mind something like the Minnesota program—both undergraduate and graduate teaching. But when I got to Johns Hopkins, it appeared to me that that would be the wrong thing in that setting. There was already a feeling that nurses were very practical people and very helpful, but not really of academic caliber. No one else in the school offered undergraduate education, so that an undergraduate program in nursing would have been something different from anything else in the school. I felt that it would drain off a lot of the energy that was needed to develop a graduate program, particularly since it didn't seem there would be a large staff; and not to do well would discredit nursing. For all those reasons, after I had a chance to look at the situation on the spot, I recommended to Dr. Stebbins that we not engage in an undergraduate program, that we not have a department of nursing, but rather have a nursing presence in the school, responsible directly to him, with free access to talk to anybody about nursing. He agreed. It was an opportunity to work with an outstanding public health figure, Dr. Stebbins; it was an opportunity to develop a new program. At the beginning I was not at all sure it was worth the time it would take for a very small number of nurse students, and I felt we would have a very small impact on nursing over the country with only about ten nursing students a year. Yet we could not get a large number of nurses without overbalancing nurse representation in the program at Johns Hopkins. So we decided that we could have a relatively small and highly select group and that nurses would not be treated differently from other students in any respect. There would be no such thing as a course in epidemiology in nursing, or a course in biostatistics for nurses; nurses would have to be able to manage the total program comfortably or we would advise them to go somewhere else.

We also decided that some nurses shouldn't be there, because they needed or wanted more intensive nursing input than we were prepared to provide. My feeling about not having a high impact shifted when it became apparent that the influence of the nursing presence, with one or more people on the faculty with reasonable academic distinction, affected the other faculty and nonnurse students as well as the nurses enrolled.

GS: Was it difficult for a person such as yourself to attain a full professor rank in public health?

RF: I think it's increasingly easy now. There were very few full professors in the 1950s and the 1960s, mostly people who had been there many years; an associate professorship there was worth a professorship anywhere else, at the point that I took it,[6] and other people who were doing work as important as mine were also associate professors. There I didn't feel I was being discriminated against. If I had chosen to have a department, I would probably have had full professorial rank within a short time rather than several years later. What would have bothered me was if that rank had prevented me from doing anything I thought needed doing, and it never did.

Main Contributions

GS: What do you consider to be your main contribution to nursing?

RF: If I were asked what my contribution was, I would say that in teaching it's primarily the development of a multidiscipline, multidepart-

[6] She returned in 1971 as a Professor Emeritus.

ment kind of responsibility. I learned this first at Minnesota from Dr. Anderson, who felt that nurses and physicians both need to know a lot about nursing in order to do their jobs. They need to know different things, but for some part of what they learn it should be together. I think that perhaps that's the thing I'm proudest of: that I feel just as comfortable, and feel that we do just as much in the nursing courses, with nonnurses as we do with nurses, and just as comfortable teaching public health or administration as nursing. I think my greatest satisfaction in teaching has been that, especially at Johns Hopkins, where it's been possible to do very individualized work, it's been possible to teach on the basis of developing individual people. The thing I abhor, and think I've avoided, is a maternalistic approach to students. I see much too much of that in nursing. It is very debilitating to the student and inhibiting for the faculty member who falls into that trap. I've never felt that my emotional satisfaction in life came from the development of students. But I felt that my teaching satisfaction came from getting students to the point where they would argue vociferously with me when it wasn't really popular, as it is now, to argue with a faculty member. A point I feel keenly about and worked hard at is keeping teaching relevant to the "real world."

Another satisfaction came from a continuing effort to relate academic work to the realities of service, through constant interchange with field agencies and experimenting with teaching approaches that offered more opportunity for students to deal with service problems.

Organizationally I think what I'd like to feel that I've done is work toward simplification. For example, I once worked on a committee [of the N.L.N.] that developed a statement called "What People Have a Right to Expect of Modern Nursing," which has just been reprinted. This put in simple, concise terms the concept of a "patient bill of rights" as seen by a group of patients, students, nurses, and physicians. I think that at the league we did a great deal to simplify the structure and administration, and that I had some small part in this.

GS: Could you pick out your main contributions to the area of public health in general?

RF: Perhaps I was one of the early people to think that administration, per se, is very important to people in health positions. I wouldn't see administration as a be-all and end-all or as having extraordinary complexity. It was for that reason that I wrote with Ed Holmes a book on administration. This has not been revised because Ed has since died, and also the need for that kind of a book is now less. But I do feel I've made a contribution to getting that content incorporated into public health and recognized as a valid area. Now it's fully recognized. Another contribution may be to show that people in any specific category or discipline have a contribution to make to planning and administration. I think one of the big problems with Health Maintenance Organizations right now is that they have far too little nursing input, and as a result they are very medically oriented and hence limited. They cannot do the job that's set out for them unless they have much, much more in the way of nursing input. I don't mean a nurse-practitioner trained by a physician in a few medical techniques, but more nursing in the overall planning, the management of patients, the decision about what constitutes proper care: nursing contributions at the decisional and policy levels. I think the Johns Hopkins and Minnesota Schools of Public Health did present the nurse as a different kind of collaborator. This meant that in the education of nurses, we had to keep the content that they need to be that kind of collaborator, which meant that we couldn't follow the then-popular line of thinking that anything that was not "nursing practice" was therefore inappropriate for nurses to be engaged in or to learn about. It seems to me that every nursing position in community *health* involves some administrative activities that are not nursing and that are shared with a good many other workers. I think I did my share to get personnel in public health to accept nurses as full collaborators and to help prepare at least some nurses to participate intelligently in this role, through education of nurses and nonnurses and through organizational activities.

I tried not to limit myself to nursing considerations or to the place of nursing in any particular decision, but to act as a general public health worker, without reference to my discipline, as comfortably as I could act as a nurse in other contexts; it's a matter of balancing the two.

GS: You also stated that you were active in organizations such as the A.P.H.A., which is not a nursing organization.

RF: Yes. I've been elected to office and been active as a member in several organizations.

GS: In public health, then, you found support from the Public Health Association?

RF: I think one of the most fascinating things about the A.P.H.A. is that, for many years, it has not been dominated by the medical group, and has been willing to give recognition and offer participation in the overall decisions of the organization to all professional and action groups. For this reason it's a particularly satisfying organization to work with. I've always felt that the Association was dealing with real problems and real people, and had changed as the times changed.

I might say definitely that my contribution was not, either at schools or in organizations, in the area of research. I've been very interested in promoting research and in helping other people to do it. But I have always felt that my contribution was in presenting a philosophic point of view: what I call "think pieces" as differentiated from definitive research. This was obviously a great handicap at Johns Hopkins, where research is considered a primary function for everybody; but as they came to accept me without a department, they also came to accept me without research. The same thing happened when I was President of the National Health Council. I thought it was possible to move away from some of the clichés and away from some of the things we'd been doing in sort of an involved way. I think sometimes the simplification took the form of an attitudinal stance, such as subjecting every new program or every new potential to a single question: "How will this affect the goals that we're trying to reach?" In some instances, a good activity in itself might interfere with the goal by overbalancing the program in one direction or another. It's at points like this that I've felt sometimes, in discussion or as a board member or as a president conferring with the staff or organizing staff, or in interagency things, I could help. I don't mean that I could have done it unless there were people like Anna Filmore and Marion Sheahan at the League, or staff at the National Health Council that were supportive.

GS: What other strategies did you use?

RF: A real belief in the importance of communication. I learned early that belligerence very seldom pays off; that firmness is one thing, belligerence another. Some belligerent people have gotten a great many things done. If you can do what you need to do by reasoning together, as the Quakers would say, rather than by fighting it out, you're that much further ahead on implementation because you can go ahead without having to fight battles at the same time. On the other hand, if the only method is confrontation on disagreements, then you have to count the cost. The important thing is to know where our points of disagreement are. You have to present what you have to say in a reasonable way, even though it is nonsupportive to another group or another organization.

I think my main contribution definitely has been in education. In carrying out my educational responsibility, I have perhaps held to a closer association with the practice or service setting than was usual. This was particularly true at Minnesota, where for the first time I was involved in multidiscipline teaching, and where I was dealing with a group of nurses who had considerable responsibility in rural areas. As a part of the exercise of teaching, I exchanged services with people who were running services. I would help them by working in their in-service education programs at their request. In turn, they would help the school by offering certain kinds of field experience to students. I think we were able to move from a kind of dumping process—of having students simply exposed to six weeks or eight weeks of nursing experience in the community—to developing a very thoughtful approach on the part of the students, in analyzing what they expected to see and what they could learn. At the same time the student adviser, with whom we spent a considerable amount of time, saw how this fitted into the total education program of the students and the students' obligations to the agency. My feeling then, as now, is that student experience that becomes too focused on the learning aspect is relatively inefficient; that in general the students learn much more if they become members of the working staff in every sense of the word, even if they don't get away exactly at four o'clock, even if they miss a class once in a while. It may be more important that they see how far nursing can be carried to meet the demands of a situation than it is to learn a little bit more in the academic sense. At Minnesota, where I also had a joint appointment with the State Department of Health as a consultant without salary, we had very close ties, and developed even closer ties, between what went on in the field and what went on in school. As part of the exercises the students did, they would develop a plan for county nursing and have to face up to the fact, as they developed the plan, that they had only a little over 2000 hours a year to deal with, and that all the things they wanted to do simply wouldn't fit into that kind of time frame. In making the adjustments we then would invite in people from the field to criticize these plans.

GS: On the international scene, what do you consider you have contributed?

RF: I did serve on technical committees—and one always works very hard at those—but it's hard to identify any particular input. I did do a survey of the W.H.O. nursing operation some years ago, which may have had some effect on practice. In developing the recommendations, we tried to develop them along the lines of indicating what needed to be done and what conditions had to be met to do what was needed, and then we recommended. The survey was late getting in, as are most reports that I do, but it had some virtue in that it got down to practical problems which turned out to be philosophically grounded. In other words, I think the report did turn the attention of administrators and nurses to some of the practical problems of getting the job done and the philosophic base on which decisions rested. This is one of the most time-consuming things I have to discipline myself to do: to move from an abstract and philosophical idea, which is unlikely to influence anybody except a few scholars, to a practical presentation. I think I helped with some of the management and planning problems.

Through serving on task forces or technical committees I was able to help develop broad funding documents such as the Technical Reports of the W.H.O. As a consultant I could deal with day-to-day problems and try to help develop new approaches. My forte was trying to hold reports and plans to reasonable levels, while classifying the basic philosophy on which discussion should be made.

Major Issues

GS: *What do you see as some of the major issues in nursing?*

RF: One of the immediate major issues, I think, is to move to some redefinition of nursing practice. It seems to me that the purpose of nursing is pretty much unchanged, and has to do with improving the capability of individuals to handle or prevent illness and promote health. This is particularly important in view of what's happening with definitions of care and with the development of the general practitioner specialist in medicine. It's my belief that we have to settle for a good bit of ambiguity with respect to this differentiation of practice, but that we ought to be clear about the basis on which we are taking a particular stand.

GS: *What is your reaction to your critics who would say that the people who advocate nurse-practitioners are a sellout to nursing?*

RF: Of course I disagree. I think if nursing maintains a narrow approach, it's going to become terribly expensive and pretty ineffective. We need some way in which we can get a primary health referent for every family in this country, and it's my opinion that it will not occur through the further development of the family physician. It seems to me that the family physician is overprepared for many things families need in health care. Another very real issue is what should be done with respect to the organization and management of the multidiscipline team. First, I think the hierarchical concept under which such teams are usually set up is no longer useful for the kind of services we're expected to render. Secondly, I think there are great difficulties in defining the responsibilities of the individual members so they feel content within some kind of reasonable framework, and at the same time allowing them to interchange responsibilities when that is necessary for purposes of economy or effectiveness in dealing with patient care situations. Another problem is what is going to happen about the organization of medical care in general. I feel that if everyone is to have a primary health referent, someone to whom he or she can turn, this health referent has to be one of a large group of professionals, readily available psychologically as well as physically. For this reason it seems to me that we are going to have problems as we move with H.M.O.'s, since they tend to be centered in a medical environment which has a different set of resources than those needed for health care. The issue is: Who is going to take the leadership or maintain control of the health programs, as differentiated from medical care programs? I tried—and failed several times—to get funded to see whether the public health nurse could be this referent. I think she could.

GS: What kept you persistent in your ideas?

RF: Well, because I still think it is possible. I think that an average community health nurse, bolstered by a cluster of helpers with various capabilities, could study and work with the total population, providing health monitoring and health services with the help of laboratory backup. I think it could be done cheaply, and it's the only way I see that we can really get to complete coverage of this country. I don't see how the H.M.O. could ever get itself down to any kind of reasonable cost. I have to add that now I think we are way overboard in our costs for community nursing as well. We have a big job to do to take a very careful, hard look at the way we're organized, and see whether a serious downtrend in costs can be effected.

GS: What are your views on either lowering the costs or getting more for the cost?

RF: With respect to cost, there are a good many things that need to be looked at. One is the allocation of personnel. When each member is seen as having a narrow, specified responsibility, there's a great deal of wasted time because staff can't interchange activities and carry dual responsibilities. Task assignment, rather than case assignment, so that two people are involved in direct care, would increase costs substantially. And yet most teams are set up on a hierarchical basis, and frequently the team leader is the one who is responsible for the case load. It seems to me that it's quite possible for every worker, including aides, to be responsible for a case load, with the public health nurse or supervisory nurse stepping into a backup rather than a controlling position. I think one of the real problems we're going to have to face up to is what we're going to do with the education system, which of course has to come after we decide what we're going to do with nurses and members of the nursing team. The present situation of degree-oriented labels as prerequisites for getting certain types of work certainly doesn't seem to be working too well. I believe that advanced education, beyond the baccalaureate and into the doctorate, may be necessary for both research and administration, as administration becomes more technically oriented; but, on the other hand, I think that it's going to be even more important to be able to reach all nurses with continuing education where they are, on their own terms, and with respect to what is needed in a particular area. This is a much bigger job. The present idea of simply transferring some of the teaching maneuvers from the university to the field, and calling it continuing education, has got to stop. Continuing education, it seems to me, should have its own flavor and depend much, much more upon the inputs of the individuals who are, hopefully, being educated! We could have a good, basic, vocationally oriented nursing—not in the subacademic sense—and also a lot of modules of education that could be plugged in at points where people need them. Then a person who happens to be in a situation where there are a good many psychiatric problems could find somewhere a module in psychiatric nursing and be brought up to date. Or the person who is interested in genetic counseling could quickly be brought up to date in that field and be given the needed help. There'd be more and more opportunities for self-learning, and some education might be in regionally oriented learning centers. It seems to me there are lots of ways it could be done, but it ought to be a kind of on-tap service available as necessary to build up skills. In addition to that there should be opportunities for continuing education that is directed toward enlarging one's perception and conception of what the whole health job is about. This might well be interdisciplinary, but in any event it should be focused not on what is being done, or how it's being done, but rather on why it's being done—on questions such as "How do you use operant conditioning in the moral sense?" "Do people have the right to have babies at will, or should that be considered a privilege?" This sort of question, which can't be resolved by any small, plug-in module, is important.

GS: What would you consider to be the one thing you did that gives you that extra thrill?

RF: I think mostly it's the contact that I had with students, and the feeling that, as you see them get out into the field and perform, you realize they're doing things very differently than you would do them; but they're doing them exceedingly well and with some kind of consciousness of why they're doing what they're doing. As you see this, you have the feeling that you have contributed something to the continuity of nursing by preparing individuals who can, in fact, do it with their own style and in their own way and produce more than we could ever think of producing. I think the most exciting award I ever got was the Pearl McIver Award. Pearl McIver was one of the great people in nursing, a simple and giving person whom one would be very proud to be associated with. The other one was the Bronfman Prize, because it showed recognition of nursing's contributions to public health and was the only Bronfman Prize awarded to a nurse.

My feeling is that nursing in the future is going to be organized in and around clusters of people who will have differing capabilities; they'll include specialists and people at the subprofessional and professional level, and they will work probably on a case assignment arrangement, whereby one member of the cluster will give primary care to the family and the other member of the cluster will provide backup support. This would permit us to use people in gerontology, for example, who are particularly good at working with elderly people, and perhaps a nurse-midwife for those families in which there were growing children and in which the primary health preoccupation of the family is with childbearing and child rearing. I think this could be inexpensive in cities; how it could be arranged in a rural area would be a little more of a problem. But this would permit a case load in which the individual worker gave total nursing care to the family with the backup of the rest of the team. It would also allow for the use of specialists without undue cost. We need a system by which we can categorize patients with respect to the kind of nursing they need. I don't mean by the number of sheets they're apt to have changed or things of that sort, but rather how well that individual or family or community, or the three in concert, can manage the situation they have to face, and how much assistance they're going to need, and what kind of assistance. If some such categorization system could be worked out, it would be clear what type of person within the cluster might be used to provide the primary care.

GS: How do you define public health nursing, and what are your comments about it?[7]

[7] For a succinct recent discussion by Dr. Freeman on the future of public health nursing and community health nursing, see Ruth Freeman, "Alternative Role for Nurses in the Delivery of Health Services," paper presented at the Minnesota Public Health Association meeting, May 3, 1974. (To be published.) In brief, she believes that the future is most unpredictable and that alternative roles must be taken by the community health nurse. She sees the management of stress as the number one health care problem. "I see no real change required in the *purpose* of community health nursing. This might be defined for our use today as: to enable individuals, families, groups and communities, singly and in concert, to cope with their health problems and threats to health in such a way as to maximize the realization of their human potential. It is in the *ways* in which this purpose is realized that the very substantial change must come. The future of community health nursing practice lies in a creative adaptation to trends such as an increasingly powerful knowledge technology; a lagging social technology; and changing life styles. I believe we can and will move in changing to new levels of service and new excitement in practice."

RF: This is a very difficult thing to define, and frequently, rather than define it, I suggest that we define the purposes and modalities, because the boundaries of practice are so fragile that they overlap with those of a great many other professional groups. In general I think public health nursing is one of the human services that are directed toward increasing the capability of people, whether singly or in groups, to deal with their health problems and with threats to health in such a way that their overall capacity to realize their capabilities is improved. In doing this they use a variety of modalities, only some of which are medical; the remainder may be sociologic, educational, or epidemiologic. I think probably what was meant by "stream of ideas" is that, over a period of years, I have developed certain philosophic basic thinking and have turned out what I call a series of "think pieces." Some of them had to do with the relationship of voluntary, professional, and official agencies. Some had to do with where I thought nursing was going, with the place I saw for the consumer and consumer inputs into services. For a while I have focused on administrative principles and problems.[8] I wouldn't go so far as to say I had disciples, as you suggest, but there are a good many people, especially poststudents, who have been kind enough over the years to let me bounce ideas back and forth with them.

I don't think any working wife can make it unless she has a supportive husband. Without this it's imposible to concentrate and to move ahead with any degree of security. This doesn't mean that you needn't plan your time so as to allow for family responsibilities, but rather that you can plan it together and there is no resentment of necessary absences from usual household chores and responsibilities. When a husband is excited about your career as well as supportive, as mine is, it extends the boundaries of thought and accomplishments to a much greater degree.

Writing

GS: *You've done a great deal of writing, starting rather early in your career. You've written several books and many articles. Do you like to write?*

---

[8] See Ruth Freeman, "Changing Times: Changing Practice," unpublished paper presented at the Alabama Nurses' Association, Oct. 24, 1974. See also Ruth Freeman, "The Expanding Role of Nursing," *International Nursing Review*, vol. 19, no. 4, 1972.

RF: Writing is not easy for me. I feel compelled to do it. I like it when it comes out right and says what I intend to say. In the last few years what writing I have done was done under great time pressure. There were dozens of articles that should have been written in the last three years I was at Johns Hopkins; but we were so pushed by survival and adjustment problems in schools of public health in the general fields of medicine and nursing, and by day-in, day-out administrative responsibility, that I could only do what had to be done.

In the beginning I felt what was a compulsion to share things that happened because I thought, "This is kind of important." Lately I've felt guilty at not writing what should be written.

GS: *Did you feel pressured to publish?*

RF: No, not at all. I never felt it applied to me. It's interesting; I guess it's like being a nurse: I thought all the things nurses went through because they were nurses didn't apply to me, because I never paid any attention to them and assumed they wouldn't. I wrote entirely from inner compulsion. When I discussed lack of publications with Dr. Stebbins at one point, feeling very guilty about it, he said, in effect, "You have to make that decision yourself; no one is going to push you. We'd much rather have you write less and write it the way you want to." When I retired, I found that I had a tremendous amount of catching up to do on my own thinking. For three years I've been floundering around, trying to get my own thinking straight again.

GS: *In what way would you say your new book is mainly different? You changed the title. Otherwise, what's the difference, conceptually, from the former book? (Public Health Nursing Practice, 1950)*

RF: The old book dealt more with direct patient care. Later I felt that the idea of nursing a community had not even begun to be appreciated, and I still don't think it's implemented at all. Nurses in public health are nursing individuals—sometimes families though by no means always—but nursing individuals in the context of their family and the family in the context of the community; but they are not nursing the community. I don't know if that difference is clear, but it's very clear to me. When you are nursing the community you are as concerned for example, with neighborly support and its development as you are with the ability of a mother to support her children, because they're both imperative in the survival of communities. I think the fact that we have so little sense of community is partly because nobody took seriously that the basic stepping stone to that is neighborliness. I don't think we can afford to live without it. When sociologists tell me that it's disappearing, I say, "You're telling me a trend; you're not telling me what needs to be true, because it doesn't have to disappear if the people decide that it can't disappear." My conviction is that it cannot disappear and that we are moving toward it now for the first time, very slowly, not only in nursing but in general. As I looked at this, it seemed to me that the important thing is to look at nursing populations and nursing communities within which we nurse families and individuals. No less devotion, and no less imagination, and no less time is needed for family care. We need to give equal billing to each responsibility.

GS: Has the book been influential?

RF: It's been influential—certainly with nonnurses. My books have been widely translated and used.

GS: How about the number of people reading the new book as compared with the first one?

RF: This has been much higher. But that, I think, reflects the fact that many more nurses are going on to education in educational institutions. I don't think that means that the book is any better; I think it means that more nurses are reading more. It is interesting that older books in supervision and administration are still being sought, although they are out of date and out of print.

I think at the time each book came out, it probably was set a little ahead of the times, but not too much. This in one of the things I'm now doing with this revision: not looking at what I'd like to see, but what I think is possible.

GS: Isn't writing that book a big job?

RF: It's a nasty job. Most people who decide they want to write a book, as you well know, don't have any idea of how much slogging work goes into it. From my standpoint, having more time in retirement, the "paring down" is much more painful. I don't have time to do a lot of articles or speeches that I'd like to do. What I have to do is to push forward with the book and then do the articles. Once in a while I give a speech and get some of the things off my mind. Of the material I have, of the references and ideas, if I use 15 or 20 percent, that's a lot.

GS: Are you going to stop now? Is the edition of the book that complete?

RF: No. What I want to do is several short pieces that are on my mind. This is my last go-around with the text.

I write for my own amusement and edification. Then I have to rewrite it so that it becomes a communicating, useful document. In doing that I have to give up some of my most cherished phrases and whole batches of content that are irrelevant to the purpose and the needs of the people for whom I'm writing, or which need to be put into a totally different context.

Earlier I gave some thought to having a coauthor, who could then take over. But, from working with Dr. Holmes, I know that it takes at least three times as long for any author to work with a coauthor as it does to write yourself; and I didn't have the time. Otherwise you get a book which is very jumpy and has no consistent philosophy. Ed Holmes and I spent six months of intensive work, meeting once a week for a whole day, talking about what we thought public health was all about, before we ever put pen to paper.

GS: What was his reason for wanting to write a book?

RF: He felt that we needed one, and we both felt that if it was going to be a joint effort, it should not be jumpy, that it should have a consolidated, agreed-upon philosophy. It was only when we got that done that we began to write. Then each of us would block out each chapter and send it to the other one in a sealed envelope, not to be opened until the other one had finished writing, so that we each had the benefit of the other's thinking; and then we decided which of us would do the final writing. The end result was that we got a book that I think hangs together pretty well. But the time cost was fantastic. You don't halve the work; you double it or triple it.

There are several nurses in different parts of the world who are looking at the possibility of a different type of collaboration with *Community Health Nursing Practice.* The original text would be retained with respect to principles and general content. However, all examples, references to national figures,and so on, would be done by a local or national coauthor. This would allow for validating the principles while at the same time giving the reader a more useful source of reference. I think this is a new concept.

GS: If you had to pick, out of the five books that you have authored, the one that you think has been the most influential, which would it be?

RF: I think probably, in terms of influence on practice, the very first

Public Health Nursing Practice was the most influential. It had a much lower sale; it reached far fewer people; but at that time it did reach people who were in the field.

Changes in Public Health Nursing

GS: *In your career, which has spanned many years, what have you noticed that you consider to be some of the biggest changes in public health nursing?*

RF: Well, I guess probably the thing that I see most in public health nursing is a short of shifting kind of allegiance and a struggle for identity between nursing and public health, instead of a willingness to accept the ambiguity that goes with being part of both.

Another thing I've seen, especially in Ms. Fitzpatrick's history of the N.O.P.H.N., is how adaptive community health nursing has been throughout the years. It moves with the things that are needed, but I'm not sure that we're moving with enough decision right now. I feel that part of the problem is that we haven't recovered from our binge of rebellion against being associated with any other professional group. We don't have a clear enough idea of what our inputs could be. I'm a bit disappointed with the development of nurse-practitioners.

GS: *I was going to ask you about that.*

RF: I think it's a great idea, but I have real reservations about the way it's developed. The emphasis has been entirely medical in far too many instances—on saving doctors' time, taking on doctors' functions, on using the stethoscope, and so forth. While much is said among nurses about expanded nursing, and while some courses are so directed, in far too many instances the nurses are talking to themselves. Often other team members still have no idea of what nursing is beyond technical interventions.

A Highly Desirable Worker

GS: *Would you say that you actively sought most of your positions?*

RF: No, I think they came my way. I had a feeling that it would be well to move out of New York City. I had gotten that far; but I hadn't really done anything definite about looking for something. I think in another few years the urgency would have been so much greater that I would have felt I needed to look. But no; the only job I ever looked for was the first job I had, as a staff nurse at Henry Street. That was a very simple thing. I went in to see Marguerite Wales and she said, "Well, I think you'll do just fine." That's all there was to it. But otherwise it's been largely a matter of someone seeking me out.

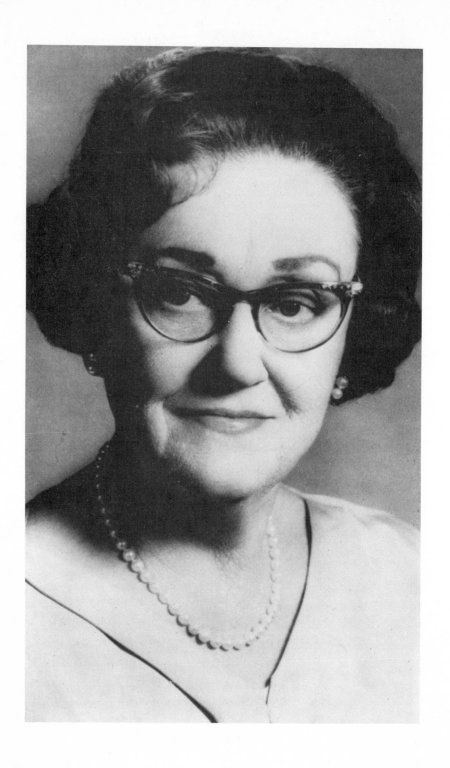

4

. . . From the beginning, her boundless energy
and consummate ability have made her
outstanding as a teacher and administrator,
challenging as a speaker, productive and
effective as a writer, enthusiastic and inspiring
in conference and consultation. In all times and
all places she has planned, participated and led
in the significant advances made by nursing as
a professional career.[1]

[1]Citation, Mary Adelaide Nutting Award of 1965, presented to Lulu
Wolf Hassenplug in ceremonies at the National League for Nursing
Convention, San Francisco, 1965.

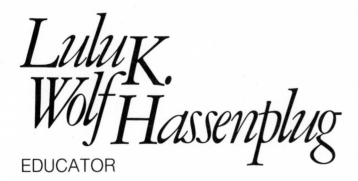

Lulu K. Wolf Hassenplug

EDUCATOR

*L*ulu K. Wolf Hassenplug was born in Milton, Pennsylvania, on October 3, 1903. She received her nursing education from the Army School of Nursing in 1924, a bachelor of science degree in nursing from Teachers College, Columbia University, in 1928, and a master of public health degree (Rockefeller Fellowship) from Johns Hopkins University in 1947. She attended the University of London, England, under a Florence Nightingale International Foundation (F.N.I.F.) Award and graduated "with distinction in the whole course."

Among her many awards and honors[2] are two honorary doctor of science degrees: from the University of New Mexico (1964) and from Bucknell University (1965). In addition to the Isabel Hampton Robb Scholarship, she received two Rockefeller Travel Grants for study of nursing in the United States, Canada, Europe, and the Orient. Lulu Hassenplug was named Woman of the Year in Education by the *Los Angeles Times* (1958). The Vanderbilt University School of Nursing, where she served as Professor of Nursing for ten years, established the Hassenplug Videotape Series and Media Collection in her honor in 1974. This special collection was sponsored by the Class of 1942. In 1975 Arizona State University presented her with its first Distinguished Achievement Award Medallion for her distinguished service to the College of Nursing.

Her elected and appointed positions in professional organizations and on national advisory councils are too numerous for inclusion here. She has been a member of the Board of Directors, National League for Nursing (N.L.N.). Currently she is serving as a member of the Advisory Committee on Physician's Assistant Nurse-Practitioner Programs, California Department of Consumer Affairs.

Lulu Hassenplug is the author of over sixty articles on nursing and nursing education, and has written two textbooks on nursing and collaborated on another.[3]

Lulu Hassenplug's experience has been as Instructor of Nursing, Piedmont Hospital, Atlanta (1925–1926); Educational Director, Jewish

---

[2] The Gold Key of Alpha Tau Delta for "Outstanding Service to Nursing" (1959); honorary membership in Sigma Theta Tau for "Leadership in Nursing Education"; the Mary Adelaide Nutting Award for "more than a quarter of a century of creative, constructive contribution to the development of Nursing as a professional discipline within the system of American Higher Education" (1965). The California Nurses' Association created the Lulu Hassenplug Award for "distinguished achievement in leadership in nursing education, innovations in curriculum and contributions to standards of excellence" (1969). Award from U.C.L.A. at its Golden Anniversary for "distinguished service to the University" (1969).

[3] *A Study Guide Testbook in the Principles and Practices of Nursing*, The Macmillan Company, New York, 1930; with M. R. Smith et al., *The Principles of Nursing Care*, J. B. Lippincott Company, Philadelphia, 1937; *Nursing*, D. Appleton-Century Company, Inc., New York, 1947.

Hospital, Philadelphia, (1927–1930); Associate Professor, Medical College of Virginia, Richmond (1930–1938); Professor of Nursing, Vanderbilt University, Nashville (1938–1948); Dean and Professor, School of Nursing, University of California (1948–1968); and consultant in nursing education (1968 to the present).

Her involvements in community service and university activities have included helping to create the Western Council on Higher Education for Nursing (W.C.H.E.N.) and charter membership in the Western Council on Mental Health Training and Research. She has been consultant in nursing education for a number of universities in the United States and for the University of Cali in Colombia, South America (1967–1968). She was a member of the Surgeon General's Consultant Group on Nursing, the Defense Advisory Committee on Women in the Armed Services, and the Department of Defense Nursing Advisory Committee.

Lulu Hassenplug is best known for her innovations in baccalaureate nursing education. She maintained that nursing students should be like all other college students, and at the time (the 1940s) this was radical thinking. Until the 1940s nursing students were expected to live in a nurses' residence and do the work of the hospital for room, board, and tuition. In addition, she believed that preparation for public health nursing should be an integral part of all baccalaureate programs. One of her citations stated: "As a great teacher, you have taught by both precept and example. As a scholar and effective administrator, you have caused such innovations in collegiate nursing education that the stature of your profession has increased greatly."[4]

Comments on Early Career

GS: Could you comment on your early career?

LH: The Army School of Nursing turned out to be the right choice for me. In some ways it was an experimental school, and since I was not too certain I wanted to be a nurse, the school fitted my needs as an experimentation. I never really planned to be a nurse. For as long as I can remember, I wanted to be an actress. Home talent productions had given me an opportunity to sing and dance in musical comedies at an early age, and by the time I had played the part of a French-speaking countess in the high school play, I was certain I'd be a great success in the theater. At seventeen one is sure of many things!

My sister had gone to the college of her choice; my brother was a

---

[4] Citation, honorary doctor of science degree, Bucknell University, June 6, 1965.

student at Penn State University; and it never occurred to me that I would encounter opposition when I announced my plans for college. To my surprise, my father thought I was too young to go "far away" from home, and suddenly he thought he couldn't afford to pay for my schooling. He said he'd rather see me enroll in the university near my home; but what he really meant was that he didn't want me to go *on the stage*. Since he had upset me, I decided to upset him by becoming a nurse—an occupation with no status at that time and one which he thought was far beneath me and my capabilities.

Of all the programs I studied, the Army School of Nursing seemed to be the best for me. It provided board, room, laundry, and a stipend of $30 per month; and every weekend was free. This meant I could be financially independent of my father and could attend the theater every Saturday in Washington, D.C. My mother was a great help, supportive in every way. My father was really upset. I was getting away from home with the theater at my doorstep. My high school sweetheart, Harry, rode the first 15 miles on the train with me—an unexpected, much-needed, and long-remembered gesture on my behalf.

Six weeks after I was established at Walter Reed Hospital as a student nurse, my father told me if I would come home he would finance the cost of my education at *any* college I chose; but by that time I was enjoying my work as a student nurse, and had about decided to complete the program. I left the door open, however, for there were many things about nursing as it was taught and practiced in those days that I thoroughly disliked. The discipline of the armed services—in this case the Army—plus the discipline of the subculture of nursing irritated me beyond words. I never could understand why nurses stood up when doctors came into the room, and I rebelled at performing nursing care procedures in a certain way when I could create shortcuts that were better. The pecking order of the military made absolutely no sense to me. And it still doesn't!

I spent considerable time in the Chief Nurse's office explaining my behavior and my need to think for myself, and to this day I wonder how it was that I was allowed to continue in the school, for I really was a chronic irritant for my teachers and superiors. My classmates were great. I developed the practice of taking two of them home with me at holiday times so my father and mother could be assured that they were indeed "ladies." We still keep in touch; one was matron of honor when I married Harry.

As soon as I completed the program, I entered Teachers College, Columbia University, to secure a baccalaureate degree. At that time I still wasn't too sure I'd continue in nursing, but because all my teachers had told me I should become a teacher, I thought it was worth a try.

After a year I took a position as Instructor of Nurses at the Piedmont Hospital in Atlanta, Georgia. I'd always wanted to see the South, and the Director of the school, Helen Ziegler, assured me I'd have every weekend free. This was indeed an unusually good year, socially and professionally. I had lots of dates, three proposals of marriage, was introduced to the taste of corn liquor and mint juleps, picked oranges off the trees in Florida over the New Year's holiday, and made my first speech at a nurses' meeting.

Since I was the only nurse teacher, I taught every nursing course in the curriculum and did the best I could to guide students in the clinical setting. This was exhausting! I studied hard to stay ahead of some very able students, and I often sought the help of interns and seasoned medical men. With the aid of a few affluent physicians I got a library started, and I stopped the practice of having a nurse chaperone the physicians' lectures. That, I thought, was utterly ridiculous. At the end of the year I was certain I'd like to teach nursing if I could learn more, so I returned to New York to complete my work for the baccalaureate degree in nursing.

Beginnings of Leadership

GS: What would you consider your first leadership position?

LH: I probably began to exert some leadership in the nursing community during the three years I taught at the Jewish Hospital in Philadelphia—now the Albert Einstein Medical Center. As Chairman of the Program Committee of the Philadelphia League of Nursing Education, I was instrumental in providing programs which eventually drew as many as five hundred people. Chairing these meetings and leading discussions of controversial topics dealing with obsolete hospital and public health rituals, as well as stereotyped nursing care activities, gave me a chance to exercise my histrionic ability and considerable stimulus to do so. In these endeavors I received help and encouragement from such leaders as Jessie Urquhart, Director of the Jewish Hospital Nursing School; Stella Goostray and S. Lillian Clayton of the Philadelphia General Hospital Nursing School [Ms. Clayton was also President of the American Nurses' Association (A.N.A.) at the time]; and Maude Muse and Isabel Stewart of Teachers College, Columbia University.

GS: What would you say you accomplished during this period of time?

LH: I was very close to students in those years, and their reactions to me were a great satisfaction and stimulus. In a way we were peers, for

I was in my early twenties. I tried to counsel those who did not like people out of nursing, and this was very difficult to accomplish, since students were needed to staff the nursing service. I think I helped some students learn that reading and studying were an integral part of the nursing care of people, and that all of us ought to try to develop a kind of divine discontent which would help us do tomorrow something better in the way of nursing care than we did today.

Some students helped me introduce ward classes and demonstrate new procedures. Others taught me important lessons about Jewish customs and health practices, and still others helped me to discontinue the practice of standing when physicians entered the classroom to teach. The generalized complaints of all of the students regarding their heavy reading assignments at the Central School of Nursing at Temple University led me to write my first article for publication. This article appeared in the *American Journal of Nursing* (*A.J.N.*), Volume 28, under the imposing title of "Time and Intelligence Study." Mary Roberts, editor of the *Journal*, wrote me, in answer to my question as to why it had not been published *immediately* after she received it, that she had delayed its publication until she could have my graphs "checked for accuracy." I remember how chagrined I was by her comment, since I thought I had learned how to make graphs accurately in one course at Teachers College. Obviously I had little knowledge of how a magazine was put together for publication.

GS: Anything else?

LH: I wrote a study guide testbook on nursing that wasn't much good, but it seemed to be the thing to do at the time. Short-type examinations were in vogue.

I guess I also thought I was making a contribution to nursing by helping nurses join and participate in nursing organizations. When we had good programs, nurses came to the meetings; and eventually some of them began to ask themselves, "What can I do for the organization?" instead of "What does the organization do for me?"

GS: Did you feel during this time and later on that nursing was really going in any particular direction? Did you see the direction?

LH: I don't remember feeling anything much about particular directions. I was disappointed in what nursing was accomplishing most of the time. I wanted to see nurses giving good nursing care in the home as well as in the hospital, and not always as private-duty nurses. I wanted most of all to have students become students when they entered schools of nursing, rather than employees of the hospital. I thought they should be learners and have time to learn; and as long as they were included in the time slips for nursing service, I thought this was impossible. The late twenties was not a good period in nursing. We were preparing too many nurses in too many poor schools, and most of them went into private duty.

During the thirties I taught at the Medical College of Virginia. These were the Depression years, and, as registered nurses couldn't find positions, many were hired to staff hospitals at very low salaries. This meant that we did see less pressure put upon students. The Social Security Act made possible grants for nurses to secure preparation for public health nursing, and this was a great step forward. With fewer students in basic nursing programs and better staffing in hospitals, we began to strengthen nursing curricula and spend more time with students in the clinical situation. During these days I taught registered nurses as well as basic students, and in the process I learned a great deal.

For one thing, I decided all over again that *public health nursing should be an integral part of all basic nursing programs and that students must have a stronger knowledge base in the sciences and humanities upon which to build their nursing care practices.* And, probably because I believed this so intensely, I thought I could see nursing going in this direction.

The 1927 *Curriculum for Schools of Nursing* was revised in the period 1934–1936; and when it was printed in 1937, it recommended two years of college as a prerequisite for the nursing major. I had helped with that revision, and I had also spent one year studying nursing in England and visiting nursing centers in the Scandinavian countries and a few other countries on the continent of Europe. And the more I saw of nursing schools and nursing services, the more I was convinced that we needed to move all nursing education programs into the educational system of the country and make nursing academically respectable.

The English system, which had been so highly touted by some of our nursing leaders and medical men, seemed to me to be archaic in 1936–1937. Undoubtedly this was why both Mary Roberts and Isabel Stewart cautioned me to remember that I would be a visitor in England while I studied there and to be careful that what I did and said would reflect favorably "upon the American nursing profession." Both of these nursing leaders were on the committee which selected me for the first Florence Nightingale International Foundation fellowship, and, as they told me later, they were indeed fearful of what I might say, since I was "outspoken and frank." I *did* tell Daisy Bridges (who was in that same 1936–1937 class) what I thought while we sipped sherry late at night, but of course I never expressed any of my disillusionment to the English matrons over tea and crumpets. After all, they were my hostesses; tea was one of their best meals (sometimes including sherry); and I was more or less hungry for good food that entire year. The best food in London was found in the best hotels, but women without male escorts were not welcome in these hotels unless they were registered guests. It took me until near the end of the year to meet the proper escort—one who drove a Bentley—but at least I got a chance to see how the other half lived before I sailed back to God's country, and I ate some excellent food in beautiful hotels.

I wouldn't take anything for that year in London—with the abdication, proclamation, and coronation; and the meeting of the International Council of Nurses (I.C.N.). It made me more aware of people and their needs, and as I traveled to the Scandinavian countries and visited nursing centers there and a number of the European nursing programs, I vowed I would do a better job of entertaining nurses from other countries when they visited the United States. There's nothing quite so illuminating and valuable as travel and study in a country different from your own. And I cherish my continuing friendship with many of the classmates I had that year.

At Vanderbilt

GS: What a year! And then you went to Vanderbilt University?

LH: Yes, after spending one year more at the Medical College of Virginia and after a stormy year with myself—trying to decide whether or not to get married. In those days I still thought about marriage as an either-or proposition. Either I got married and gave up nursing or the other way around. My ambition won out, and I decided to go to Vanderbilt because I believed that at long last I could function in a program that was in and of the university. I wanted to build a curriculum and teach nursing in a university setting, and the opportunity to do that came when Helen Ziegler, with whom I had been associated in my first teaching position and again at the Medical College of Virginia, asked me to go with her to Vanderbilt. I went! But there must have been times when Helen wished I hadn't. I was impatient and moved fast, and she was a Georgia woman who took her time.

Following publication of the Goldmark Report, the Rockefeller Foundation had appropriated funds to four schools of nursing to put the recommendations of this report into practice. Vanderbilt University School of Nursing was one of these schools, which had as their mission the preparation of better nurses in a shorter time and the inclusion of preparation for public health nursing as well as the nursing care of the sick in hospitals. By 1930 the Vanderbilt School of Nursing had become an independent school with its own dean, and by 1936, under the leadership of Shirley C. Titus, admission to the school required two years of college. Upon completion of the three-year nursing program, the student received the bachelor of science in nursing.

I went to Vanderbilt with great expectations. At long last, I thought, students will be free to learn nursing. But, though the school was located on the university campus, students in nursing were not treated as students in the other schools on the campus. They were required to live in the nurses' residence. The hospital provided them with board and laundry, and they were really counted upon in the university hospital nursing service to help staff the hospital.

This was quite a blow for me, and I decided to change it as soon as possible. That was in 1938. It was not until 1948 that I was able to bring it about. In the meantime it was possible to develop a new kind of program and to try to make nursing content worthy of collegiate credit. Here again I enjoyed a close relationship with nursing *and* medical students, and, when World War II became a reality, I found myself counseling both medical and nursing students and helping them arrange their marriage plans to coincide with the tours of duty in the armed services, internships, clinical nursing assignments, pregnancies, and the like.

The war helped to speed up many changes which our faculty and many other nurses had been trying to bring about. Students were finally allowed to live outside the nurses' residence, and more and more of them married while they were enrolled in the school. Faculty moved into apartments and homes in the community, and, as soon as they did, I imagined I could see a difference in the way they acted. They got to know the families in their neighborhood; they talked to the garbage collectors, stockbrokers, working mothers, spoiled children, neglected children, Sunday school teachers, businessmen, and businesswomen; and they developed a whole new outlook on life, love, and the pursuit of happiness.

Larger classes were entering our nursing program, and all of us were stimulated to find better ways to do more and to do it faster. Julia Hereford and I published an article telling how we had established academic credit values for nursing courses, and Lucy Dade helped me explain to *A.J.N.* readers how we managed to teach larger classes in the clinical setting—most of which was necessitated by the passage of the Bolton Act.

Emphasis in the curriculum shifted from care of the sick to *nursing for health*, and we actively sought the help of our colleagues in preventive medicine, sociology, bacteriology, and social welfare to bring this about. Wayland Hayes helped the students get the feel of what sociologists and anthropologists call "culture," and in the process some of his knowledge rubbed off on me and other nursing faculty. Together we learned about culture traits in ourselves as well as our patients, and we were able to relate them to specific patterns of behavior. Some of our nursing conferences were *painfully* humorous. Had I known at the time I was experiencing an "encounter group," I might have understood why I was not so shocked by the behavior of us leaders in the late forties, when we met on three different occasions to consider how *One Thousand Think Together.* Too bad we didn't do videotapes of those meetings. But then, maybe it's for the best that we didn't. Tapes aren't always helpful.

Most of us teaching in Vanderbilt's nursing program in the early forties were trying hard to make students more self-reliant in using numbers to determine facts, draw conclusions, and solve problems. Consequently we were grateful to Dr. Faye, Dr. Keller, and Dr. Densen for contributing their time and statistical know-how to achieve the goal. We all felt rewarded when finally our work paid off and students began to ask, "What does this mean? What happened as a result of what I did for and with patients?" We expect this kind of accountability and responsibility from professional health workers today, but even now we don't always get it, and in those days it was indeed a novel idea.

Another idea which materialized in 1944–1945 was joint accreditation of baccalaureate programs by the National League of Nursing Education (N.L.N.E.) and the National Organization for Public Health Nursing (N.O.P.H.N.). Today the earmark of all baccalaureate programs accredited by the N.L.N. is that the graduates of these programs have preparation for nursing in all settings, but in 1944–1945 only the Skidmore College of Nursing, the Vanderbilt University School of Nursing, and the Yale University School of Nursing held this distinction.

Into Public Health

GS: What was your next move?

LH: My next move took me to the Johns Hopkins School of Public Health and Hygiene for some long-overdue graduate education. It was a good year of hard work and fun. I was the only nurse and one of two women in a class of 125 physicians and statisticians, and that alone was a delightful learning experience. My undergraduate work had all been in nursing programs, mostly with female classmates, with the exception of the summer I studied play production at Bucknell University. Yes, I finally got to the university my dad selected earlier for me, and I got involved in the theater.

During the year at Johns Hopkins I determined to return to Vanderbilt and make one more try at freeing students from the obligation of staffing the nursing service of the hospital. I had never liked that "earn while you learn" or "learn while you earn" slogan that was used during the cadet nursing program. One night when I was arguing the pros and cons of "working one's way through college," Julia Hereford said, "College students work their way through college; but they do things for money, like wait on tables when they are not in classes." For one reason or another, that bland remark gave me the idea that students of nursing could be students while in class and clinical settings, but plans could be made for them to work for pay during other periods of the day or evening. To this day I can't figure out why it took me so long to get this idea.

In short order we planned the schedule, reviewed it with Dean Ziegler, and then sold it to the hospital director and the administrator of nursing service. In essence the plan gave the hospital the assurance of student-staff coverage for every evening on the seven to eleven o'clock shift and for Saturdays and Sundays. Each student was scheduled to work for twelve hours each week as an employee of the nursing service in return for her room, board, and laundry. Schedules were set; replacements or backups in case of illnesses were planned; and a stable student work force was accepted to become effective July 1, 1948. To my knowledge this was a first in nursing schools, and for a while it worked. When the hospital administration eventually found (as we had anticipated) that the twelve hours of student work did not really cover the cost of food and lodging, students finally began to pay for their maintenance and live where they chose. The article titled "A Laboratory in Clinical Experience," published in the *A.J.N.*, Volume 49, recounts the highlights of this development.

I mention these articles, published some thirty or forty years ago, not for the purpose of blowing my own horn, though that could be part of it, but to indicate some historical trends and directions in nursing's development.

GS: Why did you leave Vanderbilt?

LH: I was becoming more and more impatient because things weren't moving as fast as I thought they should. I wanted to get a graduate program started, and to do this we needed a larger budget. Chancellor Carmichael, with whom I had worked before going to Johns Hopkins, had now left, and the new chancellor was moving with great caution. I began again to search for the right place to earn a doctorate, and I again argued the pros and cons of marriage; Harry agreed to wait one or two more years while I *looked* at U.C.L.A.

University of California at Los Angeles

GS: Is that what brought you to California?

LH: Yes! I guess it was the challenge to build a school of nursing on a university campus where no school had existed before. I had been approached twice before to consider the opportunity at U.C.L.A., but at those times they were considering only a baccalaureate program for registered nurses. This time, when I was asked to consider the opportunity, it was quite different, and Esther Lucile Brown thought it was a great opportunity.

A new medical school had been approved and funded for U.C.L.A.; a dean had been appointed; and I was asked to become chairman of a newly established department of nursing in the College of Applied Arts. Funds for a nursing program had been included in the funds for the medical program—which, as we all know, is not the *best arrangement.*

I questioned Provost Dykstra as to why a school of nursing had not been established and a dean appointed. His answer was, "We don't know what kind of a program we should have, and we want you to come out here and tell us what to do about nursing." I said, "Oh! I can tell you where to go and it won't take me a year to do it!" His answer indicated he had expected some such comment, since he had thoroughly investigated me.

As it turned out, it took me a year to study the situation on the campus, in the developing medical school, and in the community, and to assemble a nucleus of faculty that could come up with a plan for the school of nursing. The regents of the university authorized the school as one of the professional schools of the Center for Health Sciences in 1949, and this action paved the way for the development of undergraduate and graduate programs in nursing.

GS: What were some of the things you wanted to do in this new school of nursing?

LH: The thing I wanted most to do was to create a bona fide school of nursing. No such school had been developed anywhere at that point in time. According to my plan there would be a curriculum structured along the lines of other baccalaureate programs on the campus. Students would be enrolled as other students were, and would be free to marry and to live where they chose. There would be *no nurses' residence* (how I hated them and what they did to nurses!) and no set time to complete the program, other than credits required for the degree.

The entire program would be structured within four academic years—eight semesters—and the registered nurse students would be fitted into the program according to their demonstrated knowledge and skill, and would meet the same standards for admission and graduation. The focus of the program was to be *care of people*, and *learning* was to become the common endeavor of faculty and students.

Faculty were to be appointed, as were all other faculty on the campus, on either a nine-month or an eleven-month basis; they were to meet the same criteria for appointment and were to receive the same salary.

GS: Could you find faculty with this preparation in 1949?

LH: As a matter of fact we couldn't. Few nurses had earned doctorates at that time, and those who had were not really oriented to clinical teaching, research, and publication. No one in that first faculty group held a doctorate, and none had made significant contributions to nursing research. "How then," the Appointment and Promotions Committee asked, "could nurse faculty hope to attain professorial rank and tenure in a distinguished university?" "How indeed?" we thought! As faculty members we had been admitted to the university's community of scholars, and we knew we had to adopt some of the characteristics of a scholar's way of life if we were to hold our positions. We also knew that nursing needed the university far more than the university needed nursing, but we hoped we could make nursing an important university discipline eventually, just as we hoped the graduates of our program could improve the *practice* of nursing.

GS: Could you get faculty appointed to professorial rank in those early years of the program?

LH: Yes! But the appointments had to be made at the assistant professor level, primarily. Later, as a few of these faculty demonstrated their scholarship and published the results of their research, they were promoted to associate and full professorships.

GS: Did you have any particular problems getting the program established?

LH: More than we had anticipated, I guess. We had no recipe for revolution, but at times we thought we were in the midst of one. The program was to be offered within four academic years; it was to meet the standards of the university for a baccalaureate degree with an upper-division major in nursing (at least thirty-six units of nursing) and at the same time meet the requirements of the state for examination and licensure of a professional nurse. The state requirements called for a thirty-six-month course in nursing with a specific number of weeks in clinical services.

Before we could initiate our program, the faculty spent hours helping to develop and secure the adoption of a new set of state regulations. This took more doing than you can imagine, but we made it, thanks to the help of some very liberal-minded members of the Board of Nurse Examiners. There are such, you know!

And, now that I think about it, we also had a few heated discussions with some members of the N.L.N. Accreditation Board, since this new program did not use *number of weeks spent in each clinical area* as the measure of competence in practice. At the same time some of our public health nursing specialists held fast for sixteen to twenty weeks in the senior year in public health nursing, and our program was not so structured, as you might know.

GS: Once the program was approved, did you encounter difficulty putting it into operation?

LH: We sure did! We had developed behavioral objectives for competence in practice (that was a great step at that time), but we soon found that the way we were planning to conduct our nursing laboratory sessions in hospitals and health agencies left much to be desired. Our laboratory sessions were far too long, as the students had been telling us, and did not produce the results we were after. We learned the hard way that practice which is a confirmation of a theory or hypothesis has a substantive content and is deserving of university credit, whereas practice which is focused on the learning of a technique does not. Even today some of us can't tell the difference.

The crowning blow, and the one which most of us found difficult to accept in 1955, was the discovery that students were subjected to considerable repetition in nursing courses and that medical-surgical, pediatric, psychiatric, and the like, were *adjectives denoting geographic areas of the hospital rather than well-defined areas of nursing knowledge.*

Discoveries of this type were very *anxiety-producing,* for they required us to *rethink the content of our entire nursing program.* On more than one occasion we lost faculty because of these painful discoveries. Other faculty, who viewed these experiences as challenging, remained, but even they fled to a mountain or beach resort occasionally to have it out with themselves and their peers, heal their wounds, or get a fresh approach to a problem.

GS: Did you have problems with the hospital or health agency, the nursing personnel, or the doctors where the students had their clinical practice?

LH: Oh, yes! But that was to be expected! After all, whoever heard of beginning clinical nursing experiences in 1950 at eight instead of seven o'clock in the morning, even if the nursing faculty and students had to drive 30 or 40 miles from the campus to the clinical setting and back to the campus again for course work in the afternoon? Who could imagine that faculty and students in nursing would decide not to wear caps? And the idea of wearing street hose rather than white hose while on duty! Only they don't call it ''duty''; they call it ''nursing laboratory practice.'' Obviously our students, who could live where they chose and be married if they wished, were a new breed of student nurses; and I think they were regarded as being wealthier than most nursing students, since they paid for everything themselves, just like other students in the university: books, fees, housing, food, and laundry.

GS: *Had you interpreted all this before the students had their clinical experiences?*

LH: Oh, many times. We had held a variety of meetings with the nursing and medical personnel who were to be involved with our teaching program, but it takes time to accept anything new. Nursing service personnel had been accustomed to having students do the *work of the ward*, and even though these students were not in the time slips as nursing service personnel, they were still *expected* to function as if they were. After all, this was the way the staff had been trained a bit earlier, and why should anyone do it differently? Why, indeed? When our students completed their nursing care activities and sat down to read the charts of their patients or confer with physicians or other health personnel, their behavior was judged to be out of line or downright unprofessional. And if these students had mothers who were registered nurses, I had a lot of phone calls to this effect.

GS: *And the physicians?*

LH: Physicians, who were accustomed to complete acquiescence from student nurses—and we had lots of them—were taken aback by their questions, and a few seemed to undergo a considerable degree of shock when our students preceded them through a doorway or failed to rise from their chairs when the physicians approached them or entered a classroom. All physicians, of course, did not behave in this fashion; a number of the younger men accepted the students and contributed to their learning in the clinical setting. On those occasions when faculty in nursing became role models for students taking over the responsibility for the nursing care of a group of patients for a short period of time, medical and nursing personnel, as well as social workers and the like, became active participants in the clinical teaching program.

Suffice it to say we lived throught the "agony and the ecstasy" of changing the system of baccalaureate education for nursing practice in the early fifties. Today this pattern of education has been emulated in practically all of our university and college programs. We continue to hear about problems in the acceptance of the "degree nurse," but well over 25 percent of our new graduates are now coming from baccalaureate programs and—God being willing—more will do so in the future!

GS: *Weren't associate degree programs established about this same time?*

LH: They were! The junior college programs, as we called them then, were developed in the early fifties. I was a member of the advisory committee for that Cooperative Research Program, probably because I was "agin" them. I tried unsuccessfully to get the name of these programs changed to "vocational nurse programs" so that we would eventually have only two programs for nursing when the diploma schools were discontinued, but I lost the battle with Louise McManus. Who didn't lose when arguing with Louise? Now we have associate and baccalaureate degree programs preparing nurses for the same license to practice, and this continues to create more problems than it solves. And of course we still have the traditional diploma programs, which I thought would—and said *should*—be out of existence by 1973. How long, Catalinus! How long!

GS: *What of the present one-year program?*

LH: The practical nurse programs and the California vocational nurse programs, which are the one-year programs, should be developed into two-year associate degree programs which should be called *vocational nursing programs*. This would leave us two types of nursing programs, and as things are developing now, I believe these would more than supply our needs for licensed nursing personnel.

GS: *Where do the diploma graduates fit in this plan?*

LH: Wherever they want to fit and can qualify. We have created all kinds of mechanisms for testing the knowledge and skills of registered nurse students who wish to enter college and university programs, and these equivalency tests make it possible for potential applicants to validate their previous knowledge and skill. And of course we are now seeing baccalaureate programs set up solely for diploma graduates.

GS: How soon after the U.C.L.A. school was established did you develop the graduate program?

LH: Contrary to what most people believe, both programs were planned as soon as the school was established. We awarded the first master's degree in 1952, two years before the first baccalaureate degrees were awarded in 1954.

GS: Were you active in the junior college movement in California?

LH: Quite! As an integral part of the University of California, the faculty accepted the philosophy that its three major functions were teaching, research, and service. In the early years—say the first five—most of our energies went into program development, teaching, and public service. The faculty contributed to the work of the committee appointed to make a "Restudy of the Needs of California in Higher Education," and it was mainly through our efforts that the report, published in 1955, included the recommendation that education for nursing be moved "into the total structure of higher education" according to a statewide plan. Later, when a coordinating committee was created in 1956 to help develop this plan, a resolution initiated by the U.C.L.A. faculty went before this committee to ask the California Nurses' Association to introduce legislation to make possible junior college programs for the preparation of technical nurses. Such legislation was passed the following year.

GS: So you and the faculty were active in state nursing organizations?

LH: Yes. And when it was necessary, we got involved with the legislature. I spent hours traveling back and forth to Sacramento when we were trying to get the law passed to create schools and licensure for vocational nurses. The faculty as a whole concerned itself with regional planning for improvement in nursing education and nursing service. When the opportunity came, they helped to launch many of the new ventures under the aegis of the W.C.H.E.N. I chaired the committee that made it all possible.

GS: Did some of this regional work help your own school?

LH: Yes, in many ways. Perhaps the most helpful activity, which was a direct outgrowth of the faculty's participation in the work of the graduate seminar, was the proposal we prepared in 1954 to study the undergraduate and graduate programs in nursing and the possibilities of education in *nursing at the doctoral level*. The proposal received support from both the Commonwealth Fund and the Rockefeller Foundation in 1957. The study covered a two-year period, and was conducted by Dorothy Johnson, of the U.C.L.A. faculty, and Eleanor Bernert Sheldon, a sociologist employed on the grant. Assistance was provided by faculty teaching in graduate programs in the schools of nursing in the western region and by consultants from the local area and throughout the country.

An important by-product of this intensive study of nursing content was the stimulation it provided to all W.C.H.E.N. member schools to delineate and refine nursing content at the undergraduate and first-year graduate levels.

GS: What about nursing research? Did the study reveal much?

LH: Actually, it revealed how little nursing research was being done. A considerable body of literature in nursing research was examined, and it revealed what most of us knew: namely, that nurses were more inclined to focus their attention on the *occupation of nursing* than on the *patient.* Since most nurses had received their doctoral preparation in schools of education at that time, it was not too surprising to find their dominant interest to be of an educational rather than a clinical nature.

GS: What happened when the study was completed?

LH: Well, the study led to our initiation of an experimental two-year post-master's program in nursing research.

GS: Not a doctoral program?

LH: No, and for two very good reasons. On the one hand, we did not have enough faculty with research training who could qualify for appointment at the tenure level. The budget of the school made possible this level of appointment, but in the late fifties there were very few nurses available for appointment with doctoral preparation and demonstrated research skills. On the other hand, the systematization of nursing knowledge was not well advanced, and the training required for research in clinical nursing had not yet been studied critically. Thus it seemed wiser for us to initiate an experimental two-year post-master's program in nursing research rather than try to establish a doctoral program.

GS: Did you have many faculty with doctoral preparation?

LH: The first one to hold a doctorate was appointed in 1957. Another was added in 1958 and two more in 1959. I had made a concerted effort to identify talented young faculty and graduate students and to encourage them to secure a Ph.D. in one of the sciences, and while this plan was beginning to get results, the prospects of having them return to the school seemed far in the future.

GS: Were any of the faculty doing research and publishing?

LH: Yes. Some had made a beginning, and others were quite conscious of the importance of participating in the creation and extension of knowledge through research.

Two faculty members had sought and received a grant from the U.S. Public Health Service (U.S.P.H.S.) to evaluate the nursing performance of the graduates of the basic program. Another group, under the leadership of Virginia Crenshaw, Marjorie Dunlap, and Mary Meyers, had received a grant from the N.L.N. (Selantic Fund) for the development and evaluation of a color film concerned with *Pain and the Alleviation of Pain.* Dorothy Johnson's studies and writings about the philosophy and science of nursing were being published, and Harriet Moidel had received a fellowship award from the U.S.P.H.S. to work on a project focused on the "Nursing Care of Patients with Myocardial Infarction."

A number of faculty had participated in an interdisciplinary research project cosponsored by the School of Nursing, the Institute of Industrial Relations, and the Graduate School of Business Administration on the U.C.L.A. campus. Their work culminated in a report titled "Tenderness and Technique: Nursing Values in Transition," written by Genevieve Rogge Meyer. Jo Eleanor Elliott, a participating member of this project, was coauthor of an article published in *Nursing Research* under the title "Varying Images of the Professional Nurse." Jeanne Quint Benoliel made her start in nursing research as a participating member of this project.

Actually the faculty was doing quite a little in nursing research, curriculum evaluation, and revision in the late fifties, but, as might be expected, they complained about lack of time to engage in scholarly pursuits and also lack of help in their undertakings while on the job.

This was not new to me. After my first five years of being dean I had asked the administration for a full-time faculty member to provide research consultation. But, since faculty were supposed to be able to generate their own research and secure extra funds through the University Research Fund or from outside sources to conduct their studies, I was not successful in securing a regular budget item for this kind of expertise.

Now that the faculty had made a beginning in research and seemed interested in doing more, I had to respond with some other kind of help. Accordingly I prepared an application for a Faculty Research Development Grant early in 1959, and by late summer it had been approved for five years. The grant was made by the U.S.P.H.S. Division of Research Grants through the Division of Nursing.

GS: What was the nature of the grant or project?

LH: It was aimed to promote, develop, and increase the research activities of the faculty in nursing. It provided a full-time research consultant, full- and part-time nursing research personnel, and part-time research consultants on an on-call or continuing basis.

GS: Was it successful? Did the faculty do a lot of research?

LH: My report of this project, published in 1965, gives the story in some detail, and copies of it are available in the library at U.C.L.A. It isn't easy to say how successful it was because it takes some time to change attitudes and, in this case, to reorient nurses to believe that *thinking* is as important as *doing.* Certainly, discernible progress was made toward reaching the goal of the project. Faculty did become more and more interested and productive in research activities as the project progressed. During the last two years they were seeking consultation on a regular basis, were requesting "released" time for the preparation of research designs and articles for publication, and were using research assistants and readers in a productive fashion. And as the faculty created a climate for research, it spilled over into student activities with the result that we created a nursing care research laboratory. Eventually, joint research projects were generated by faculty and nursing service personnel and by faculty in the Schools of Medicine and Nursing and graduate students.

Dorothy Johnson and Margo Smith McCaffery did an extensive study on "Crying in the Newborn Infant"; Laurie Gunter, Clara Arndt, and others studied "Three Types of Nursing Care Assignments"; Margaret Kaufmann reported the findings in relation to "Autonomic Responses as Related to Nursing Comfort Measures"; and Mary Meyers, who had been a major contributor to the pain project earlier, completed and published her research on "The Effects of Types of Communication on Patients' Reactions to Stress."

The establishment of the Nurse-Scientist Graduate Training Grants programs in 1963 provided an additional incentive for faculty to seek the preparation they needed for teaching and research in nursing. Thus a number of forces within the profession of nursing as well as within the school and the university helped to stimulate faculty to do research to add to the body of knowledge in nursing.

GS: You mentioned the undergraduate program. Were any changes made in the graduate program during the period?

LH: Yes, there were. Actually, in the year 1965–1966 the faculty completed its study and revision of the program and received approval to offer two master's programs. One was designed to educate the nursing specialist and the other to contribute to the development of nursing scientists. The primary aim of the master of nursing (M.N.) program was to develop professional specialists with a high level of competence in a field of nursing. Along with this goal the program also provided opportunities for students to gain knowledge and skill in the functional areas of teaching, consultation, and supervision. The primary aim of the master of science (M.S.) program was to develop scholars who would be prepared to contribute to nursing knowledge and to the knowledge of human behavior. The program included course work in nursing and in the basic sciences, required research training and a thesis, and was meant to be a foundation for doctoral study.

The idea of creating two master's degrees was to prepare nurses better for their stated goals and to take into account each student's dominant motivational orientation and type of intellectual ability.

These two programs were offered for the first time in 1966–1967. Half of the 114 enrolled students chose the new program (M.N.) in preference to the master of science degree. Both groups stated they were well satisfied with their choice of program, and both were reported to be doing exceptionally well.

GS: Do they still have these two programs?

LH: No, they do not. I think the M.S. degree program was terminated in 1970–1971.

GS: Why? Was that after you left?

LH: Yes, it was about two or three years after I had retired from the school, and I think there was a question as to whether or not there were enough faculty with research training available to handle the thesis guidance, and also whether the school could afford two programs at the master's level.

Threatened Closure of U.C.L.A.
School of Nursing

GS: Is it true that the medical school tried to take advantage of your retirement to phase out the school, or was it an administrative decision?

LH: Actually, I think it was a little of both. I wouldn't want to say the medical *school*, however, for we had many strong supporters in medicine. Everyone functioning in a university nursing program knows how hard it is to get complete medical support for university nursing education. We were no exception at U.C.L.A. In addition, we never had had wholehearted support from some members of the established scientific disciplines on the campus because it was not clear to the members of these groups how we could really be an academic discipline unless our faculty all held doctorates and were good in research. We had made progress, however, and every time our programs were reviewed (and it seemed to me they were reviewed every hour on the hour) by Academic Senate committees such as the Educational Policy Committee, the Graduate Council, and the like, we received favorable reports. During the late sixties the university was experiencing budget cuts as well as student uprisings; government grants were not as plentiful as before; enrollments in the health fields and graduate programs were high; and space was at a premium. Our offices and classroom space were closely associated with the space occupied by the medical school, and some of it seemed very desirable to the dean of the medical school and one of his faculty who was also director of the hospitals.

GS: Do you think they wanted your space?

LH: I know they wanted some of our space, particularly my suite of offices. But of course they wanted other things, too, like control of the school. Attempts to control the nursing school had been made by the first dean of the medical school, so I guess we might have expected these attempts to continue, particularly since the Chancellor of the University was also an M.D. It probably did look easy to accomplish, as I had informed the Chancellor that I had decided to take early retirement.

In retrospect, I know I made a mistake by giving him a year's notice to find a dean to replace me. Instead of creating a search committee to find a new dean, he utilized that year to marshal forces and plan to phase out the School of Nursing. In some ways it was the most shocking and painful experience of my nursing career. In other ways it was the most rewarding, for the support we received to maintain the school was beyond anything I could have imagined.

The faculty and the secretarial staff worked hard to help me get the word to all baccalaureate and higher degree programs, to nursing organizations, universities, nursing service personnel, and the like; and no sooner had these communications reached their destination than letters of protestation (and what letters they were!) went to the newly appointed President of the University, members of the board of regents, and the Chancellor and Vice Chancellor on the U.C.L.A. campus. Soon the *Los Angeles Times* and other local papers were printing letters of protest, and every so often the U.C.L.A. Vice Chancellor, who had issued the plan to phase out the school and replace it with a *hospital training program*, had to answer letters of protest by communications to the *Los Angeles Times*.

While some of our faculty were also adding their comments via the *Los Angeles Times*, I met hourly with representatives from the U.C.L.A. nursing service, with graduate and undergraduate students, with nursing groups who came to the school for information, and with representatives of the U.C.L.A. student organizations and the U.C.L.A. *Daily Bruin* (the students' paper and a powerful force on the campus). Suffice it to say we had 100 percent support from all of these groups, and through the efforts of local nursing service directors and alumni, an office was established in Westwood Village, where the university is located. This office was called the Citizens' Committee for Nursing, and it was there that an aroused community and a goodly number of our strong supporters from the community, from the medical school, and from the other disciplines on the campus made their protests known and circulated them to sources of power.

I postponed my retirement for about five months—until I could see that there would be no phasing out without an opportunity for the school to defend its programs in an orderly fashion before the designated committees of the Academic Senate. By that time I was reasonably certain that the school would continue, and of course it has.

GS: How did all this affect you? Were you crushed?

LH: Maybe I should have been, but I really wasn't, probably because I was looking forward to a more leisurely life with Harry, whom I had married in 1953, and I didn't have much time to dwell on my own feelings. I kept thinking how wonderful it was to have so much support from nursing all over the country and from international groups. I had been a member of the board of the National League for Nursing for a long time, had served as Chairman of the Council of Baccalaureate and Higher Degree Programs for four years, and had worked with and for the Western Council on Higher Education for Nursing since its creation; and all of these groups, along with the American Nurses' Association, supported us 100 percent. The nursing journals carried our story as we provided information, and that kind of support was a great sustaining factor as we all fought for the preservation of university nursing education. The loss of the U.C.L.A. School of Nursing would have had marked repercussions throughout the country, and all of us were determined that that should not happen.

Retirement

GS: Since your retirement from U.C.L.A., what have you been doing?

LH: I've continued to function in nursing in a more leisurely way as a speaker and consultant, and I've served as a member of the State Advisory Committee on Physician's Assistant and Nurse-Practitioner Programs in the California Department of Consumer Affairs.

GS: What is your opinion of the nurse-practitioner movement? Do you think this is a sellout to nursing?

LH: The nurse-practitioner movement, which got under way in 1965, could never be a sellout to nursing in my opinion. Actually it has served to reorient many nurses to the *care of people* by preparing them for more responsible practice roles. Professional nurses have always assumed some of the functions performed by physicians—at physicians' request and with the patients' consent, when the physicians were not available. Now that the need for nurses to do this has been recognized by both the medical and the nursing professions *and* by the public, we are providing this type of preparation in some of our collegiate programs and through continuing education in nurse-practitioner programs.

This development is not proceeding without some confusion and controversy within both the medical and the nursing professions and between them. This is to be expected, perhaps, since changes in the professional work areas of nursing are bound to affect the work areas of medicine. But in time physicians and nurses will appreciate the fact that patients are receiving the appropriate, continuing health care they need because nurses are prepared to function as primary care givers as well as specialists in clinical nursing in acute and chronic care settings.

Not all nurses will want or need to function in these more demanding roles, but for those who do, we must see that their preparation includes a strong base in anatomy, physiology, pathophysiology, and pharmacology, and well-developed interviewing skills, and a systematic approach to history taking.

To deliver health care that is appropriate and effective and to offer it where patients can reach it by public transportation, we must do a better job in our outreaching health centers, our inner cities, our physicians' offices, our ghettos and barrios, and with our American Indian populations. And we must try harder than ever before to view health and illness within a social context and from the consumer's point of view.

GS: What do you see ahead?

LH: The challenge we face as we enter the last quarter of the twentieth century is to put to work what we know to deliver health care and then to help people understand what services exist to help them and how to use them properly. Nurses and physicians particularly (working with other health professionals and nonprofessionals) must come to grips with this problem, and their educational programs must include experiences aimed to provide this kind of knowledge and understanding.

GS: Is this your view of nursing practice? Patient care?

LH: Yes! The old image of nursing was *care of people*. I now see it becoming the *new* image of nursing. And that's what I've always thought and taught. This is a great time for nurses and for nursing. To quote Emerson, "This time, like all times, is a very good one if we but know what to do with it." I'm certain the present generation of nurses knows what to do with what it's got and has the legislative know-how to get it done.

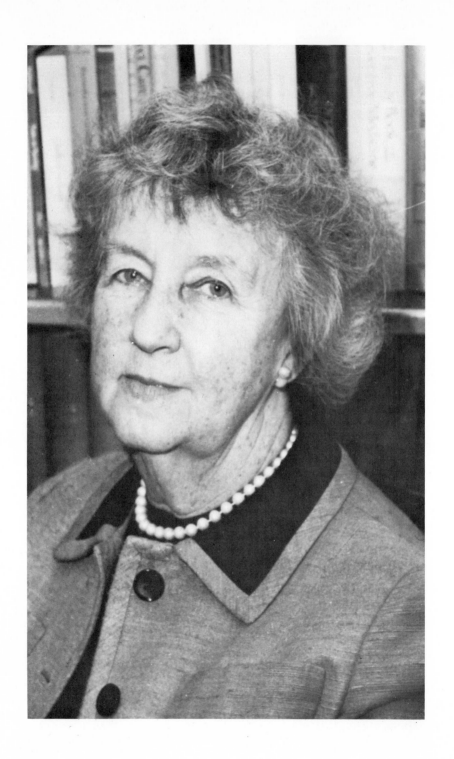

5

. . . for distinguished and exemplary service,
nursing leadership and social consciousness in
furthering the worthy cause of Nursing and
health care.[1]

[1]American Nurses' Association, June 1974.
[2]"This is what I would like to be called." Virginia Henderson to
author in an interview in her office at New Haven, Conn., Oct. 22,
1974.

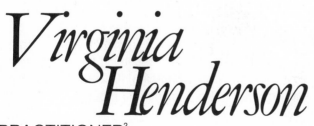

Virginia Henderson

PRACTITIONER[2]

*V*irginia Henderson is widely known as a nurse who is outspoken on the "practice of nursing." She has made many contributions to the nursing profession, and she is recognized for her definition of nursing, her *Textbook of the Principles and Practice of Nursing*, her monograph *The Nature of Nursing*, and her timeless contribution through the *Nursing Studies Index*.

Virginia Henderson's definition of nursing is:

The unique function of the nurse is to assist the individual, sick or well, in the performance of those activities contributing to health or its recovery (or to peaceful death) that he would perform unaided if he had the necessary strength, will or knowledge. And to do this in such a way as to help him gain independence as rapidly as possible. This aspect of her work, this part of her function, she initiates and controls; of this she is master. In addition, she helps the patient to carry out the therapeutic plan as initiated by the physician. She also, as a member of a medical team, helps other members, as they in turn help her, to plan and carry out the total program whether it be for the improvement of health, or the recovery from illness or support in death.[3]

Virginia Henderson was born in Kansas City, Missouri, in 1897. Her mother, Lucy Minor Abbott, was a strong and lovable character who had a potent influence on all who knew her. She was the daughter of William Richardson Abbott, whose school for boys was well known in the South. Virginia Henderson's father, Daniel Brosius Henderson, was a lawyer who, his daughter says, was an "idealist." There were eight children in the family, four boys and four girls, of whom she was the fifth.

Early in his law practice, Daniel Brosius Henderson became so concerned about the American Indians and the injustice done them that he decided to devote his practice to them. This necessitated a move from Kansas City to Washington, D.C., because his work involved claims by the Indians against the United States government. The family lived in nearby Virginia most of the time.

In 1918, with the United States involved in World War I, Virginia Henderson decided that she ought "to do something to help either the sick people of this country" or those returning "maimed by the war." She read about the Army School of Nursing and thought that was the

3 *The Nature of Nursing*, The Macmillan Company, Collier-Macmillan, Ltd., London, 1966.

answer. But she said it wasn't because she had always wanted to be a nurse; actually, that idea had never occurred to her.

She graduated from the Army School of Nursing in Washington in 1921. Her first position was as staff nurse at the Instructive Visiting Nurse Service in Washington. Although she had wanted to stay in nursing practice, she was persuaded by Ethel Smith, the head of the State Board of Nurse Examiners in Virginia, to accept a teaching position in the Norfolk Protestant Hospital. She thinks she was the first full-time instructor in a school of nursing in Virginia. After five interesting and satisfying years she decided that if she was to be an educator, she needed special preparation. She went to Teachers College, Columbia University, where she earned B.S. and M.A. degrees in nursing education. From 1929 to 1930 she was a teaching supervisor in the clinics of the Strong Memorial Hospital in Rochester, New York. She returned to Teachers College to join the faculty and stayed there until 1948, conducting courses focused on clinical practice and the analytical process.

In 1953 she joined Leo Simmons in making a national survey of nursing research.[4] In 1959 she took over the direction of the *Nursing Studies Index* project. Started as an effort to make an annotated bibliography of nursing research, it grew into a four-volume annotated index of the analytical, historical, and biographical literature on nursing from 1900 through 1959. This twelve-year task was financed by the U.S. Public Health Service (U.S.P.H.S.) and sponsored by the Yale University School of Nursing.

Virginia Henderson says she wrote *The Nature of Nursing*[5] to show how she came to regard the nursing function and how the concept has affected her idea of nursing practice, research, and education. She suggests that her most lasting work may be the *Nursing Studies Index*.[6] The publication in 1963 of one volume of this *Index* preceded the publication of the *International Nursing Index* and almost certainly influenced the decision of the National Library of Medicine to collaborate with the *American Journal of Nursing (A.J.N.)* in the publication of the *International Nursing Index*. The *Nursing Studies Index* had demonstrated that there was a body of literature on nursing that was not

[4] With Leo W. Simmons, *Nursing Research: A Survey and Assessment*, Appleton-Century-Crofts, Inc., New York, 1964.

[5] Op. cit., p. v.

[6] *Nursing Studies Index: An Annotated Guide to Reported Studies, Research in Progress, Research Methods and Historical Materials in Periodicals, Books and Pamphlets published in English*, J. B. Lippincott Company, Philadelphia, vol. IV (1957–1959), 1963; vol. III (1950–1956), 1966; vol. II (1930–1949), 1970; vol. I (1900–1929), 1972. Prepared by the Yale University School of Nursing *Index* staff under the direction of Virginia Henderson.

available through the use of existing indexes. The Interagency Council on Library Resources for Nursing, organized as a coordinating committee by the *Nursing Studies Index* staff, has stimulated the development of various library tools and services. Virginia Henderson stresses that the *Nursing Studies Index* was a group endeavor, that at one time there were seven workers on the staff, and that one member of the staff, Elsie S. Mowe, deserves much of the credit for the consistency of the *Index*.

Virginia Henderson is now, with Gladys Nite and twenty collaborators, completing the sixth edition of *Textbook of the Principles and Practice of Nursing.*[7] The first three editions were written by Bertha Harmer, a Canadian nurse. This text, considered a classic, has been translated into Spanish, and is to be translated into Japanese. *The Nature of Nursing* has been translated into Japanese and Hebrew. *Basic Principles of Nursing Care,*[8] which she prepared for the International Council of Nurses (I.C.N.), has been translated into over twenty languages. Among her numerous awards and citations are two honorary doctoral degrees.[9]

Virginia Henderson is an attractive woman who has a delightful sense of humor and an individualistic, artistic approach to life.[10]

Army School of Nursing

GS: Could you please comment on the Army School of Nursing?

VH: For me it was an outstanding experience. I loved nursing from the day I went into it. The Army School of Nursing was in many ways remarkable and ahead of its day in what it offered students. It was the brainchild of Annie W. Goodrich. She thought, as many people did, that World War I might last a long time and that many nurses ought to be prepared by the Army so that these graduates could supplement the civil nurses then available to go into military service. Hospitals and other health services were terribly understaffed. You may have heard of the flu epidemic that in 1918 was enough to scare the life out of everybody. It was really horrifying. There wasn't a thinking person who didn't real-

---

[7] Bertha Harmer and Virginia Henderson, *Textbook of the Principles and Practice of Nursing,* 5th ed., The Macmillan Publishing Company, New York, 1955.

[8] *Basic Principles of Nursing Care,* International Council of Nurses, London, 1960 (revised in 1969).

[9] The degrees are doctor of laws, University of Western Ontario, London, Canada, 1970, and doctor of science, University of Rochester, Rochester, N.Y., 1972.

[10] For example, she likes to design rooms and clothes and to spend her spare time making a variety of objects.

ize that the care of the sick in this country and the care of the military were big problems. So that's why I went into nursing. It was not because I wanted to be a nurse. However, I was fascinated by nursing from my first day as a student. The faculty and students in the Army School of Nursing were exceptional, I think. There were, I believe, 10,000 applicants for that first class, and not more than 2000 were taken. In the Walter Reed Unit there were many college graduates and vivid personalities. I remember a Phi Beta Kappa law student and a student of landscape architecture, for example.

The Definition of Nursing

GS: When did you first come up with your definition?

VH: I came up with the necessity of being clear about the function of nurses when I revised the *Textbook* for the first time in 1939. I also remember refining it during the time that Ester Lucile Brown was making a study of nursing that resulted in the report *Nursing for the Future.*[11]

Esther Brown held regional conferences in connection with this study, and at one of them a group of us formed a committee to present the necessity for clearly defining nursing. The discussion in this group helped me clarify my own thinking, but I believe the definition presented at the end of the conference was my definition—the one that guided me in the revision of the *Textbook of the Principles and Practice of Nursing.* Elizabeth Porter was a member of the small group and was the person who gave its report to the conference. I remember that at the time Lucile Petry Leone said, "That's a beautiful definition, and I recognize Virginia's hand in it" (or something of that sort) but she said, "That's not all there is to nursing." I think it really is all there is to the *unique* function of the nurse if you interpret it broadly enough. In the definition [quoted above from *The Nature of Nursing*], the statement "if he had the necessary strength, will or knowledge" puts no limit on what might be included. And helping a person gain independence as rapidly as possible is a tall order. Actually it's a tall order to maintain our own independence. Few of us are as healthy as we know how to be because we haven't the will. Few of us have the knowledge we need to keep healthy. Newborn babies lack the knowledge and the strength to get up and get what they need, so they are always dependent. The limitations that we all live under keep us from being as healthy as we could be. So, to supply what someone else needs to be healthy, when we can't even

[11] Esther Lucile Brown, *Nursing for the Future*, Russell Sage Foundation, New York, 1948.

supply our own needs, suggests to me that it's quite a difficult thing to do. As a footnote I might add that "independence" is a relative term. None of us is independent of others, but we strive for a healthy interdependence, not a sick dependence.

GS: Do you still hold to the same definition today?

VH: Yes, because I've never found one that is more satisfactory. But my interpretation of it has been modified. I still think it is the nurse's function to help people carry out the therapeutic plan prescribed by the physician; I still believe the physician is best prepared to prescribe therapy but I have been forced to conclude that physicians are often unavailable or have so little time to give to the patient's problems that they fail to prescribe effectively. Therefore I believe the nurse in many instances must help the patient with therapy.

A colleague once challenged my definition of nursing and gave me hers as "putting the patient in the best condition for nature to act upon him." This sounded strangely familiar, and I soon recognized it as Florence Nightingale's statement in *Notes on Nursing.*[12] If you have read this priceless little volume, you may notice that Florence Nightingale says nothing in this connection about carrying out the doctor's prescription or therapeutic program. I have come to the conclusion that she had little confidence in physicians, and I can easily understand it because the medicine practiced in her day was generally questionable. She said in *Notes on Nursing* that sickness was a "reparative process" and that the art of nursing as practiced in her day interfered with the reparative process; I believe she thought the art of medicine was equally, if not more, guilty of interference with nature.

The military medicine she saw practiced was especially lacking, and it was certainly nature and nursing—according to the Nightingale pattern—that accounted for the change in the mortality statistics after she took charge of nursing in the Crimean hospitals.

Somebody has said that the body is a three-million-year-old self-healing machine. I am more and more impressed with the ability of living things to adapt and adjust. I therefore accept Florence Nightingale's definition, but it does not seem to me to be in conflict with mine.

GS: How does your definition differ from Florence Nightingale's?

VH: I think mine says more specifically what nurses do to help patients with their natural functions, and it also says that they work with

_____

[12] Florence Nightingale, *Notes on Nursing: What It Is and What It Is Not,* Dover Publications, Inc., New York, 1969.

physicians. If the definition is read in its entirety, it says that when physicians are not present—in emergencies—nurses assume responsibility for treatment. Today, in writing about the function of nurses, I put more emphasis on the responsibility they must take for helping patients and their families with health management when physicians are unavailable. I don't limit these occasions to emergencies.

GS: Is there anything you would like to add to that?

VH: I might add that since the I.C.N. has used my definition in its basic documents, I must assume that it is a clear statement and has meaning for nurses around the world. This does not say that it is a definition that will stand for all time. I believe nursing is modified by the era in which it is practiced, and depends to a great extent on what other health workers do.

The I.C.N. Pamphlet, the Textbook and The Nature of Nursing

GS: What is the thing for which you consider yourself best known?

VH: People have used this expression to me so often that I hope it has some validity. They say, "Your name is synonymous with good nursing care." My name was first associated with the description of nursing in the 1939 revision of Bertha Harmer's *Textbook of the Principles and Practice of Nursing*; then with the description of nursing in the little pamphlet *Basic Principles of Nursing Care*, which I wrote for the I.C.N. I don't know whether you are old enough to remember Amos and Andy. These radio comedians used to talk about putting something "in two nutshells." I find that the smaller the publication, the more people read it, and therefore the better known it is. Of course the more languages a book appears in, the wider the audience. So the little I.C.N. booklet is the thing that most people have read. Many people seem also to have read *The Nature of Nursing*.

GS: Which of your publications came out first?

VH: The textbooks; I revised Bertha Harmer's text in 1939, again in 1955, and now, with others, I'm doing it for the third time. The little I.C.N. booklet was first printed in 1960. That's the one I think is best known or, rather, the most extensively known, because it's been published in so many languages. *The Nature of Nursing* came out in 1966.

Writing *The Nature of Nursing* happened this way. I was asked by

Eleanor Hall to give the Claire Dennison Memorial Lecture at the University of Rochester School of Nursing. I wrote a paper that was too long to read, so, thinking it a pity to waste all the effort that had gone into writing the paper, I sent it to the *American Journal of Nursing*. The editor, Edith Patton Lewis, liked it but said it was too long to publish. She said the *Journal* would publish it in two or three installments but would prefer to edit and publish it in one short article. I agreed, but still had material that I thought might be of interest to the profession, especially because it showed how a definition of nursing affected curriculum revision and how it affected research. In the longer version I suggested a way of regulating nursing research in an institution, how to get the cooperation of people involved, and the kinds of research that I thought were needed. All of this I hoped might be helpful, so I submitted the manuscript to The Macmillan Company. The editor at Macmillan, Henry Van Swearington, said the manuscript was my "epitome," sort of the essence of what I had been talking about for many years. Florence Wald, dean of the Yale University School of Nursing, once said she thought of what I had published up to that time, it would last longest.

GS: There must be a demand for the Textbook *if it's going into so many editions.*

VH: Yes, it seems to be a useful book, for there is still a demand for the 1955 edition. The *Textbook* happened this way. I was a young instructor in the state of Virginia. At that time there was no state league for nursing education in Virginia, but there was an educational section of the State Nurses' Association. I was chairperson of this section, so I was, in effect, head of the league for nursing education in the state. That brought me to the attention of publishers because, when we had conventions, I had something to do with the exhibit of books and educational supplies of all sorts. The publishers came to know me and, thinking I had something to offer, tried to persuade me to write a textbook. I used to say that I would not write a textbook on nursing because I couldn't improve on Bertha Harmer's text, which I was using then in teaching basic students at the Norfolk Protestant Hospital. Later, when Ms. Harmer (whom I had never met) died, The Macmillan Company approached me on keeping up the Harmer book. I had no real desire to take over this formidable task, but I had no excuse to give to myself or Macmillan for not making the effort. I accepted quite unwillingly. I don't really like to write; even now I don't enjoy it as so many people say they do.

GS: Why is that?

VH: Because it is very hard work, and the reward is long delayed. I like to make things and see immediate results, and I think that's one reason I enjoyed active nursing. I liked to go into a situation that looked to me ugly because of illness, sickness, disability, or disorder, and see if I could turn that around and help the patient and the family make something that was bearable or even constructive. Nursing seemed to me to be as creative as painting a picture. But to write a book! There you are, closeted in a room by yourself with a lot of inanimate materials. You don't get your reward for years, maybe not then. It really does not appeal to me. It's tedious; it's laborious. Also, you are stuck with anything you put into words. If it's a mistake, it stands; whereas with things that aren't put on the record, it's just a little bit easier to correct your errors. My father used to say, "Virginia, have you ever considered the Persian proverb 'Would that mine enemy would write a book!'?" My father also used to remind his children that we were "slaves of our spoken words; our unspoken words were our slaves." We are even more the slaves of our printed words.

GS: Do you find you have to discipline yourself when it comes to writing?

VH: I think writing's the greatest discipline there is. I can remember saying to an uncle of mine, James P. Southall, who was a very fine writer, that I found it hard to express my ideas. He said, "Virginia, you're not honest when you say that. You *can* express your ideas if they're clearly formulated in your mind. It's thinking that you're having trouble with, not the process of putting your thoughts into words." I am sure he was exactly right. It's thinking that's so hard; it isn't really the writing.

GS: You've considered writing as being your unique contribution to nursing. Anything else you want to add?

VH: Well, I suppose so. I believe something goes before writing. I would hope that the process of nursing that I developed in my practice of nursing and in teaching nursing is really what counts. I couldn't have described nursing effectively if I had never practiced effectively. So I think the effort I made after I was taught how to nurse, to work out a constructive way of helping patients, is the basis for the writing I've done. Even though I had, probably, as good teachers as there were in this country at the time, I had to "put things together" for myself. Because I was prepared at the Army School of Nursing, I say that I had outstanding teachers. Annie Goodrich was Dean of the school; she was ahead of her time as a nurse educator, and she had the confidence of people all over the country. Those she asked to teach accepted if they could, I imagine. At any rate, the faculty included illustrious names like

Effie J. Taylor, Mary Roberts, Harriett Gillette, and Sally Johnson. Nevertheless, I was taught nursing with very little, if any, opportunity to see expert nurses practice. We were taught in classrooms and expected to make our own applications in the clinical unit. I came to see that what had been emphasized in the teaching of that basic course, as I perceived it, was not enough. I may have failed to absorb what my teachers were trying to tell me, but I finally concluded that much of what I had been taught in the hospital setting was not what I believed was good nursing care at all. The best nursing care that I saw in a hospital was given on the Boston Floating Hospital, where each of us could devote our time to three babies. That was good hospital nursing in many ways and the only hospital where I saw case assignments practiced, but the experience that impressed me was public health nursing. There I came to see that what you did *to* a patient didn't help so much as what you got them to learn to do for themselves. I think I made a switch to rehabilitative nursing, and I hope this comes through in what I've written. I'm pretty sure it came through in teaching students in the basic program. The students who graduated from the Protestant Hospital in Norfolk, a small institution hospital, used to go to very large centers. I often got reports from people who worked with those students, and they seemed to think they were exceptional nurses. So, if there is anything useful in the books we've been discussing (and I hope I'm not claiming too much), it's because those books put into words what I developed in caring for those I nursed.

GS: What would you say the main difference would be in comparison with other books at the time? Was yours the only textbook?

VH: No, there were nursing texts throughout the history of professional nursing, though none were, I believe, comparable with the Harmer text when it first appeared. Bertha Harmer started the textbook we are discussing. While, as I said before, I never knew her, I'm pretty sure she was a very able nurse; and I'm pretty sure that her ideas and my ideas about nursing were to some extent parallel. I tend to look for reasons, for causes, just as she did. The Harmer book was the first book to stress why, not just how, a nursing procedure was carried out. She depended very heavily on Howell's textbook of physiology. She nearly always gave a good physiological review before she described method. In revising her book I rejected her heavy reliance on one underlying science and on one source. By the time I took over the text, I had had physiology with medical students at Columbia University. I had had three courses in chemistry and bacteriology and a little physics, and I had come to realize that almost everything in physiology, or any science, is debatable. So, when I revised the book, I think what may have been unique was that I said here are representative opinions, rather than saying this is *it*. I said, for instance, "These are authoritative views on the clotting of blood or the healing of wounds or what kind of catheter causes least trauma." But then in the text I also said, "In order to act, you've got to make a choice." So in discussing nursing procedures as, for example, helping with lumbar puncture or giving an enema or catheterizing or turning a patient, I reviewed the underlying science and then gave a "suggested procedure." I always implied that there were other methods, but that at this point in my thinking, this was my chosen method. I believe this emphasis on underlying principles and on *a* suggested procedure, rather than *the* procedure, was what made the text different.

GS: Under the name of each leader there will be a subtitle. What concept or word do you feel most appropriate or the one you want under yours: researcher, administrator, educator, or what?

VH: You haven't mentioned the word I'd like used. I'd like to be thought of as a practitioner. I didn't practice very long, so it may be unrealistic to expect others to think of me as a practitioner, and inappropriate to use the term. When I graduated, I expected to be a public health nurse–practitioner. However, on taking my state board examinations in Virginia, I came to the attention of Ethel Smith. She had studied under Annie Goodrich at St. Luke's Hospital School of Nursing in New York City. She knew that I had been influenced by her in the Army School of Nursing, and she persuaded me that I could help upgrade the nursing schools in Virginia. I came from a family of educators and liked the idea that I was doing something different. My father, who said he would like to have been a doctor, encouraged my interest in nursing practice. When I went into teaching, I thought of it as temporary. On weekends I often nursed patients in the hospital where I was teaching, to make sure that I wasn't losing my ability to practice.

While I was at Teachers College, I decided to return to practice, to try to bring the spirit of public health nursing into the hospital. I took a supervisory position in the outpatient clinics of the Strong Memorial Hospital, Rochester, New York, and while I did work with students there, it was always in the clinical situation. But again I was pressured, or perhaps tempted, to go back into teaching. I was asked to join the Teachers College faculty and was offered an Isabel Hampton Robb Fellowship to complete the work for a master's degree. As you know, I stayed there for fourteen years, but I like to think that it was because I believed I was helping graduate nurse students focus their studies on nursing practice and introductory research on nursing methods. During the forties I worked with students in the advanced course in medical-surgical nursing, which included clinical practice. I was with students and patients two days a week in the hospitals of New York City, and I did some volunteer staff nursing in addition. Actually I've enjoyed nursing everywhere I've had a chance to practice it. For friends I accepted several private-duty maternity cases soon after I graduated. While I enjoyed the home delivery and the care of the mother and baby, there was no way during the twenties to practice privately and lead a normal life. I never considered this field seriously. Up until the time I left Teachers College, I expected to return some day to active participation in nursing care. Unfortunately (or maybe fortunately?), since then I've been caught up full time in research and writing, but it has been by accident rather than intent.

The Index

GS: *How did the* Nursing Studies Index *come about; how did it develop?*

VH: That's a long story but I'll try to shorten it. Following World War II there was a National Committee for the Improvement of Nursing Services (N.C.I.N.S.). Marion Sheahan was chairwoman, and there were many distinguished people on it. Questions were always coming up in the committee proceedings that led someone to say, "We need a study on that." Often another member would say, "We've had several studies along those lines." The Committee came to realize that the reports of many studies were lost, or were little used, and that a great deal of effort was being wasted because the nursing literature was undocumented. To try to use it was like sailing in uncharted seas.

Leo W. Simmons, a social scientist, was studying patient care at New York Hospital at this time, and in speaking at various meetings he had shown an understanding of nursing—appreciation of its potential value and some of the difficulties nurses faced. He was asked by the Committee to compile a bibliography on nursing research, to identify the major studies reported and the types of studies that were needed. The Committee probably thought this could be done in a few months, certainly in less than a year, and that it would have the bibliography to use in its work. Actually the Committee was disbanded long before there was a substantial publication from the indexing staff.

Leo Simmons asked me to join him and another social scientist in making this survey of nursing research. At the time I was finishing the fifth edition of the *Textbook of the Principles and Practice of Nursing*, but accepted his invitation as soon as I was free.

The survey was conducted under the sponsorship of the Yale University School of Nursing; it was funded by the U.S.P.H.S. Our first task was to develop a classification under which we could list reports of students and needed studies as we identified them. In order to find out what research had been reported and what was needed, we traveled to centers in about three-fourths of the states and we reviewed the literature. Fortunately for me, I did most of the field work and most of the review of publications. The field work was a particularly rich experience. It gave me an understanding of nursing and other kinds of health work in this country I would never have had otherwise. I interviewed more than 500 nurses, doctors, social scientists, educators, and students, asking them what research they had done, what they knew about, and what they thought was needed.

After the field work was completed, we undertook a rather extensive review of the literature and built a bibliographical file that came to be known as the best source of information on nursing research in the country. Students at Yale used it, and visiting scholars consulted it. While much of the material in it was cited in Leo Simmons's and my report, *Nursing Research: A Survey and Assessment* (which was not published until 1964), people in the Division of Nursing in the U.S.P.H.S. (Ellwynne Vreeland, Helen Tibbitts, Margaret Arnstein, Ava Dilworth, and Faye Abdellah) all saw the value of a bibliography on research. Florence Wald, Dean of the Yale University School of Nursing, also saw the need for it. It was thought that the whole bibliography should be published separately from the *Survey and Assessment* report.

In 1959, after Leo Simmons left Yale to be Director of the Institute of Research and Service in Nursing Education at Teachers College, Columbia University, I was asked to direct what came to be called the *Nursing Studies Index* project. This project, started as a relatively unambitious two-year task, grew into a systematic survey of books, pamphlets, and journal articles on nursing from 1900 to 1960. The Committee was also charged with the responsibility of recommending a way to provide for a continuing index. It took twelve years to complete. The staff grew from two to seven persons at one point, although in the last stages Elsie S. Mowe and I were the only workers.

To coordinate the indexing project with related work, the Yale *Nursing Studies Index* staff organized in 1960 a coordinating committee that, since the first meeting, had functioned as a national Interagency Council on Library Resources for Nursing. The *Nursing Studies Index* project had a distinguished Technical Advisory Committee, and with its approval we enlarged the scope of the *Index* to include the analytical, historical, and biographical aspects of the nursing literature. The staff included librarians, and we covered the contents of the best nursing libraries on the East Coast and used the published shelf list of the Case–Western Reserve University Nursing Library. From 200 to 300 journals were scanned, and in Volume II of the *Index*, for instance, more than 300 publishers of books or periodicals are represented in the thousands of monographic citations. The fact that the citations are annotated and the fact that periodic and monographic literature citations are interfiled make this, for any field, a rather unusual publication. The *Index* covers only publications in English, but because of the far-flung British Commonwealth, a person who wants to take a historical approach to almost any nursing problem can find a fairly adequate and ready-made bibliography by consulting the *Index*.

Indexes are very expensive to prepare, and publishers make no money on them. We were therefore delighted when the J. B. Lippincott Company of Philadelphia agreed to publish the *Nursing Studies Index*. We think every health science library—certainly every nursing library— should have the *Index*. It is irreplaceable and invaluable to all those who take the historical approach to understanding and trying to solve the problems of nursing.

GS: Have you been content with your work?

VH: Yes, I suppose on the whole I have. But, as I told you, I wanted to remain a practitioner. As it is, I've mostly taught and written. I've been asked to consider deanships, and I've been asked to consider other administrative posts which would have given me certain advantages over the work I've done, but I've wanted to stay close to nursing. I've always taught the practice of nursing or research in nursing. That's what I thought I could do best. And since I was more interested in research than most nurses seemed to be (for years nobody was interested in nursing research very much), I felt as if I was sort of a pioneer. This sounds pretentious and is actually untrue, for Florence Nightingale was our first researcher, and many leading nurses saw its value. Adelaide Nutting, Annie Goodrich, and Isabel Stewart all recognized the need for it, so I can't say that any of us since has pioneered in research. Those people I've mentioned were the pioneers. Isabel Stewart tried to develop an institute for research at Teachers College during the thirties. But the rank and file of nurses didn't see how important Florence Nightingale's work was because she could and did back up her recommendations with data. That's the chief reason she was effective in changing military medicine and health care in India.

But to go back to how I happened to do the *Index*. It was first designed to regularize or make publishable the file that we had built up during the *Survey and Assessment of Nursing Research* under the direction of Leo Simmons. It came to be something quite different because, I'm sure, in the back of my mind there had always been the hope that a complete search of the literature could be made. In teaching research methods, I had been keenly aware of the need for a guide to the nursing literature. Now we have an Interagency Council on Library Resources for Nursing, which promotes all sorts of nursing resources. It has representatives of the following organizations: American Hospital Association; American Journal of Nursing Company; American Library Association; American Medical Association; American Nurses' Association; American Nurses' Foundation; Canadian Nurses' Association; Catholic Hospital Association; Medical Library Association; National Association for Practical Nurse Education and Service; National Federation of Licensed Practical Nurses; National League for Nursing; National Library of Medicine; National Nursing Archives, Mugar Memorial Library; National Student Nurses' Association; Seventh-Day Adventist Hospital; Special Libraries Association; U.S. Public Health Service, Division of Nursing; Yale University School of Nursing, *Nursing Studies Index* project.

The Council's recommendation to the national nursing organizations that they consider the production of an index to the nursing literature carried weight. Similar recommendations had been made before by an ad hoc committee; nothing had come of them, but this time something happened.

We now have the *International Nursing Index*, which is the counterpart of the *Index Medicus*; we have an abstracting service in the publication *Nursing Research*; we have a nursing archive at the Mugar Memorial Library at Boston University, which has already collected an impressive body of material. I believe the profession has, as Dr. Bayne-Jones said in referring to the indexes, "come of age professionally." In this era an occupation can scarcely be called a profession if it has no control of its literature.

GS: The Nursing Studies Index *ends in 1959. Is this the last of this project?*

VH: Yes, although it is a pity that the work wasn't continued until 1965, when the *International Nursing Index* began.

Perhaps I should stress that indexing is complex work, that it requires a substantial outlay of money, and that it involves group effort. The need for an index to the nursing literature has been recognized throughout the history of professional nursing. If you had searched the literature, you would know that people like Ethel Bedford Fenwick in England and Adelaide Nutting and Isabel Stewart in the United States recommended the production of an index. All thoughtful, scholarly nurses throughout the development of nursing have realized that we needed some way of getting at what was published. It's a crime, the amount of time that people have had to spend throughout this century trying to find what was written about nursing and nurses before the existing indexes were developed. I think an index would have been developed eventually without my efforts. I may have pushed the event ahead a little bit, but I dislike the idea of taking credit for this accomplishment. But since you asked me what I believe my contribution is, I might suggest that improving the use of library resources is certainly one of them. The work with which I am connected that will last longest is the *Nursing Studies Index*, simply because it is a record of nursing as published in the English language over a sixty-year period.

The *Index* isn't the publication for which I am best known. When I was given an honorary degree at the University of Western Ontario in 1970, it wasn't even mentioned. Too few people know the value of indexes; too few people use them; too few know of their existence.

During vacations in Europe in the sixties, I set up meetings at the I.C.N. and at the World Health Organization (W.H.O.) to discuss nursing indexes and the need for them. Although the meetings included distinguished people, few took seriously the question of whether international agencies should sponsor an index. Some persons said frankly that they didn't know what I was talking about. I think I'm not talking off the top of my head when I say that there are still leaders in nursing who don't see the need for indexes and don't use them. People in administrative positions tend to send others to find the information they need. Real nurse scholars who write and who use the literature are few in number, although I believe the number is increasing rapidly. It has been said that "People who think, don't want power; and people with power, don't think." This is a commentary on human nature rather than a criticism of nursing.

GS: You're saying, then, that you feel that the Index *will be the one that will survive longest?*

VH: Yes. I think it will survive on the library shelves longer than any other publications with which my name is associated. Nobody with good sense who runs a library will throw away the record of nursing as published in English from 1900 to 1960.

Some Issues and Opinions

GS: What are some of the major issues in nursing and your own particular role in them; and where do you think nursing is going?

VH: We were asked—a group of us—to discuss this a few years ago. So you can find a very carefully structured statement on trends and a discussion of the issues in the *American Journal of Nursing.*[13] One of the things I believe I said was that I thought a national health service was coming that would provide health insurance for all citizens in the United States. I think that has to mean a democratic accessibility to health care so that one person has got about as good a chance as another of getting the help needed and good health care.[14] I believe the only way that health care can be made universally available is to give nurses a much broader and more responsible role than they now have. I think we could learn a lot from the British nurses, who are encouraged not only to make suggestions about health care but also to question what the doctor is prescribing. This was stated by British health officers in *The Greater Medical Profession*, a report of a 1972 Josiah Macy, Jr., Foundation conference.[15] I think those who spend the most time with the patient—I won't say regardless of their preparation, but assuming that they have a professional preparation—are most likely to know what help their patient needs. Therefore I think that as long as the nurses, of all professional workers, are the ones who spend most time with patients, they are probably going to have the most important contribution to make to health care. In my judgment, far more attention is going to be paid in the future to what nurses think patients need than we now give it. I think the role of nurses is going to be a more responsible one, that they are going to be given more authority. They must have legal backing for this, so all nurse practice acts are going to change rapidly, and the medical practice acts too. I believe that most people see this necessity, and it seems almost too obvious to mention.

I've just been trying to write about the settings in which nurses function. I'm not a bit sure that what we now call private-duty nursing and independent nursing practice aren't going to merge. Right now the nursing indexes are confused about these two terms. Sometimes indexes put items under one heading and sometimes under the other. So even now it's really hard to distinguish the two settings.

You asked me a little while ago what I thought about the term "practitioner." I like the term but not the way it is used. So many use practitioner to mean a nurse with specialized preparation. I think all nurses ought to be considered practitioners and ought to be considered clini-

13 "Illustrious Past, Challenging Future: A Salute to the American Nurses' Association on its 75th Anniversary," pp. 1773–1880.
14 This includes providing better health care for presently neglected groups of persons, for example, the aged—those in their own homes and those in so-called nursing homes—and all those in jails and prisons, who are perhaps the most neglected.
15 Royal Society of Medicine and Josiah Macy, Jr., Foundation, *The Greater Medical Profession*, The Foundation, New York, 1973.

cal unless they are proved otherwise. I think it ought to be the exception when a nurse is *not* a practitioner and an exception when she *doesn't* know something about clinical nursing.

A trend most people recognize today is toward what is called "the ladder concept," developing health curricula that make it as easy as possible for students to change from one to the other. Continuing education is another, more or less accepted, idea. The health worker who ceases to be a student is lost in today's world.

GS: What is your view on the physician's assistant?

VH: I don't question the physicians' right to prepare people to share their work, but I doubt whether people in this country accept the idea that one professional worker "assists" another professional worker. The very term means that the person who is being assisted has to assume teaching and legal responsibility for what the assistants do. I fail to see how physicians can successfully assume these responsibilities, and I doubt whether short-term courses can adequately prepare workers for the kind of work physicians' assistants are now doing. I also question dead-end programs. It is important that all health workers be continuing students. I would like to see the professional degrees that people earn inform the public on their preparation for what they are doing. In Europe for many years people have been able to get a bachelor's degree in medicine, or a master's degree, or a doctoral degree. I think the public should be told how much the individual has invested in preparation for practice and let it go at that, instead of tagging workers with all sorts of names, the significance of which the public must learn. I would like to see all professional workers prepared in colleges and universities. They could then say they have a bachelor's, a master's, or a doctoral degree in a declared field. I see nothing wrong with saying any medical worker is a specialist in maternal-child care or a specialist in psychiatric care or a specialist in medical and surgical treatment or is any one of the subspecialists.

GS: Do you think that all nursing education should be in college?

VH: I certainly do. Since it is an accomplished fact for professional nursing in a number of states, it seems less and less debatable. But unfortunately the hospital schools for professional nursing have passed on their faults to the schools of practical nursing. The President's Commission on Higher Education in 1948 proposed that there be two categories of nurses: those produced in the junior colleges, which would be the equivalent of practical nurses; and those produced in the senior colleges, which would be the professional nurses. A group of nonnurses wrote the report, I think, and that's the conclusion they came to. I believe it's perfectly sound. I believe that's an opinion many people hold, and it has been around since 1948—actually much longer, for individuals came to these conclusions long before they were given out by agencies and organizations.

GS: Did you agree with the Position Paper for nurse education which the American Nurses' Association (A.N.A.) came out with in 1965?

VH: Yes, I did. At the time, the A.N.A. stressed that the position was not a new one. Actually it is somewhat the same position I've just stated as that of the President's Commission on Higher Education. It's interesting that the report of that Commission seemed to have little impact.

GS: Why would you say it didn't create as much furor?

VH: I really don't know. But when a report comes out in seven volumes, there are few nurses in the country or others concerned with nursing education who will read the report in its entirety and find the recommendations that affect nursing. Actually the Commission was only an advisory body, and wasn't charged with implementing its recommendations.

GS: Is there anything you care to add at all?

VH: No, I believe not. I realize that you have a difficult task. In one day you are trying to get enough information to write a biographical sketch. There are at least three persons besides yourself involved in today's task: the person I think I am, the person you think I am, and the person I really am. The person I really am is what you're trying to get at, and I don't know how to help you except by answering your questions as honestly as I can, especially the questions about the work I've done, since the only value this interview has in my eyes is pointing out such usefulness as this work may have for others interested in what Annie Goodrich used to refer to as a healthy citizenry.

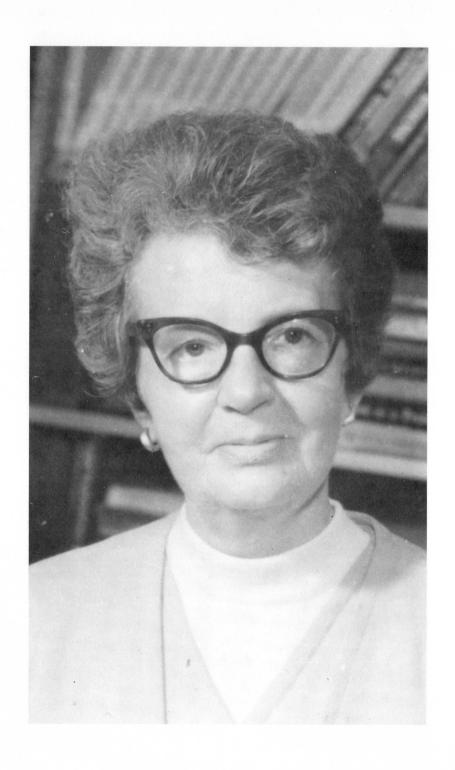

6

Eleanor C. Lambertsen has demonstrated the quality leadership which ANA (American Nurses' Association) had traditionally advocated and sought in its efforts to carry out the purposes for which the Association was founded. Dr. Lambertsen has directed her interests and talent to the organization and delivery of nursing care services, which are ANA's primary objectives. She is nationally and internationally recognized as an articulate spokesman for nursing, an accomplished professional writer, a researcher, an educator, an administrator, a social activist, an authority on the organization and delivery of health care services, and a very strong advocate of the professional organization.

Although her contributions are many, it is their uniqueness which we believe deserves the recognition and appreciation of ANA. The strength of her relationships with members of other disciplines; her involvement with state nurses' associations; her proficiency in nursing service administration, and her professional leadership and inspiration in nursing education; are each significant in themselves. In combination they result in a breadth and depth of professional insight which is outstanding.[1]

[1] From American Nurses' Association Award, 1970.

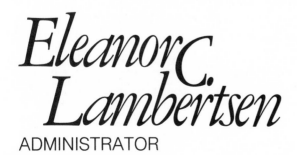

Eleanor C.
Lambertsen
ADMINISTRATOR

*E*leanor C. Lambertsen is renowned as a nursing leader who has made significant contributions on an interdisciplinary level. She developed nursing service administration along with team nursing. At the present time[2] she is a Senior Associate Director for Nursing Service at The New York Hospital and Dean and Professor of Nursing at the Cornell University–New York Hospital School of Nursing.

Dr. Lambertsen received her diploma from Overlook Hospital School of Nursing in 1938; her B.S. in 1949, her M.A. in 1950, and her Ed.D. in curriculum and instruction in 1957 from Teachers College, Columbia University. Her doctoral dissertation was entitled "Education for Nursing Leadership."

Her vast professional experience has included administration and teaching at Teachers College. She was with the American Hospital Association (A.H.A.) from 1958 to 1961 as the Director of the Division of Nursing and Assistant Secretary, Council on Professional Practices.

Her professional activities are extensive. She has held a number of elective offices; has been an active member of many associations; and has been appointed to various boards, commissions, and committees. In addition to government assignments, she has been given international assignments and has served as a consultant to agencies, associations, and journals.

Dr. Lambertsen has received numerous awards and honors.[3] She has conducted many research projects and studies and has published 2 books and over 150 articles.[4]

Early Background

GS: Did your family influence your career choice?

ECL: I was born in Westfield, New Jersey, on January 2, 1916. My

---

[2] July 1975.

[3] Among these are the R. Louise McManus Medal, May 1971; Honorary Citizen of Tel Aviv Award, 1970; honorary doctor of science degree, Alfred University, New York, 1969; and Honorary Fellow, the American College of Hospital Administrators, 1971.

[4] To cite only a few key publications: *Nursing Team Organization and Functioning*, Teachers College Press, Columbia University, New York, 1953; *Education for Nursing Leadership*, J. B. Lippincott Company, Philadelphia, 1958; "If Nursing Has Changed, So Have Doctors and Hospitals," *Modern Hospital*, November 1962; "Evaluating the Quality of Nursing Care," *Hospitals*, November 1965; "Reorganize Nursing to Re-emphasize Care," *Modern Hospital*, January 1967; "Use of Sabbaticals for Research Training," *Nursing Research*, July–August 1968; "Research in Nursing: The Task and the Tools," *Focus on the Future*, S. Karger-Basel, New York, 1970; "Preparation of the Nurse Practitioner," *Chart*, March 1971; and "Licensure for Nursing Practice," *Journal of the New York State Nurses' Association*, Fall 1970.

mother died in childbirth of eclampsia with the fourth child. My father remarried when I was age thirteen. My stepmother was a typical house-wife and good stepmother. There were no children from this marriage. My own mother was rather unusual for her time in that she was a high school graduate and had been in business. She met my father when she came to Fanwood, New Jersey, for a holiday. She had a long-lasting impact upon me, for she was an avid reader and valued educa-tion. She and my father discussed and shared family affairs with me and my older brother. Her death was tragic for all of us. She died at age thirty-two. It was her hope that I would be a schoolteacher.

My father was in business, not self-business. Following my mother's death he devoted himself to his family. The entire Lambertsen family—aunts, uncles, cousins—had close family ties, and these continue to exist. We are really a clan.

I finished high school during the Depression. My brother Chris was planning to study medicine; this had been his dream all his life. He is now an internationally renowned scientist. I was not interested in teach-ing as a career, although I was encouraged by the high school principal to do so. I was a member of the honor society and debate varsity, editor of the school newspaper, and a member of the dramatic society. Fol-lowing graduation I spent the summer, as usual, at the shore with my grandfather. I met a nurse and for the first time became interested in nursing. Without informing my family, I wrote to schools of nursing and selected the one that enrolled students in February. I didn't want to interrupt a long vacation period. That, if you can imagine, is how I selected Overlook Hospital School of Nursing in Summit, New Jersey. My grandfather in particular was quite vehement about my decision. My father, after much discussion, supported my decision.

GS: Did you like nursing?

ECL: Very much, very much. I just wasn't the type of person, I guess, to have a comfortable existence in nursing at that period of time. I had not had any guidance in high school about nursing. It was never men-tioned as a career choice for those majoring in the college preparatory courses. The nurse I mentioned previously only knew about diploma programs, and I only wrote to diploma programs and therefore selected one. I can still remember the first morning in the school. Our Director of Nursing was British and a graduate of Roosevelt Hospital School of Nursing in New York City. The entering class of fifteen were all to report to her office in uniform; if I recall, it was about 6:30 in the morning. I had never been up at 6:30 in the morning except to watch a sunrise on a mountain or to watch the fish boats come in. We were all standing; she was sitting at her desk. There were a couch and chair in her office so I

just invited myself and others to sit down. I was immediately repri-
manded and asked why I was sitting. I said I was tired and also thought
sitting down was appropriate. She informed me in no uncertain terms
that she doubted I would ever finish. We became very close friends
after graduation. I could sense as a student that she was fond of me,
but I was called to her office rather frequently.

GS: What was your nurses' training like?

ECL: We were assigned to the wards the first day, and cleaned and
cleaned until we learned how to do simple nursing duties. We had the
typical probationary period of study for that era with concentration on
nursing arts and sciences taught by one nurse. The emphasis was to
prepare us as quickly as possible for ward duty. The two nurses who
taught us nursing arts and sciences had master's degrees from Teachers College, Columbia University. I know that was rare for that time and
I was influenced early by both of them. The lectures for the clinical
areas were typical, also: doctors' lectures followed by an interpretation
by a nurse. We affiliated for three months of medicine and three months
of pediatrics, with a few weeks of psychiatry, at the Jersey City Medical
Center.

Summit, New Jersey, was an affluent community, and the community
took a great deal of interest in the School of Nursing. In retrospect one
might say it was one of their favorite "charities."

The doctors were, in general, a well-prepared group, many of them
board specialists. The first group practice in the United States was located in Summit, with members of the group holding appointments in
medical teaching centers such as Presbyterian and The New York Hospital in New York City. The doctors outside of the group formed an
association and called themselves the Independent Group. There was
rivalry, and we sensed this as students. But the doctors were interested
in students. A great deal of my education came from my association
with these men. They were always interested in explaining or teaching,
and I was always asking questions. Perhaps one of the greatest influences on my life as a nurse, interested in multidisciplinary approaches
to health problems, was my early relationships with doctors who were
interested in a student nurse eager to learn. Our classes seemed to
stress "what to do," but I was encouraged by them to ask "why." You
just couldn't raise questions with nurses on the wards. That was not
considered appropriate behavior for students! In 1933, a year before I
entered the school, the National League for Nursing (N.L.N.) published
A Study of the Use of the Graduate Nurse for Bedside Nursing in the

Hospital. Student nurses were the labor force. We did purchase our own uniforms and books, but received room and meals and a $5-a-month stipend.

When I graduated in February 1938, two of the fifteen were offered positions. And we were both informed that if we didn't do well, there would be others to take our place. It was also at this time that private-duty nurses were working for room and board. It was still the Depression and there was no work for them. This was really one of the beginning introductions of graduate nurses for staff nursing positions. At that time students and graduates were assigned for a twelve-hour tour of duty with two half-days off a week. If you were a student on night duty, you were required to go to day classes regardless of when they were scheduled.

Overlook Hospital— As Director of the School of Nursing and Nursing Service

My first assignment was as staff nurse on nights. Within the first year I became the assistant night supervisor, and the following year the night supervisor. I am not certain of the year, but in either 1941 or 1942 I was informed by the newly appointed Director of Nursing that I was to be responsible for teaching nursing arts and medical-surgical nursing. I had enrolled summers in courses in premedical science at Rutgers University and later in courses in nursing at Seton Hall College, but I had never taught.

On New Year's Eve 1945, when I was dressing to go home for the holidays, I was called and asked to come to the hospital immediately. The president of the board of trustees and the director of the hospital told me the director of nursing had been fired, and I was now principal of the school and director of nursing service. Needless to say, my New Year's Eve was rather dismal. I had wanted to resign and continue my education. It was the war period, and I was unacceptable for the military because of a knee injury and wore a brace for several years. Because of the cadet corps, teachers were considered frozen. The president of the board of trustees was the president of Merck and Company and another significant influence in my life. He met with me regularly, and through him I was invited to attend the meetings of the board of trustees of the hospital. This was another unusual assignment for a nurse at that time. Today this is all too rare an experience in the majority of hospitals. Through him I was introduced to, and became involved in, civic affairs.

The experience as principal of the school and director of nursing was invaluable. For early in my career I became interested in the federal government through my experiences with the Student Nurse Cadet Corps. It was at that time, if you will recall, that there was strong emphasis upon raising the standards of diploma programs—of arranging programs so that students could complete their education in two years and be assigned to a senior cadet experience. It was the beginning, really, of looking at what could be done educationally in two years, with the third year resembling an internship.

The board of trustees was highly supportive of the school. In the early forties, students spent one semester at Rutgers in Newark, New Jersey. Ella Stonesby had introduced a preclinical science program for hospital schools of nursing, and our school was one of the first to enroll. Students enrolled in the basic sciences, including psychology and sociology, at the time they were enrolled in nursing arts at the home school. I introduced a one-month public health experience and transferred the pediatric affiliation from Jersey City Medical Center to Babies Hospital, Presbyterian Hospital in New York City. The students also had a three-month affiliation in psychiatry. Very little time was being spent in the home hospital. The State Board of Nurse Examiners was a vital force in nursing education in New Jersey—a vital and positive force. Two very important people were responsible, Edith June Holden and Bernice Anderson. Once a month a Principal's Day was sponsored by them. Today we would call this a program of continuing education. Each meeting focused upon some area of education that was significant: student evaluation, objectives of programs, student affiliations, teaching methods, and so forth.

I was the youngest of the group, and the first time I appeared they didn't know quite what to do with me. The women were well-known figures in nursing; one saw them at conventions, read their articles. I felt as though I was with a group of professors, but they adopted me. I called them when I had problems, was encouraged to visit them, and received help. But the most significant person at this time of my life was Bernice Anderson, and she has continued in this role. She was always available, interested, and a critic in the most positive sense. We had at this time, or I had available to me, a group of women who were courageous leaders in nursing, interested in improving nursing education and in working together. They were interested in grooming young leadership, and in these beginning days for me I developed contacts that have been not only influential but lasting, people who opened many doors and opportunities. It was through Bernice Anderson that I experienced the significance of organized nursing and the potential of key leaders for effecting change.

GS: And you don't think that's the way it is today?

ECL: I don't think it is. There is too much selfness now, too much concern for individual situations, too much competition. At that time I didn't sense competition. It was more "let's help you in any way we can"; it was a sharing; it was a very different era. I don't like to just say I'm looking nostalgically to the past, but I do think there was a cohesiveness among the nursing leaders, not only state leaders but national leaders as well.

GS: Sounds to me like they were working for the ultimate goal of nursing.

ECL: They were, and for grooming young leaders.

GS: What would you say there was about you that the early nursing leaders and other leaders perceived in you as a potential leader?

ECL: Oh, I think I've always been an outgoing kind of person. I get involved; I get involved deeply. I became extremely interested in my time at Overlook Hospital in what the nurse's role was in patient care and the relationship of nurses and physicians as colleagues. The setting was such that it promoted this. We worked hard, but I was not aware of any concept of doctor-nurse conflict. The nature of the setting—the community support and interest—was conducive to positive work relationships and to learning.

One positive example, perhaps, was that when I resigned in 1947 to enroll full time at Teachers College, Columbia University, the medical staff and the board of trustees gave me a check for $5000 for my education.

GS: You obviously have been successful working with physicians and with hospital administrators.

ECL: The same situation exists today. I don't think anyone gets anywhere just being purely verbal. I think you have to demonstrate that you are interested in, and knowledgeable about, the welfare of patients. The status of the nurse should be unquestionable. I have a strong concept of self and I am proud I am a nurse. I have not felt that nursing was under anything; I have felt that it had a significant contribution to make and one did not have to be defensive. Equally important is the appreciation that others, hospital administrators and physicians, have problems and also have significant contributions to make. I believe that all my life I have kept in touch with the broader relationships of nursing. I have remained a generalist and I am not threatened by the situations I have encountered. I happen to believe that doctors and hospital administrators are under as much stress as we are.

Teachers College (1947–1949)

GS: Was there anything significant about your student days at Teachers College?

ECL: Teachers College was viewed by everyone as the place to receive a degree. The world's greats in nursing education were, or had been, on the faculty. The alumni were in power positions.

When I enrolled to complete requirements for a baccalaureate degree, I wanted one course, a course in budgeting. The remainder of the requirements I accepted, but it was difficult for me to understand the reaction to what appeared to me to be an essential requirement. I had had an overwhelming experience with the financial records associated with the Cadet Corps. The early experience with government financial forms and prodedures led me to believe there must be a simpler way. I continue to believe today that there must be. The course never was available until I developed one with the controller of Teachers College, where I became involved with the W. K. Kellogg project in nursing service.

When I finished my undergraduate major—teaching and supervision in medical-surgical nursing—I had decided to enroll in the major in hospital nursing service administration. In 1949 the veterans were enrolling in large numbers. It took days to register. The second day I had progressed to third in line for advisement and program approval with the adviser of the major. Bernice Anderson was at the next table (we enrolled in the library) as adviser for the major of administration in schools of nursing. She saw me and said, "What are you doing in that line?"—or words to that effect. The next day I found myself enrolled in the education major. She was a persuasive woman and at that time I really didn't see much difference. Most of the positions were combined positions. I was still oriented to a future as director of nursing and director of a hospital school of nursing.

Teachers College (1950–1958)

GS: What next?

ECL: Following completion of requirements for a master of arts degree in administration in schools of nursing, under the advisement of Professor Bernice Anderson, I decided to enroll in field experience in public health nursing in Harlem under the sponsorship of the Visiting Nurse Service of New York. I had taken all electives in public health to qualify for the position. I realized this preparation was vital for anyone in education. During the summer R. Louise McManus, Director of the Division of Nursing of Teachers College, Columbia University, wrote and asked me if I would be interested in a position at Teachers College. I later learned that Bernice Anderson had recommended me. The division had received a grant from the W. K. Kellogg Foundation to develop programs in nursing service. My assignment primarily at that time was to work with Mildred Montag and Amelia Leino on a project for development of the concept of team nursing. A pilot unit was initiated at Women's Hospital in New York City. In 1951 a grant for development of junior college programs was awarded to the division, and Mildred Montag became director of this project. At this time the Department of Hospitals of the City of New York arranged for the facilities for a new hospital, the Frances Delafield Hospital for the treatment of cancer, to be affiliated with the College of Physicians and Surgeons of Columbia University. I became responsible for the study and organization of the hospital on a team basis, and a year later became director of the entire W. K. Kellogg project.

R. Louise McManus became another great influence on my life. She was a visionary and a scholar as well as a great person. The team concept, the junior college program, clinical nurse specialists, and so many other major concepts in nursing were her ideas. She had the capacity for developing people and providing them with the personal and professional resources required to be creative and innovative.

Mildred Tuttle, Director of the Division of Nursing of the W. K. Kellogg Foundation, became interested in my work and appointed me to the Nursing Advisory Committee of the Foundation. Once again I had the opportunity to be associated with significant leaders in nursing. It was then that I first met Lulu Wolf Hassenplug. Others on the committee were equally significant, but Lulu remained a constant inspiration and friend. Because of the interest in team nursing, I had the opportunity for a great deal of national consultation and visited many other universities as well as hospitals. By this time we had extended the research to Memorial Hospital for Cancer and Allied Diseases, and were conducting a number of short-term courses a year to prepare nursing service and nursing educators.

In my manual on team nursing, published in 1953, I revised the organization chart of the traditional nursing service department and started with the patients, wherever they were, defining the objectives for their care. The whole philosophy of team nursing that I described in my publication was that one reversed the order of the organization chart and started with defining the objectives for care and programs for care. Then you defined the functions of the personnel: the direct caring people, the team leader, and the other mix; then the head nurse, then the supervisor, and finally the Director of Nursing Service. As I assumed responsibility for the majors in supervision and nursing service administration, the concepts were further refined, and I did more and more consultation in organizing departments of nursing service throughout this country and Canada.

GS: Where did you get the idea to reverse the chart?

ECL: I believe I was largely influenced by my education at Teachers College as well as my prior experiences. I was exposed to Virginia Henderson and Francis Reiter at the undergraduate level as well as to Mary Maher. The philosophy of the major in medical-surgical nursing at that time at Teachers College was patient care–oriented. R. Louise McManus was also influential. Her assumption of the functions of nurses as a spectrum, ranging from the simplest activity to the most complex function, formed the theoretical framework for team nursing and the associate degree educational programs. I am now in the process of developing a paper on team nursing *revisited,* because of the current emphasis on redefinition of nursing practice. R. Louise McManus's functions identified diagnosis of the nursing problem of the patient as the basic premise in 1947.

As I became more involved in the project, and others visited the demonstration center, the philosophy was more and more shared with others. I was invited to take part in surveys of hospitals with hospital consultants or consultant firms, as well as architectural firms, for design of patient care units. One such experience was as a consultant to the group of United Mine Workers hospitals in Kentucky and West Virginia. I was fortunate in that I had a base in two areas, nursing education and nursing service, throughout this period. I rarely worked summers at Teachers College, but accepted opportunities to conduct workshops in other universities and hospitals or participated in consultation.

GS: Is there anything you wish to add about your team nursing concept at that time?

ECL: A lot of people have distorted the concept. The concept started out, as I said, with the McManus assumptions of the functions of nursing. The whole emphasis was upon the leadership role of the professional practitioners of nursing in planning, providing, and evaluating nursing care. The concept was that of professional practice.

GS: You were talking about how the concept has been distorted.

ECL: Well, it has been distorted. I still have people call me up or write and say, "We tried team nursing yesterday but it didn't work"! What they fail to recognize is that it is an intellectual process—that the team leaders have to have a background in the concepts, the content, the principles of nursing if they are to be capable of identifying the patients' problems, plan the care, communicate with other members of the health team, and constantly evaluate this care. It became another administrative position in the minds of many with the emphasis upon the mechanics or management of things. They have forgotten completely—nor did some ever appreciate—the concept of team nursing and utilization of nursing service personnel for safe, efficient, and therapeutically effective nursing care. They ignore the nursing care plan, the team conference, examples of which were published in *Education for Nursing Leadership.* It is the ability to draw upon principles and to draw inferences that is requisite. I still get uptight with critics who never did understand. If care plans are not written, perhaps it is because the individual does not have the knowledge. If conferences appear to be a waste of time, perhaps the team leader is incapable of drawing inferences from the communications shared by the team members.

One reason I came to The New York Hospital–Cornell Medical Center was that I wanted to be in another situation where I could again concentrate upon the examination of the roles of nurses in practice.

I was one of three nurses who originally approached Elliot Richardson, then Secretary of Health, Education, and Welfare (H.E.W.), to encourage him to look nationally at the contribution of nursing to the national health scene. I was then a member of a group that met several times. He finally appointed a committee to study extended roles for nurses, and the report *Extending the Scope of Nursing Practice* was published in 1971. The first year as Dean of the Cornell University–New York Hospital School of Nursing, I submitted a proposal to the National Center for Health Services Research and Development for the preparation of family nurse-practitioners (PRIMEX). Two contracts were awarded in 1971, one to Chapel Hill and one to our school. At the same time the Department of Health of the City of New York approached the Dean of the Medical College and me and asked if we would consider preparing pediatric nurse associates for the child care stations in New York City. This we have done and with tremendous success, I think. We have also just completed our first program to prepare public health nurse epidemiologists.

Once again I believe it is because of the many associations I have been fortunate to make that I do not have difficulty in securing laboratories or hospitals and other service agencies willing to participate in programs. This has been an exciting period, and there is a tremendous similarity to my work with team nursing. It is again an extension of the McManus assumptions. While team nursing was predominantly within the hospital setting, we are now concentrating upon our roles external to the institutional setting.

On Writing

GS: *Do you like to write?*

ECL: Yes, I write easily. Whenever I have to present a paper or I get uptight about something, I write, and I do it for publication. I hadn't written a thing before 1953 except teaching materials or reports. Once again R. Louise McManus was an influence. I became upset because I found people publishing my materials as their own. I think this is something that continues to distress me to no end. I was very free with the duplicated materials that I was using, and time after time I found them coming out under other people's names. And, as a young person, I became upset. One summer Ms. McManus said to me, ''Now instead of taking another appointment somewhere, I want you to write a manual on team nursing." I'd never written, and I just assumed that since she said I could do it, I could do it. You also have to know salaries at the time. I was given $300 for that two-month period to write. I also paid for my own secretary and typing. I went home and stayed home and wrote. I set up the sun parlor at my home and remained there all day and wrote the manual. When I returned for the fall registration period, R. Louise McManus asked to see me, thinking, I later found out, that I might have made some progress. I said, "It's finished." It was finished and typed. She sent it to the editor of the Teachers College Press, and it was published without any changes. Another thing that did help was that I accepted, after I left the American Hospital Association, the discipline of a monthly column in *Modern Hospital;* and I did that for about ten years. I like to write.

GS: Could you say something about your work habits in writing? Do you find that you set aside a certain number of hours a day?

ECL: Oh, I think you have to be disciplined. I think a great deal about what I am going to write. I mull it around before I sit down to write, but my writing now just has to be done on weekends or at home. I have no time in my work to write. I do a lot of writing there, but it's accreditation reports, grants, staff documents, that kind of thing; my own writing is done here at home. My writing has also led to international involvement, for much of it has been published in other languages as texts or in official journals.

International Level

GS: Could you say something about your involvement in nursing internationally?

ECL: My first international experience was in South America—Brazil and Chile—in 1954. The W. K. Kellogg Foundation sponsored a group of nurses from Brazil and Chile to be prepared for strategic nursing service positions. They were my advisees. When they returned, I spent four months with them as well as with other W. K. Kellogg trainees. During this period I conducted conferences, consulted in hospitals and schools of nursing, and also lectured in the School of Hospital Administration in Brazil. Since I had also taught in the hospital administration program of the School of Public Health of Columbia University, I had met a number of Hospital administrators from South America.

I was one of the first to learn that the King Edward's Hospital Fund for London had started a fellowship program for hospital administrators to visit and spend some time studying the system in Britain. This was in cooperation with the A.H.A. I was on the program of the International Hospital Association meeting in Chicago and met the person in charge, Frank Reeves. I asked him why this same opportunity wasn't available for nurses. I have always acted this way when I feel nursing should be represented. I just telephone or write whenever I feel a committee or other activity should have nursing representation. In this instance my comments were made at a social affair, and I had no idea he had been planning to invite me. While I was in London, the nurses in Britain spoke about the fund's sponsoring international seminars for hospital administrators and physicians. Frank Reeves and the trustees of the Fund were interested, and I then participated in planning an international seminar for invited nursing leaders from Britain, Canada, and the United States.

I spent my sabbatical as a visiting Professor at the University of Tel Aviv in Israel, and have continued to accept invitations each year for short-term assignments in various countries. This year I spent two weeks in Japan and two weeks in Australia.

At the American Hospital Association (1958–1961)

GS: What next?

ECL: In 1957, I finished my doctorate. I had been employed at Teachers College, and I decided I needed some other experience. I had been there seven years (1950–1957), and was quite frankly looking at moving into another educational setting. I had been offered (at that time there were fewer doctorates) sixteen positions.

GS: How did you ever make up your mind?

ECL: I'll tell you how I made it up. I didn't. Somebody else made it up for me. I knew I wasn't ready to be a dean. At that time I was looking at a professorial position in a school of nursing, though I was offered any number of deanships. I was also interviewed for the position of General Director of N.L.N. I could not accept the position because I knew that my major area of interest was nursing service and education, and I could not in good faith accept a position such as this, knowing that I could not commit myself for any length of time. At the same time I was approached by the A.H.A. Dr. Edwin L. Crosby was planning to create a Division of Nursing within the organization and was seeking candidates. When someone from the A.H.A. came to interview me about the position, I gave them names of other people; I was not the least bit interested. I did not realize that I had been recommended by such people as Marion Sheehan. A number of key nursing leaders also came to see me and said, "You're young enough at this stage; it is important for a nurse with your background, your interests, to move into the American Hospital Association and help shape a program and be a person who can effectively relate to nursing." I got all kinds of advice and pressure from all over, and also support. The position was viewed as strategic by these women; they also knew where nursing should go. I also held the position of assistant secretary of the Council on Professional Practices.

GS: And they helped.

ECL: I was encouraged to take the position and I saw the significance of it. As they discussed with me the opportunity that existed in this position, I felt responsible, particularly since for seven years I had been involved in the W. K. Kellogg project in nursing service administration. Little did I realize that a major portion of my time would be spent resolving issues of accreditation of hospital schools of nursing by the N.L.N.

Throughout my tenure at the A.H.A. I had complete support from organized nursing and individual leaders of nursing as well as from Dr. Edwin L. Crosby and the other administrative officers and trustees. This does not imply there were not organizational conflicts; there were. In this position I represented nursing in every or any situation and became more involved with national organizations, both federal and other professional organizations.

Also, at the time I went to Chicago I had friends in the American Medical Association (A.M.A.), and I continued to maintain contacts with this organization as well as others located in Chicago.

GS: There must be something about you personally that would make these many different professionals recommend you. What would you say objectively it is?

ECL: Well, I think I have been a student of organizations all my life. I keep in close touch with social change, social legislation; I believe I had one of the best residencies one could have had in the study of social organizations in my years at the A.H.A., although my work at Teachers College contributed to this. Dr. Edwin L. Crosby was the kind of administrator who respected strong and aggressive leadership. I don't think I'm hostilely aggressive, but I have made it my business to be informed and to take a stand on issues. I believe that at many times one has to look at all sides of a question, but then make a decision. I do believe that I have been able to influence decision making and that certain people recognize this. I might add that some of my stands have not always been popular with some nurses or hospital administrators.

My experience with the A.H.A. was invaluable and resulted in my being recommended for a majority of multidisciplinary national commissions, councils, and conferences. It was during this time I was appointed to the Surgeon General's Consultant Group in Nursing, which resulted in the legislation for the first Nurse Training Act.

At one time I had considered hospital administration as a career, for I was offered a scholarship in the field. This was during a period of upheaval at Overlook Hospital. A Citizens' Committee in 1946 took strong action against the then current hospital administrator, following numerous complaints of physicians, nurses, and patients. A consultant was employed, and during the consultation strongly recommended that I consider hospital administration. I was unofficial, acting hospital director with the president of the board of trustees. But at that time the financial management began to change. Blue Cross was entering the field, and I wasn't interested in finances of a hospital. Now I am a board member of Blue Cross–Blue Shield of Greater New York.

Contributions to Nursing Service and Nursing Education

GS: What took you back to Teachers College at Columbia University?[5]

ECL: I had been at the American Hospital Association for only one month when the president of Teachers College visited me in Chicago. He had been out of the country when I resigned and then had had a major health problem. He informed me that I had been considered as the person to succeed R. Louise McManus when she retired. No one had informed me and I doubt now that I would have remained, for I

---

[5] Dr. Lambertsen was on the faculty of Teachers College from 1950 to 1958, before going to the American Hospital Association. She returned to Teachers College in 1961, assuming faculty and administrative positions.

believed I needed other experiences. I had also, by this time, accepted the premise that one had an advantage for bargaining for conditions of a position if one was not currently employed by that organization. I had this on the good advice of someone I highly respected in the academic world.

My experiences with the issues and problems of leadership in nursing education and nursing service during my employment at the A.H.A. and my increasing involvement with policy and legislative programs of H.E.W. influenced my decision to return to nursing education. I was at that time primarily interested in graduate education.

I was interviewed again for several positions as dean, but my primary interest was Teachers College. The national and international status of the Division of Nursing Education, the historical heritage of the student body were determining factors. I was also planning to marry, and my husband and I agreed that New York City was the area for both of our careers.

When one reacts to contributions to nursing education and nursing service, my reaction is that it has primarily been through my students. The advantage of being on the faculty of Teachers College was that of influencing, and being influenced by, graduate students from all over the United States and from abroad. I was, for example, adviser for students from other lands during my first period at Teachers College and continued this responsibility when I returned. One innovative program was a Learn-Earn program for students from other lands. The program was developed collaboratively by the American Nurses' Association and the Division of Nursing Education. I was appointed adviser. Whenever I attend an International Council of Nurses (I.C.N.) meeting or travel abroad, I continue to meet significant leaders of nurses in other countries who were enrolled in this program.

Upon my return I continued to teach and advise in the major program preparing for leadership positions on the master's level for nursing service administration. I also continued to supervise and participate directly in the field experience of students. In this way I maintained a continuous association with a wide range of hospitals. My appointment was Director of the Division of Nursing, with an enrollment of approximately thirteen hundred students, and Director of the Institute of Research and Service in Nursing Education. I also held the endowed Chair of the Helen Hartley Professorship.

I became deeply involved in doctoral advisement at a time when the nature of dissertations for the doctor of education was being reexamined. There was clearly a need for an emphasis upon the theory of nursing as well as the theory of the teaching-learning process. It is, or should be, a humbling experience to be a sponsor for a doctoral candidate. So many of our students searched throughout the university for educational opportunities. I like to believe that my association with other key leaders in the university helped to remove some barriers.

One major innovation was the award of a grant to prepare nurse-scientists on the Ph.D level. It was a breakthrough for our division. Columbia University's program at the Ph.D level was classic. A nurse was at a disadvantage because of the liberal arts requirements at the undergraduate level. But through the cooperation and leadership of Dr. Elizabeth Hagen, Professor in Educational Measurement of the department of psychology, a program was approved. The grant provided for prerequisite liberal arts requirements and I believe was one of the major innovative programs promoted by the Division of Nursing of H.E.W.

Another area I believed I helped to foster was that of continuing education. A grant from the National Institute for Mental Health was awarded to develop a program in continuing education for nurses in mental health–psychiatric nursing. Teachers College and of course the Division of Nursing had offered a number of short-term courses and work conferences for practitioners and administrators. But this grant was the first in the Division of Nursing Education, since the W. K. Kellogg nursing service project, to develop through systematic study a continuing-education program for nurses practicing in a major clinical area.

What I had envisioned when I returned to Teachers College was a total university endeavor that would in some coordinated way develop a system of education from the baccalaureate level to the doctoral level for leadership positions in nursing as well as other health-related fields. A beginning was made in 1968, when Teachers College was reorganized and I was appointed Director of the Division of Health Service, Science, and Research. The reorganization brought together in one organizational unit the departments of nursing education, health education, and nutrition education. Recognizing the distinctive educational requirements of students preparing for leadership positions in health services, sciences, and education, the college sought through this reorganization to clarify the nature and scope of intra- and interdepartmental courses and programs, to appraise college and university resources available or essential to program development, and to more effectively utilize faculty ability and experience.

I realized at the time of the student rebellion at Columbia and the resulting response of the various faculty groups that this concept was, to be mild, far from acceptable to some of the tenured members of the faculty of the division. I have retained extensive records of that particular stage of my history.

I had formally resigned prior to the reorganization, but had been requested to reconsider. I extended my resignation for two years, and was granted a terminal sabbatical the spring of 1970. I had accepted the position of Dean of the Cornell University–New York Hospital School of Nursing prior to leaving for Tel Aviv, Israel, but the college administration withheld the announcement. It was their judgment.

In May 1971 I was awarded the R. Louise McManus Medal by the Nursing Education Alumni Association of Teachers College.

I believe also that other areas of involvement in both nursing education and nursing service were the opportunities I had to be appointed to numerous committees of the American Nurses' Association, the National League for Nursing, the New York State Nurses' Association, and the Division of Nursing at the federal level.

Hospital Administration

What I want to stress is that a great deal of my becoming knowledgeable about hospital affairs came through my exposure to key leaders in the hospital field. All of my professional experiences led to a commitment that one had to work in a multidisciplinary world and that one had to employ every strategy to resolve problems in the beginning before they became unmanageable. Nursing services are part of a complex structure, and to influence the structure constant study and appraisal of the system is essential. I take pride in having received, in 1963, the American Hospital Association Trustee Award for outstanding contribution to nursing and the hospital field. In 1971 I was made an Honorary Fellow of the American College of Hospital Administrators.

Dean at Cornell

GS: As a dean at Cornell, what problems did you have?

ECL: The major problem was that of faculty development. Other problems were curriculum revision and development of an organizational structure. I believe the dean is a leader in curriculum development and faculty development. I have always been fortunate in identifying people with particular talents. I also believe that it takes one year to become oriented to a new situation and that major changes are not indicated until one is familiar with the available personnel resources and one has gained a rather thorough understanding of the new situation. My style of administration requires an associate who can assume responsibility for the internal administration. I perceive the role of dean as external—program development and liaison at the medical center, state, and national levels. The current associate dean, a graduate of the school whose career has been in various positions in the department of nursing service and the School of Nursing, is a rare find. We have formed an ideal, for me, administrative team.

GS: Now, when you're still the Dean, do you have anything to add?

ECL: Yes. The position in this center has provided numerous opportunities for establishing positive relationships with the chiefs of the medical staff and faculty, with nursing service personnel, and with the hospital and center administrative staff. In addition, the president of the university maintains an apartment in the city and I have ready access to him, since he spends time in our center. One major accomplishment has been the joint continuing-education programs sponsored by the School of Nursing, the Medical College, The New York Hospital, and community agencies such as the Visiting Nurse Service of New York and the Department of Health of the City of New York. The university approved a Division of Continuing Education of the school in 1971, and an assistant dean was appointed. A medical center such as this offers unlimited opportunities. We have demonstrated as a school that we can meet community needs. We offer courses in pharmacology, in physiology, in coronary care, and so on, and they are oversubscribed. Our program is geared to the practice of nursing, and the response has been overwhelming.

Continues as Dean While Assuming the Position of Associate Director

GS: What brought about your assuming the additional administrative position of associate hospital directorship of The New York Hospital?

ECL: The Director of Nursing had announced her early retirement. As Dean I had been involved, at the policy level, in long-range planning and development of the Medical Center. We are, as are all voluntary institutions, reexamining our future and long-range goals. Issues such as the distinctive nature of educational programs for nursing, medicine, and allied health; reimbursement; the impact of national health insurance; planning an ambulatory care center; developing plans for a new hospital; the priority programs of a teaching-research-referral hospital—these and other similar problems have been the concern of the center administrative staff. I had been involved in these deliberations. Nursing service as well as nursing education was perceived to be a significant factor.

The first I was aware that I was being considered for the position was at a luncheon meeting. We meet once a week at lunch as well as other times during the week. The President of the center, the Dean of the Medical College, and the Director of the hospital had evidently been conferring and also had approached the president of the University. I was asked with very little prior discussion if I would accept responsibility in addition to retaining my responsibility as Dean.

Although the position had been a dual one prior to my appointment as Dean, I was assured the position was to be viewed in a different perspective. I debated with myself and others for one month. But I came to realize the exciting opportunity. I do not view this as a dual position nor do I recommend it as a form of organization for all other settings. I consider that I hold two positions. I would be the first to say that if we were in a financial position to offer a graduate program, I could not retain the two positions. We have a natural setting for a graduate program with the resources of the Medical College and the Graduate School of Medical Sciences and the rich clinical resources of the hospital and affiliating agencies.

I assumed responsibility July 1, 1974, and still view the opportunity as challenging and exciting. It is a rare opportunity to be involved in the affairs of nursing service and education in a medical center at this state in time.

GS: *To me that sounds like a tremendous responsibility.*

ECL: It is. It's a huge one. It is a huge one because of committee involvement in all phases of program development of the center in addition to operating responsibility and program development in nursing service and nursing education. Our center is unique in that we have a joint board consisting of members of the board of governors of the hospital and the board of trustees of the university. Both Presidents are members and rotate the responsibility of chairman. I attend these meetings as well as meetings of the medical board and meetings of the board of governors of the hospital, as do the dean of the Medical College, the director of the hospital, and the president of the center. The

Center Management Committee, under the direction of the president of the center and consisting of the director of the hospital, the dean of the Medical College, and myself, meets constantly. I cannot enumerate the number of other deliberative committees we are expected to attend in this stage of developing long-range plans.

I have one major advantage: the resources for leadership within the faculty and the department of nursing service. In the department, for example, there are well-prepared and strong clinical nursing department heads who have primary responsibility for the clinical departments. In this situation, as well as in the school, I can devote my time primarily to policy issues and program development. My associate in nursing service has major responsibility for internal affairs and problems of the department.

GS: And you have the power to make decisions?

ECL: Yes. In the instance of the school and nursing service, there is no question that appropriate nursing personnel are involved. In the instance of the center, my input into decisions is respected.

GS: Have you thought now of maybe relinquishing your deanship with the School of Nursing?

ECL: No, not at this time. It would not be appropriate and I do not believe it would be supported by the center administration or the faculty. It may be appropriate to assume responsibility for one of the two positions at some future date. I don't know at this time.

GS: Now, is there anything you would like to add about your leadership position at the hospital-administration part?

ECL: I subscribe to what I call the triad of administration—the triad of administrator-physician-nurse. This was the philosophy I presented before I accepted the position. We are developing our organization in this manner. One example is the introduction of unit coordinators responsible to hospital administration. I have written numerous articles on the utilization of nursing service personnel, for studies continue to demonstrate that from 25 to 50 percent of a nurse's time may be spent in institutional services or the management of things rather than upon services to patients and their families.

Utilization of the talents of nursing must take priority in a center such as ours. We might well be considered one large intensive care unit because of the requirements for nursing care. The clinical nursing department heads really function as an advisory cabinet. We have been actively involved in redefining objectives of the clinical departments and functions of nursing service personnel. I view their role as being comparable with that of a director of nursing, for the size and complexity of the various services is comparable with that of a 300-bed specialty hospital.

I have also an advisory committee of head nurses elected by their peers, and I meet regularly with the clinical specialists. Recently a group of senior staff nurses was elected, and they too will be meeting with me on a regular basis. In this way I hope to have direct interaction with representative groups—groups who will work on particular problems or program areas for referral to the clinical nursing department heads. I find our progress quite productive.

Leadership

GS: *What have been some of your strategies?*

ECL: Well, I believe in surrounding oneself with experts and in delegating responsibility and authority.

GS: *Now, when you say surrounding yourself with experts, what happens when you have—I suppose at times it would be inevitable—conflict? How do you handle overt conflict?*

ECL: Conflict has to be resolved through examination of policy. As an administrator, I have to assume responsibility for ensuring that policy is endorsed. Most conflicts relate to methods or how something is to be carried out or how something should be done. I do not care what methods are used as long as there is no violation of policy. If there is no violation of policy, I encourage differences. If policy is involved and change is indicated by a significant majority, then we establish the mechanism for reexamination.

GS: *Is it difficult to change policy?*

ECL: Not if you are in a power position. You may not make policy, but you can influence policy.

GS: *What do you consider characteristics of a leader?*

ECL: First, an appreciation of the culture or the setting(s) in which you function. The power of the words you use and the way you express opinions or make comments. It has been fascinating for me to observe some highly effective leaders who might be considered low-keyed and others who know when it is appropriate to be crisp or abrupt. The ability to tolerate hostility. You have to realize that people may not be hostile toward you but to the ideas you appear to represent. In a leadership position you are not always going to be liked or even have general approval from many with whom you associate. Change is stressful, and a leader is constantly dealing with change. People respond differently to seemingly similar situations, and hostility may be ever present as a first phase of response to change for certain individuals. Having and maintaining a strong knowledge base. The ability to tolerate ambiguity. Predicting or forecasting and problem definition are constant components of a leadership role. Skills in communication and interpersonal relationships.

GS: Do you think that leadership—now I'm thinking of nursing—can be taught?

ECL: Nurses can experience it.

GS: Teach a future leader?

ECL: One doesn't set up a course in leadership in isolation. Certain skills can be learned or taught: group process techniques, communication skills, appreciation of the principles of human relationships, problem solving. But I think a major factor is the students' exposure to teachers as role models. That they realize in their relationship with teachers that the teachers may not always have the answer, but will say, "I know where to find the answer" or "We will find out together." Students should be encouraged to question, to build upon their strengths. I think one concept of human relationships we often forget is that you concentrate first upon enhancing existing traits and characteristics.

Students enrolling in schools of nursing have been exposed to beginning traits of leadership throughout their elementary and secondary school years—problem-solving skills, communication skills, application of scientific principles to problem solving, critical inquiry. I once submitted a statement of program objectives to a group of doctoral students. Their response was that these objectives could not be achieved at the baccalaureate level in nursing. The objectives were for elementary education. We cannot continue to assume that our students have an absence of traits or characteristics for leadership if our admission practices are sound.

But I agree that we need more study in the area of characteristics of success. This has been one area of interest in continuing-education programs preparing nurses for expanded areas of practice.

GS: Do you think risk taking is important?

ECL: Yes, you must have the capacity for risk taking. Risk taking involves alternatives of choice and recognizing what the consequences may be.

GS: Would you put risk taking with the other traits of leadership you mentioned?

ECL: Yes. But I have one final comment to make and that is the influence leaders have on others. My professional life has been influenced by significant leaders at every strategic period. I referred to some, but there were numerous others. Leaders breed other leaders and they accept this as an inherent responsibility.

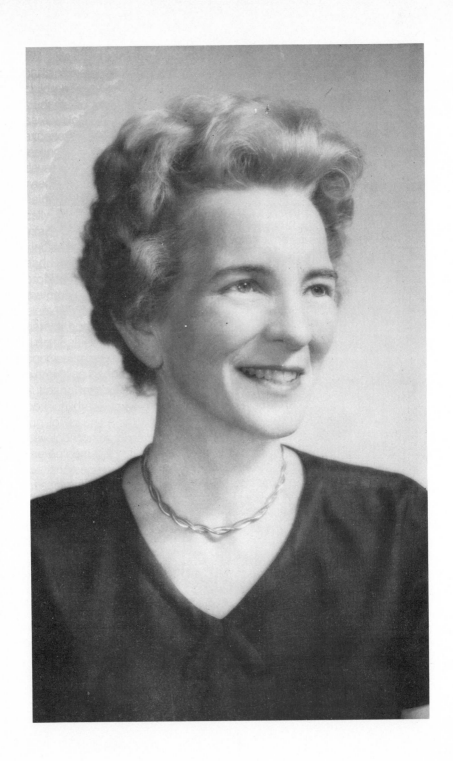

7

In recognition of her far-ranging contributions to the field of nursing in the United States over a period of two decades and for her leadership in the establishment of close and enduring ties between the Federal Government and the Nation's hospitals and schools of nursing. This has led to vast improvements in nursing education, nursing service, and nursing research throughout this country and the world.[1]

. . . inspired countless nurses and led in the raising of . . . a noble profession to ever higher levels . . .[2]

. . . a cherished colleague who has been honored time and again for unique and historic contribution to excellence in nursing . . . characteristically ahead of her time . . . never allows anyone to forget the solemnly purposeful ingredient of quality . . . a pioneer in thought and deed . . .[3]

[1]Citation from the Distinguished Service Medal from the Surgeon General of the United States, Sept. 20, 1965.
[2]Citation from the honorary doctor of science degree, Boston University, June 4, 1951.
[3]From the presentation of the Mary Adelaide Nutting Medal to Lucile Petry Leone at the biennial convention of the National League for Nursing, Minneapolis, Minn., May 9, 1973.

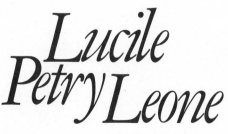

Lucile Petry Leone

ADMINISTRATOR

*L*ucile Petry Leone[4] was possibly the most widely known nurse in the United States during World War II and immediately thereafter. She directed the wartime U.S. Cadet Nurse Corps program, and after that successful experience was chosen in 1948 to be the first nurse and the first woman Assistant Surgeon General in the U.S. Public Health Service (U.S.P.H.S.). She held the position of Chief Nurse Officer with this rank until she retired in 1966.

Her previous professional experience was as a head nurse and supervisor at Johns Hopkins Hospital (1927–1929) and as a Professor and Assistant Dean at the University of Minnesota School of Nursing in Minneapolis (1929–1941); after her retirement from the federal government in 1966, she was Professor and Associate Dean at the College of Nursing, Texas Woman's College, Denton (1966–1971). She has had a lifelong commitment to teaching.

She has received eight honorary doctoral degrees and a long list of national and international awards.[5] She has been sought after for membership in a large number of advisory committees, boards, and commissions.[6] She was President of the National League for Nursing (N.L.N.), 1959–1963. Lucile Petry Leone was a consultant on nursing for the World Health Organization (W.H.O.). In 1951 she went before a conference of the W.H.O. to ask its member nations to promote wider recognition of the professional status of nursing. In later years she has preferred those invitations which afforded opportunity for multiprofessional and consumer participation. She has made innumerable speeches. She "got around" to see firsthand how nursing was progressing in meeting the health needs of people and what issues were emerging in health, in education, and in nursing, discussing proposals for action in each of these areas.

Lucile Petry Leone accepts acclaim reluctantly but warms to the idea of being loved and respected by many. She has been described as "brilliant," "modest," "ahead of her time."[7] Her contributions have

[4] Lucile Petry was married to Nicholas C. Leone, M.D., in 1952.

[5] To cite only a few of her awards: named one of twenty-five Women of the Year in 1953; granted the American Public Health Association's Lasker Award in 1953, the Florence Nightingale Medal of the International Red Cross in 1958, the U.S. Public Health Service's Distinguished Service Award in 1965, and the Mary Adelaide Nutting Medal in 1973.

[6] Among her positions: chairperson of the advisory committee of the Sealantic Fund; appointed to the board on medicine of the National Academy of Science and to the Commission on Mental Illness of the Southern Regional Education Board; member of the first advisory committee to the W. K. Kellogg Foundation.

[7] For more detail on Lucile Petry Leone's career and life, see Edna Yost, *American Women of Nursing*, J. B. Lippincott Company, Philadelphia, 1947; *Modern Medicine*, Aug. 12, 1968; "Lady With

been numerous, and she will be one of those credited with leadership in developing the role of the federal government in nursing here and abroad.

The enlarged scope of United States participation in World War II confronted director Leone with the unprecedented responsibility of recruiting and training a massive work force of nurses for immediate use in a crisis situation. According to one account, between 1944 and 1946 the Corps oversaw the education of some 170,000 cadets, who constituted 90 percent of the total enrollment in nursing programs for those years and nearly doubled the number of nursing students previously enrolled. Indeed, as the study explained, "this was a remarkable achievement, considering the competing appeals for women war workers at this time and the difficulties met in expanding the teaching, clinical housing, and other facilities needed for these enlarged quotas."[8]

She helped to formulate the first comprehensive nursing legislation, the Nurse Training Act of 1964.

Her concerns are for large wholes—"the health of everyone," "health actions in their social, economic and political contexts and the nursing contribution to these actions." But her major concerns are humanizing the care of each person and determining how health workers learn to make caring achieve its goals. She believes, as she states in her article on nursing in the *Encyclopaedia Britannica* (1975), that "nursing is an instrument of social progress."

Lucile Petry Leone has always worked in a truly democratic manner. She is always ready to assist others to develop and to grow professionally. Although her place in history as an outstanding nursing leader is firmly established in her role as the director of the U.S. Cadet Nurse Corps, she wielded great influence in other areas, for example, as chairman of the Joint Committee on the Unification of Accrediting Activities. She has always emphasized that nursing should not be restrictive in outlook; she has stressed that health care is multidisciplinary and that nursing is but one part of the whole.

She has published numerous articles in nursing, hospital, public health, medical, and educational journals. The *Encyclopaedia of Nursing*, which she helped to edit, was published by Saunders in 1952 at her insistence. Her article on nursing in the *Encyclopaedia Britannica* is

a Mission," *Public Health Service*, February 1966, pp. 8–11; and Mary M. Roberts, *American Nursing: History and Interpretation*, The Macmillan Company, New York, 1954.

[8] Isabel M. Stewart and Anne I. Austin, *A History of Nursing*, G. P. Putnam's Sons, New York, 1962, p. 221.

considered classic. In addition to her own extensive writing, she has actively encouraged others to write about their ideas and experiences.

She influenced the development of nursing research by working for the preparation of nurse-researchers, by obtaining grants for research, and by enabling selected institutions to become research centers. She helped establish scholarship programs in areas of teaching, administration, and clinical specialization and promoted attempts to formulate a theory of nursing.

Lucile Petry Leone "has enormous energy, physical and intellectual . . . warmth, humor, a great sense of timing—an even disposition—vision—diplomacy . . ."[9]

Early Days

GS:　Could you say something about your background?

LPL:　I was born in Lewisburg, Ohio, in 1902, an only child. My family had little money, but we had a rich and loving family life, always small-town. I always liked school and dreamed of Vassar. When my parents moved to Delaware, I entered the state university, where I studied in the liberal arts program and my major interests were English and science.[10] After graduating I knew that I wanted to work with people, and I admit to having a little of the "do-good" concern. I wanted to find opportunities in which science operated in human beings rather than in laboratories, and nursing became my choice. A summer job in a New York hospital before graduation confirmed its appeal to me.

After completing my nurse's education at Johns Hopkins Hospital,[11] I later went to Teachers College, Columbia University, where I received a master's degree in nursing education (1929) and still later spent another year of graduate study. I credit Johns Hopkins with my lifetime interest in clinical education and in excellence of patient care. I credit Teachers College with beginning my lifetime concern that graduate education in nursing must rest firmly on science and with exposure to "progressive education" and the teachings of John Dewey. I was happy to have close contact with Isabel Stewart, a nurse leader I loved.

---

[9] *Public Health Service*, February 1966, p. 11.

[10] She received her B.A. degree in 1924.

[11] She received her registered nurse diploma in 1927 from Johns Hopkins Hospital School of Nursing, Baltimore, Maryland.

At the University of Minnesota

GS: What was your first job?

LPL: My first real job was at the University of Minnesota School of Nursing (1929–1941), then the largest in the country. My task was to improve the clinical instruction of 500 students. I also taught a course on individualized nursing care, which gave me an opportunity to work out theories of "humanization" and a belief that "every patient needs a primary nurse." Later, I taught methods of teaching and was among the early designers of practice teaching in nursing. I also taught experimental techniques in nursing, which gave impetus to my lifelong interest in research in nursing. I believe some of the students in this course conducted experiments which could stand along with researches of today.

GS: Is there anything else you care to add about that period?

LPL: I served as both assistant and acting director of the program at the University of Minnesota. The director, Katharine Densford (now Dreves), was a valuable mentor who encouraged us all to try new ideas and pushed us toward university and community involvement, toward professional organizations, and toward individual improvement. Her idealism still influences my actions.

Washington, D.C.

GS: What brought you to Washington, D.C.?

LPL: Well, in the summer of 1941, I was teaching at the University of Washington as an exchange professor. It was exciting to be in Seattle (in the summer of 1941) because with the approach of World War II, the situation was getting acute. Japanese ships were held in the harbor, and the military camps along the coast were expanding. I had favored United States entrance into the war for many months. With my firsthand contact with the possibilities of war involving the Orient, I was overwhelmed with patriotism when I received a telephone call in Seattle from the Surgeon General of the U.S. Public Health Service in Washington, D.C., asking me to come on July 4 to be interviewed about a position there. They asked me to come for six months, and I stayed for twenty-four years. [*laughter*]

About the beginning of that twenty-four years: It's hard for us who want no more wars and have hated the war in Vietnam to realize how wholeheartedly the people of the United States threw themselves into World War II. Read histories of that time to see that few people opposed the war. Almost everyone sacrificed and worked for the "all-out war effort." Planners in all fields had to foresee how much of their resource would be needed and where the resource would come from. There were production plans and goals for everything, from iron to cotton, from health personnel to shipyard workers and farmers. Both military and essential civilian needs were to be met.

planning for increasingly scarce nursing resources began before Pearl Harbor. Nursing organizations and government agencies and defense preparatory committees worked for legislation which provided funding for refresher courses to prepare nurses to return to active practice and for tuition and subsistence for basic and graduate students. Schools participated on a selective basis, about four hundred of them.

The first federal program achieved its limited purposes. But its achievement fell short of meeting the challenges of war and its demands, which were accelerating phenomenally.

The U.S. Cadet Nurse Corps

GS: Why, aside from patriotic motives, did you accept the position as director?

LPL: As the war went into its second year, the military talked of needing 30,000 more nurses immediately. With the civilian hospitals and health agencies already facing the crisis stage in staffing, the need for a spectacular program was acute. We sensed the challenges of designing and operating a program to hit quantitative targets for nursing personnel while maintaining and improving the system for nursing education. The Cadet Nurse Corps program was pounded out at countless committee meetings; legislation introduced by Frances Payne Bolton was passed by the Congress, and I became its director on July 1, 1943. (I never saw my Victory garden again!) Everything moved very fast. The goal became 65,000 students to be admitted in the next class, mostly in September.

The Division of Nurse Education was established; the nursing staff, young nurse leaders recruited from all over the country, was quadrupled almost overnight; and public relations people, accountants, and managers were added. We had to figure out the details of how it would all work and get out instructions and forms. How to stay simple amidst such complexities? How to keep it friendly? Dr. Parran, the Surgeon

General, the dynamo behind it all, barnstormed across the country with me or another nurse, for twenty regional meetings attended by nurses and country administrators. We reached practically all schools in less than two weeks. Spirits were high. Bands and flowers and flags. Here was a program that could solve an acute problem that threatened to wreck hospitals and could provide for military needs which everyone acknowledged had to come first. Working together we might make it succeed. That was the high spirit in which the Corps began, and it was maintained throughout.

GS: What did the program offer?

LPL: The new program offered students "a free education," a chance to enter "a proud profession," and an attractive uniform to make them a visible part of the war effort. It gave schools incentives to expand. It accelerated the educational program, compressing the usual three years of instruction to thirty months, with a six-month Senior Cadet period when students could be assigned to other health agencies, including stateside military hospitals.

Here I must remind you that in the early forties, in hospitals that operated schools of nursing, about two-thirds of the nursing services were given by students. (It had been higher in the thirties.) So any increase in students meant more immediate service with more possibility for releasing registered nurses for military service, as well as more registered nurses in subsequent years.

GS: Then the students really staffed the hospitals?

LPL: Yes. It is easy to see why service by students should have been so vital to hospitals. The first schools of nursing were founded in 1875. Population growth meant more health needs. The westward march created new communities which needed hospitals. There were practically no nurses for many of these hospitals. The way to secure nurses was to start a school and use the students, and you were lucky to find one nurse to teach in it. Not until the late twenties was there a concerted effort to discuss the exploitation of students. Not until the late thirties were there enough registered nurses available for employment to start pushing down the proportion of total service given by students.

GS: Don't student nurses learn by doing?

LPL: True. Learning nursing entails a good bit of practice. But the amount and kind of practice must be determined by a student's educational needs, not by an institution's need for services. And the practice must be seen as application of scientific principle, not merely rote. Teachers and students must be free to search for and select high-quality experiences for students wherever these are—not only in one parent institution, a hospital, where there is a vested interest in keeping the students under that roof. Through the thirties, these and other qualities of education were discussed, and many sets of opinions were formulated.

Some Issues

GS: What were some of the big issues?

LPL: One big question for argument was: Who should pay for nursing education? Another: Who should control nursing education? And of course: What nature of nurse is being educated?

I think it is important for today's thinkers about nursing education to know where nursing came from: confined, controlled, narrow, provincial, ordered; illumined by intense desire to help sick people; self-abnegating; often unaware of its low image. The apprentice pattern of education persisted in nursing much longer than in other fields. The awakening of medicine to modern science and education came with the Flexner Report in 1910, stunning the world and starting a revolution. The revolution in nursing started later. World War II brought phenomenal progress in scientific medicine. It brought public awareness and self-awareness to nursing, essential to the more rapid evolution which persists today.

In 1930, there were nearly 2000 schools of nursing with a total of 80,000 students. In 1945, with the impact of World War II programs, there were 1300 schools and 127,000 students. Admissions in 1944, with the incentives provided by the Cadet Nurse Corps program, were 67,000, more than double the admission in 1935. That many more students meant finding more patient situations where students could learn. That also brought the services of students into more institutions and agencies. Less than a third of the schools had offered experience in psychiatric nursing, but by the end of World War II, more than three-fourths did so. There were several other examples of enrichment of students' learning.

Schools of nursing found neighbor colleges where students could take courses—in chemistry or anatomy or sociology, for example. This saved teaching time, often improved the instruction, and, perhaps more important, brought together two institutions with commonality of purpose—institutions which would cooperate later in establishing degree programs in nursing.

More students require more teachers. But teachers had volunteered for the military Nurse Corps in large numbers. The legislation that created the Cadet Nurse Corps also provided funds for concentrated nurse teacher preparation and for supervisors and administrators in all the fields of nursing—hospital, public health, and the like. These, too, had joined the military in high proportion. Ten thousand nurses benefited from the new federal program. An on-the-job education program was also financed. Four hundred trainees from all over the country were prepared in universities, and spread out to offer specifically designed programs to another 6000 nurses. In addition to providing greatly needed training, the program reached nurses who had not thought of special preparation or ever moved out of their local situation.

GS: You keep referring to "getting around" as an asset. How so?

LPL: I've said already that provincialism was a characteristic of nursing. Perhaps not more than for lots of other professions. Inbreeding has hurt us all. World War II put millions of men overseas. It mixed up all kinds of men living on military bases and mixed many kinds of families who traveled toward bases to live near husbands or visit them.

Nurses in the military services were involved in all this. The Cadet Nurse Corps program moved nurses around the country. The nurse consultants—the staff of the program—learned in depth about regions where they operated and shared that knowledge with colleagues everywhere.

The cadets, during the last six months of their enrollment in school, chose another institution for experience. Many chose military or veterans' hospitals, public health programs on Indian reservations, or hospitals or health agencies not related to the federal government. I remember running into two senior cadets from Stanford on the Norfolk Naval Base and one from Philadelphia on an Indian reservation in New Mexico. I even tried to plan itineraries for special consultants and members of the Advisory Committee so that they saw parts of the country new to them. Getting around sharpens understanding of differences—professional, regional, and other—in kinds of nursing needed, the youth available to enter nursing, attitudes toward education and toward science, quality of medical practice, and more. With such knowledge, sounder judgments on policy questions could be made for either a local or a national program.

Influence of the Cadet Nurse Corps on Nursing Programs

GS: What effect did the Cadet Nurse Corps program have on the educational programs in nursing?

LPL: We who helped design and administer the program of federal aid believed that decisions about curriculum should be made by faculty members of schools and that "government" should not "interfere." Obviously, the shortening of the educational program of every participating school by six months affected the curriculum, though the decision to do so, made by those who designed the legislation, was based on the need for nurses—first, more students to relieve registered nurses who went to war, and then, more nurses because those students were ready for full responsibilities six months earlier. Of course, this acceleration was a curriculum issue. But how the shortening was to be accomplished was up to the schools. I have always felt that the thinking which had to go into decisions about which experiences and learnings were essential for students, and which could be omitted or learned later, was the most significant value of the Corps. Needless repetitions and some useless stereotypes were identified. New concepts were arrived at by enough thinkers to accelerate markedly the process by which nursing is arriving at a new day.

This brings me to another point, another value of so large a program which touched so high a proportion of all schools of nursing. It brought all participating schools (1100 of the 1300 in the country) into the mainstream of action. Some staff and advisory committee members and many others were surprised—shocked would be better—at the conditions found in some of the schools. These schools were usually small, isolated in their communities, and operated on a shoestring. Now they had money (federal allotment) which was theirs to spend. They were part of a national movement to attract more students, and they were pressed to expand experience for their students; they attracted new and favorable attention from their communities. They could buy some books for their libraries, often the first in years. Then teachers and directors attended regional meetings. Overworked deans and teachers from well-known schools and staffs of nursing organizations conducted many reality-oriented workshops for faculty of schools needing help.

The nurse staff of the Division visited the schools frequently and gave staunch service, particularly to the schools which needed help in carrying out their plans for balanced instruction and clinical experience.

The financial aid, which could be stopped, became a strong incentive to improvement. An analyst who recently reviewed hundreds of reports written by these consultants commented that he believed there was evidence of improved patient care in the clinical facilities of the schools as well as improved education of nurses from their efforts.

Periodic reporting of the schools' programs and the students' progress and accounting for expenditures of federal funds were required, of course. From these reports we gained more detailed information about how the nation's schools of nursing operated than had ever before been collected. A compilation and publication of this information supported the determination of the N.L.N. to go forward with an interim classification of schools of nursing and to establish the National Nursing Accrediting Service (N.N.A.S.), which moved nursing education ahead rapidly after 1950.

While the schools complained about the work of financial accounting, they recognized the necessity for it. It was the beginning of their system of procuring, disbursing, and accounting for federal funds, continuing up till now. Most schools didn't have a budget before 1943. They were required to establish one. This move clarified issues about identity, autonomy, and interdependence of the school. Such a simple statement for such a telling concept, and such an emotional controversy!

GS: All those data: What use did they have—just keeping government records?

LPL: The data served an important purpose of indicating that a school continued to be entitled to receive funds allotted to it. But most important, data collected from all sources were used for planning, placing program emphasis, and continuing evaluation.

When war began to appear likely, needs for knowledge of our resources became acute. The American Medical Association (A.M.A.) counted and analyzed the supply of physicians. The newly formed Nursing Council for National Defense planned a study of nursing and requested cooperation from the U.S.P.H.S. Pearl McIver, of the U.S.P. H.S., was a member of the council. The inventory was a joint effort, directed by Pearl McIver, and the response of nurses to "getting counted" was phenomenal. Of the total 289,286 nurses, 60 percent were active; 9 percent were inactive but available; and 31 percent were inactive and not available. Distribution was uneven: Vermont had 1 active nurse for each 336 persons, and Mississippi 1 for each 2143 persons.

The National League of Nursing Education (N.L.N.E.) compiled annual reports of enrollment of schools of nursing and also graduation and admissions data. The U.S. Office of Education compiled data on high school enrollment. The women graduating each year were the primary source of recruits for nursing. (I'll discuss men in nursing later.)

The military services did their best to predict their needs for nurses. Civilian nursing needs were estimated by the American Hospital Association (A.H.A.), the Public Health Service, and others.

All these were balanced with lots of subtle factors and intuitive judgments into a figure for the number of new students who should be recruited for admission to schools of nursing.

This wartime cooperation in compiling data gave birth to a continuing committee, composed of chief statisticians of related organizations, to share data essential for such planning and for early detection of trends. And the value of continuous, comprehensive, factual information for planning was established.

The 1941 program of federal aid to nursing education did not do enough to meet the needs for nursing, which mounted unpredictably. The first goal for the Cadet Nurse Corps program was 65,000 admissions. This was exceeded by a few hundred students. The second successful year, ending June 10, 1945, overreached V-E Day. V-J Day came soon after the third year began, and the students recruited to enter school in the fall of 1945 were the last members of the Cadet Nurse Corps. Thus, the first substantial program of federal aid accomplished its purpose. It cost $160,326,237 of the taxpayers' money and untold effort by the schools. It was credited with providing the nurses needed by the military services and "saving the lives" of the civilian hospitals.

Public Relations Aspect

GS: Could you comment on the role of public relations?

LPL: Yes. Public relations played a large role in the development of the Cadet Nurse Corps. For example, the word "cadet" was used because at the time a military connotation was desirable, and there were, after all, West Point cadets. Cadet was a word that implied "student," "learner." I also participated, along with leading health professionals of all kinds, in many committee meetings with the War Advertising Council, and we all were stimulated by contacts with writers, artists, and others who wanted to interpret nursing in an attractive and appealing way.

GS: *What was the War Advertising Council?*

LPL: The War Advertising Council represented the major advertising agencies and coordinated public relations efforts focused on high-priority wartime programs. The council assigned one of its agency members to a chosen program, and the Cadet Nurse Corps program had the good fortune to have the J. Walter Thompson Company. Obvious publicity included full-page newspaper ads, car cards, posters, spot announcements for radio and movie theaters—all sponsored by various industries. The less obvious included the enlisting of artists for posters; testing of recruitment messages and selection of the best; getting together the style show at the Waldorf Hotel ballroom, where leading designers presented competing designs for the Cadet Nurse uniform (Molly Parnis's design for uniforms and Sally Victor's for hats won); planning nationwide convocation ceremonies for cadets in schools and groups of schools with a broadcast program including a song by Bing Crosby ("Going My Way" was the hit of the day); and securing fine writers and actors for a movie short about how a woman decided to join the Corps. Cadets appeared on many publicized occasions, from buying a bond from a prominent seller to breaking the champagne bottle at the launching of a battleship. An official song and a flag were chosen. Millions of dollars worth of publicity services were donated, and this was several times as large as the amount of federal funds used for recruitment campaigns.

GS: *Public relations, of course, has a bearing on how people view nursing. How do you yourself see it?*

LPL: I have always been deeply dissatisfied with attempts to describe the real meaning of nursing. Certainly it is not to be found in legal definitions, even the new ones, which of course were not written for the purpose of communicating what nursing means to a nurse or a sick person or a family or a fellow community worker. Nor is it found in textbooks or the abstractions in speeches (I've written many) or the theories of educators (I've used many, even formulated some). Where are the writers, artists, musicians, psychologists, and others, who can describe caring which is not caretaking? Always I have searched for this and struggled, myself, to communicate what I know is there.

As an aside, I gleaned that, to describe an art, one could speak in parables. For me, stories about people and nurses communicate best what I am striving for. I've always collected them. But I needed more when I was interviewed by the Writer's Board and others of the War

Advertising Council about what they could tell about nursing. Imagine an opportunity to talk with Robert Sherwood or Oscar Hammerstein or Helen Hayes! What would you tell them about nursing? There were hundreds of opportunities to give a quick glimpse of that human relation called nursing to someone who would communicate it maybe to millions. I'm still trying, and searching for others who try. The literature of nursing has been a major concern throughout my life.

GS: *What effect did the war have on nursing organizations?*

LPL: I remember one of my first conversations with my boss, Thomas Parran, about eliciting cooperation or information from, or establishing a communication channel with, national organizations. There was one organization for medicine, one for public health agencies, and one for hospitals (sometimes two). But for nursing, there would have been four which would be frequently involved, and three more sometimes involved! Fortunately, these had organized a Nursing Council for National Defense (before Pearl Harbor), which became the National Nursing Council for War Service. It was composed of the president, executive officers, and others from the American Nurses' Association, the National League of Nursing Education, the National Organization for Public Health Nursing, the Association of Collegiate Schools of Nursing, the National Association of Colored Graduate Nurses, the American Association of Industrial Nurses, and Directors of nursing services in federal government departments—Army, Navy, Public Health Service, Veterans Administration, Bureau of Indian Affairs, and Census Bureau—and the American Red Cross. (One of its first actions, which I have already mentioned, was the national inventory of nurses carried on with the cooperation of P.H.S.) It would take several hours to list the activities of that Council. (Almira Wickenden was its Executive Secretary, and at the end of the war she received the Distinguished Service Medal, the highest civilian award.)

The council worked on all the nursing actions during the war. For the Cadet Nurse Corps, it had contracts with P.H.S. for the uniforms, for major recruitment efforts (such as P.O. Box 88, a nationwide source of information), and for many other efforts which facilitated detailed action without some of the restrictive government regulations. It paralleled the governmental Health and Medical Committee, which, through its changes in placement, retained a subcommittee on nursing. It paralleled another activity within government: Assignment and Procurement, a manpower program which came a little later.

To answer your question: The war called on the nursing organizations for unity, for finding the places of power to express the voice of nursing; and it put nursing in a place to express itself and to keep informed of the rapidly shifting crises the war brought. Interprofessional relationships and consumers' stakes in individual and community health were seen in a bright light during the war. All this made the postwar restructuring of national nursing organizations inevitable.

GS: Do you want to add to what you have said about the effects of the U.S. Cadet Nurse Corps program on nursing education in the United States?

LPL: As I've said, one of the major effects was the realization on the part of a much larger proportion of the schools that they had an educational identity and were part of the mainstream of national development. Another was the loosening up of many old rigidities: for example, that time spent (three years) in a school indicated that learning was complete.

I should also mention one of the studies done as a part of the program. Congress became alarmed at the increase in tuition for students, particularly in those schools in universities and colleges. A conference of administrators led to better understanding on all sides. A need to know whether or not the value of student service to hospitals exceeded the cost of education the hospitals provided also emerged. This question is irrelevant today, but in the forties, it was argued bitterly. A cost analysis, carefully controlled and objective, showed that many schools did make money for their hospitals. And it raised the question: Who should pay for nursing education? Should the increased cost of high-quality education be paid as part of the patient's hospital bill? This study shed light on the need for nursing education to be financed in the same way as other higher education in this country. Financial independence from hospitals opened the way for many constructive interdependencies between schools of nursing and community health agencies (including hospitals, of course), where students experience nursing and also community responsibility for health care.

GS: When did the Cadet Nurse Corps program end, and what happened to the staff?

LPL: The last cadets graduated in the fall of 1948, but the program started winding down shortly after the fall of 1945.

The thirty-some nurses on the staff which administered the program worked with creativity and commitment, and helped the program bring to the country the values I have described, and more. They learned about the diversity of the country and learned sensitivity to its needs, and formed their own ideas about the role of government in health and in education. Almost all of them moved on to positions where they could determine policy—in government or universities or elsewhere. About half remained in the Public Health Service. One became a force in establishing federal funds for research in nursing and all that that means. Another became the principal nurse in the national development of training programs for nurses in psychiatry and mental health. Another became Director of Nursing Service in the new Clinical Center of the National Institutes of Health (N.I.H.). Others developed a role for nursing in the enormous hospital construction program. The U.S.P.H.S. expanded quickly after the war with many new programs in which there was a nursing component, and the staff of the wartime program was another source of nurse leadership.

The wartime program brought nursing to a very high degree of visibility and raised esteem for nursing throughout the country. Should it continue? We all decided that there should be no effort to continue a wartime program into peacetime. Needs for federal aid to nursing would depend on different factors not easy to predict. In a short time the most urgent need became apparent—for nurses with graduate education in teaching administration, supervision, and clinical specialties. The Professional Nurse Traineeship program was born.

The Division of Nurse Education continued after the war with Margaret Arnstein as its chief. It undertook studies, and it searched for what federal assistance could do to make nursing a productive and important component of many other kinds of planning. It later became the Division of Nursing, which continues to make a tremendous impact on nursing. Among other functions, this Division has invested over one billion federal dollars in nursing education and research.

In 1948 the position of Chief Nurse Officer was established in the Public Health Service. I was chosen for the position and also given the rank of Assistant Surgeon General.[12] The rank attracted a lot of public attention, and, while I often disliked being conspicuous, I could tell myself that it was good for nursing.

My position put me in contact with developments on most health fronts at a time of rapid progress. I tried to feed this knowledge into the decision-making processes for nursing both inside and outside government. I continued to get around and to learn the nursing and health

---

[12] Women were first commissioned in the Corps of the Public Health Service in 1944. The rank of Assistant Surgeon General is equivalent to that of Rear Admiral in the Navy or Brigadier General in the Army.

needs throughout the country. I was often the only woman or the only nurse in health councils of many kinds, or the only generalist among devoted specialists.

I am delighted with the progress in nursing, particularly in recent years. I foresee nurses creating extension health services for ambulatory patients in clinics and homes, for older people in nursing homes and their own homes, and for children in schools. I see them creating systems for disseminating health information to keep people strong and productive. All this, along with all the complex life-saving services in hospitals. Yes, nursing education and administration in all fields will be enriched, and as a result nurses will make health teams ever more effective. I see nurses reaching into the development of health programs, community action, politics, and administration of general education. We shall have more nurse seekers and finders of principles, more theoreticians, more statesmen of science—none of them content until their efforts make nursing care serve people and help them achieve health, often through their own actions. I am expecting nurse journalists who inform and who stir action for human values. And poets and artists who portray the subtleties of nurse-people interactions which are at once sensitive and scientific.

GS: Shall we pull back from the future and discuss the past a bit more?

LPL: Shortly after the war there seemed some prospect of federally financed health insurance for all United States citizens. I studied plans and programs in other countries and visited such countries as England, Sweden, Denmark, Finland, New Zealand, Australia, and Canada to learn both how their programs or partial programs worked and how nurses contributed to making them reach goals for health. [I suppose nurses in Health, Education, and Welfare (H.E.W.) are again preparing themselves in this new round of interest in national health insurance.]

International health was a major interest. I served with the United States delegations to the first and eighth assemblies of the W.H.O. in Geneva. At first I was one of a small number of women and was the only nurse. I believe this small, early recognition of nursing gave just a little extra emphasis to the role of nursing in W.H.O. Subsequently, I served on expert committees on nursing on two occasions, once as rapporteur, a real writing experience. I learned to know the chief nurse officers of other countries. I helped explain United States health and nursing to streams of visitors—nurses and others—from other lands. I helped plan and select nursing personnel from this country for missions and programs in many countries, both bilateral and multilateral.

The Cadet Nurse Corps program was the first example of nationwide planning and government action for nursing. How many nurses do we need? What kinds? How do we get them?

Shortly after the war I took brief leaves of absence to participate with a small team of private consultants in planning for medical centers in such cities as Los Angeles and Houston. We surveyed the needs in all fields of nursing employment; sized up the impact on nursing of city growth as predicted by industry, the press, education, and the like; looked at the nursing education system and the human resources available; and put nursing and nursing education into the picture of the future centers—that was experience in citywide planning. Then came statewide planning, in some states as a means of deciding whether, where, and when there should be a school of nursing in a state university. Over the next few years the Division of Nursing assisted with surveys in nearly all states and, for many, more than once. These were done at the invitation of state nursing organizations and with the participation of other professionals and consumers. (How the definition of "consumer" changes!) The nature of the surveys evolved to include focus on utilization of various kinds of personnel and took on new qualitative values. This kind of thinking laid a basis for quality evaluation and control, a current preoccupation in health institutions.

Regional planning for nursing became a strong part of the programs of the Southern Regional Education Board (S.R.E.B.), the Western Interstate Commission for Higher Education (W.I.C.H.E.), and the New England Board of Higher Education (N.E.B.H.E.). In 1967 the S.R.E.B. employed me to write a monograph—"State-wide Planning for Nursing Education." So much more could be said about the need for goal setting and planning in large wholes and collaboratively: the Report of the Surgeon General's Consultant Group on Nursing and the resultant legislation; the evaluation and planning groups in all the nursing programs of the P.H.S. and how planning moves action along.

Nursing has benefited greatly from many other P.H.S. programs. Health programs in heart diseases, cancer, tuberculosis, venereal diseases, chronic diseases, neurological diseases, and others have involved nursing in research, education, and community health action. One could philosophize at length on categorical and generalized approaches to health and on different appeals to congressional and philanthropic sources of funds. One could write books about the impact on nursing of the Mental Health Act, and other volumes on the influence of regional public health nurse consultants through the years.

Nurses in P.H.S. and in many other places have acted beyond nursing — manpower, community planning, and management in education, to name three— taking on their leadership and administrative responsibilities as health workers. Two quick examples—unrelated—from my own experience: I was the first fair employment practices officer of the P.H.S. and saw the beginnings of affirmative action; I chaired the Committee on Health of Migrant Workers, which made the first small steps toward new programs. More related were my experiences with programs of the Sealantic Fund for "disadvantaged youth" in nursing education.

The horizon for nursing expands exhilaratingly. The depth has not been sounded. So we explore depths and distances. The nugget of truth lies in the nurse-patient relation. The distant star is the health of all people.

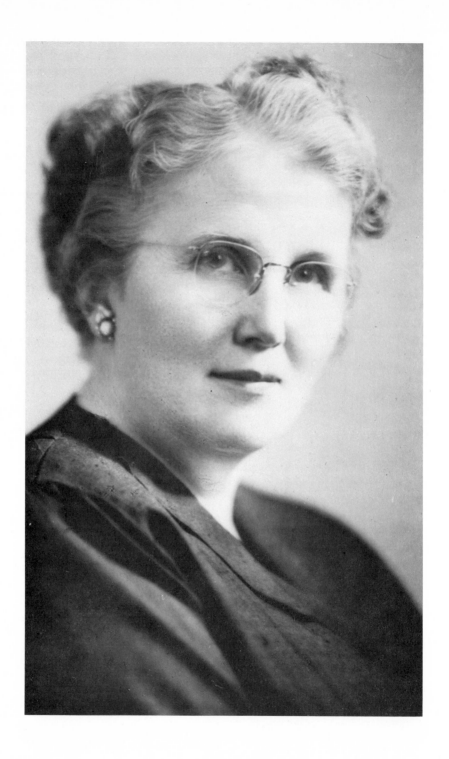

8

Dedicated to the betterment of man's condition,
she foresaw the need for professionally
educated nurses and for nursing research that
nursing practice might better achieve its goals.
A deep sense of social responsibility
characterized her participation in the initiation
and establishment of the National Testing
Service which was to become the National
League for Nursing—Measurement and
Guidance Service. She established the first
organized unit for research in nursing. . . . Her
achievements are international in scope and are
indicative of the broad sweep of her interest,
vision and leadership. . . . teacher,
administrator, dreamer, and humanitarian—the
means whereby she served society and nursing
are too numerous to mention. The evidences of
her activities are on every side. Her
contributions are immeasurable[1]

[1]From the Mary Adelaide Nutting Award Citation to R. Louise
McManus, May 1963.

R. Louise
McManus
INNOVATOR

*D*r. R. Louise Metcalfe McManus[2] is known as a leader with *ideas*. She bubbled over with original ideas and was one of the very first nurses to obtain a Ph.D. degree. She received the degree in educational research in 1947 from Columbia University in New York. The title of her published dissertation was *The Effect of Experience on Nursing Achievement*.[3] One of her areas of contribution was in measurement and guidance. She was responsible for the development of the State Board Test Pool Examinations that were serviced by the National League of Nursing Education (N.L.N.E.). This was a landmark because one set of examinations could be given in every state, with standard scores that facilitated transfer from one state to another. The very construction of the examination by experts was a major achievement. She was the originator of projects leading to experimentation and development of the team concept of nursing and the junior college nursing program idea. She set up the Institute of Research and Service in Nursing Education at Teachers College, which was one of the early attempts to involve nurses in organized research.

Dr. McManus was born in North Smithfield, Rhode Island, March 4, 1896. She received diplomas from the Institutional Management Program at Pratt Institute in Brooklyn, New York, and the Massachusetts General Hospital School of Nursing in Boston, Massachusetts. She received her bachelor's and master's degrees from Teachers College, Columbia University.

Dr. McManus was Director of the Division of Nursing Education at Teachers College from 1947 until her retirement in 1961 and Director of the Institute of Research and Service in Nursing Education, which was established under her guidance in 1953. Her creative leadership at Teachers College led to the expansion of the department of nursing, and her influence has had an impact both in the United States and throughout the world. Upon her retirement from Teachers College, she was invited to serve as a special adviser in the development of higher education in nursing in Turkey.

Dr. McManus has published extensively[4] and has been the recipient

---

[2] She married John H. McManus, a widower, in 1929, becoming the mother of six stepchildren; she and her husband had one daughter. Her husband died in 1934, and Louise McManus reared the seven children along with taking care of her aged mother-in-law and later her ailing mother.

[3] Bureau of Publications, Teachers College, Columbia University, New York, 1949.

[4] To cite a few of her bench mark publications: "Research in Nursing Education," *The Nursing Education Bulletin*, January 1928; coauthor of *The Hospital Head Nurse*, The Macmillan Company, New York, 1944; Committee on the Function of Nursing, *A Program for the Nursing Profession*, The Macmillan Company, New York, 1948; *Study Guide on Evaluation*, National League of Nursing Educa-

of numerous awards and honors.[5] She has also been extremely active professionally, serving on many national and international committees.[6]

Teachers College

GS: *Dr. McManus, will you say something about your leadership role at Teachers College?*

RLM: When I was appointed the Director of the Division of Nursing Education at Teachers College in 1947, programs for graduate nurses had been offered at Teachers College for nearly fifty years, first under Adelaide Nutting's and then Isabel M. Stewart's leadership.[7] From admitting nurses to classes set up for public school teachers, the course offerings had been expanded to full programs leading to either the baccalaureate or master's degrees and preparing for a variety of specialized positions in nursing, including teaching, supervision, and administrative functions. A growing number of nurses were coming in with baccalaureate degree from generic programs, and they, with others, sought master's degrees. The demand for graduate degrees grew faster than the distinctively graduate-level nursing programs could be set up. In many instances the same courses in nursing were taken by the baccalaureate and by the master's degree candidates, with only graduate-level courses in other departments of the college differentiating the two (baccalaureate and master's) degree requirements. As World War II

tion, 1944; *The Effect of Experience on Nursing Achievement*, Bureau of Publications, Teachers College, Columbia University, New York, 1949; "Cost Estimates for Graduate Nurse Programs," *Nursing Outlook*, vol. 4, April 1970; "Nurses Want a Chance to Be Professional," *The Modern Hospital*, October 1958; "Newer Approaches in Nursing Education," *Teachers College Record*, October 1952.

[5] Among them are the Mary Adelaide Nutting Award for Leadership from the National League for Nursing, 1963, and the first R. Louise McManus Award, established in her honor, from Teachers College, 1964. In 1966 she received from the Greek Red Cross Society citations and medals for service to nursing. The Columbia University Bicentennial Medal was presented to her in 1954.

[6] She was invited by General Marshall in 1949 to join the initial group of fifty women to form the Defense Advisory Committee on Women in the Services, and served on the committee for six years. She served as a consultant on nursing education and research many times to various sections of the federal government. She was chairperson of the Council of the Florence Nightingale International Foundation, 1950–1956; consultant to the Walter Reed Army Institute of Research, Department of Nursing, 1956–1961; consultant to the Medical Service, International Cooperation Administration, A.I.D. mission in Turkey on the project on the University of Istanbul–Florence Nightingale College of Nursing, 1956–1961.

[7] Isabel M. Stewart retired in 1947. ". . . [The] brilliant R. Louise McManus became the third director of that [Teachers College] internationally famous 'school.'" Mary M. Roberts, *American Nursing: History and Interpretation*, The Macmillan Company, New York, 1954, p. 478.

Isabel M. Stewart became the Director of Nursing Education at Teachers College in 1925, succeeding Adelaide Nutting, who retired. Adelaide Nutting had come to Teachers College in 1907 to accept a professorship in institutional management. She was the first nurse in the world to become a professor in a university. In 1910 a department of nursing and health was set up at Teachers College, and she became its chairperson. See Edward T. James (ed.), *Notable American Women*, The Belknap Press of Harvard University Press, Cambridge, Mass., 1971, pp. 642–644.

was drawing to an end, and anticipating the desire of many nurses to pursue university study, Isabel Stewart had obtained a grant from the Kellogg Foundation to conduct five studies which would aid the faculty in the further development of the curriculum. Her retirement before all the studies were finished left me with the responsibility of seeing that they were completed and the results brought to bear upon the curriculum of the Division of Nursing Education. It was soon clear that an overall curriculum study in which all faculty should take a part was needed. Additional funds were obtained to provide curriculum consultants to the faculty for that purpose. In addition, with the assistance of Dr. Eli Ginzberg of Columbia, a plan was made to invite a number of well-known specialists in the health-related disciplines of medicine, public health, and social welfare, along with several nursing leaders, to serve as members of the Committee on the Function of Nursing to explore together under his leadership what the future function of nursing *should* be. It was hoped that their recommendations concerning the proper function of nurses would help point the direction in which nursing education programs should move.

GS: What was recommended? And was there consensus?

RLM: The recommendations were not all agreed upon in every aspect. There was agreement that the report prepared by Dr. Ginzberg as committee chairman should be shared with many others trying to plan for nursing and nursing education for the future.[8] Among many of the ideas stemming from the committee's discussion that were of great value to me were the concepts of the nursing team as an effective way of utilizing varying levels of nursing skills, the spectrum range of nursing functions, and the need for an organized program of research in nursing. Each concept was more fully explored as the division's program developed and as funds became available to employ staff assigned to study, experimentation, and research. The committee saw the spectrum of nursing functions ranging from the simplest to the most complex: the functions assigned to nursing aides, licensed practical nurses, registered nurses, and nurse specialists. Preparation for such functions was seen also to range in order of length and difficulty and intellectual demands upon the student: on-the-job training for nursing aides, vocational education for licensed practical nurses, technical education for registered nurses who would routinely work under supervision, profes-

[8] Committee on the Function of Nursing, *The Ginzberg Report: A Program for the Nursing Profession*, The Macmillan Company, New York, 1948.

sional education for registered nurses who would practice independently, and graduate studies for clinical nurse specialists. It was recognized that registered nurses are often employed in leadership positions in nursing, which require them not only to continue to improve nursing care but to take on the *added* function of organized teaching, supervision or administration, consultation or research. For these *added* functions, specialized preparation including the science and art underlying the practice of these functions should be available for the graduate nurse. The directions for the Division of Nursing Education programs became clear, and curriculum development toward these goals got under way.

GS: How many students were there?

RLM: There were enrolled at Teachers College at that time over 1400 graduate nurses, over 75 percent of them candidates for the baccalaureate degree. The Division of Nursing Education was the largest in Teachers College and, in fact, in Columbia University at that time.

The nursing faculty had already questioned the wisdom of continuing to offer preparation for the specialized functions of teaching, supervision, and administration at the baccalaureate level. They also recognized that the many diploma school graduates lacked the breadth of knowledge about nursing to prepare for professional-level practice. The graduates of basic nursing generic programs coming to us demonstrated this.

Should nursing majors of the baccalaureate program for registered nurses Teachers College be allowed to broaden their preparation to an equivalent level of professional nursing competence, and should that level be established as a prerequisite for admission to any nursing program leading to a graduate degree? Plans were made to explore the concepts of the professional role of the nurse, team leader, and nursing team organization of nursing service. After some experimentation, Eleanor Lambertsen was released to write the manual *Team Nursing*. Arrangements were made with Delafield Hospital to set up a teaching demonstration center there where our baccalaureate students could have field experience in team nursing and where competence in the professional role of the nurse could be demonstrated and new learnings focused and applied.

It was soon agreed to limit the division B.S. degree program to one, with a major in nursing practice and the team nursing course its main focus. The B.S. program in nursing for registered nurses was thus initiated. Although our decision was understood by most of the nursing

faculty in other colleges and universities in and around New York City
with whom we had been meeting to discuss our concerns about B.S.
programs, many nurse educators, including members of the N.L.N.E.
staff, were very critical.

GS: Of what in particular?

RLM: They wanted to know if we were adding to the time and cost of
preparing experienced registered nurses for the many positions waiting
to be filled, by requiring first a baccalaureate major in nursing practice!
Yet only three years later the League took action that made similar
programs for registered nurses a requirement for all accredited B.S.
programs within five years.

Some of the Teachers College faculty were keen to discontinue even
the new B.S. program entirely and immediately and to offer only graduate programs. With the large number of registered nurses needing to
get their B.S. degrees in order to qualify for graduate study, it was
decided to carry on the B.S. program for them at Teachers College for
at least a five-year period and then to taper off as the demand dimin-
ished. (Actually it was carried on for several years but was eventually
dropped after my retirement.)

GS: What was the emphasis?

RLM: When Teachers College and other institutions for teacher education first developed, the curricular emphasis was upon techniques
and methods of teaching, assuming that the teacher already had mas-
tery of the subject to be taught. For many years the nursing programs,
too, concentrated upon methods with little attention to providing instruction dealing with advanced nursing content. The first course that
dealt with nursing content of scope in advance of that provided in basic
nursing programs was offered by Teachers College in maternity nursing
in the mid-forties with lecturers from the staff of the Maternity Center.
Soon advanced instruction in psychiatric nursing was offered. Impressed by the success of these early courses in clinical nursing, the
faculty recommended that provision be made in each graduate major
for advanced study including clinical nursing practice in one or more
fields of nursing. In the preparation for leadership positions in nursing,
increasing *nursing* competence should go hand in hand with acquiring
competence in other specialized functions, teaching supervision and
the like, it was believed. Under the exceptional leadership of Frances
Reiter, Ruth Gilbert, Margaret Adams, Lydia Hill, and other clinical

nurse specialists, opportunities for the advanced study in many nursing fields were developed.

Adelaide Nutting and Isabel Stewart had given early leadership by example and by involving their students in ongoing study-making and research in the Division of Nursing Education. By the late twenties an introductory course in study-making in nursing was offered as an elective. In the division's new program, the scope of this introductory course was expanded and made a requirement of all candidates for the master's degree. Eventually more and better-prepared nurse faculty members became available and were employed, and enrollment in the graduate programs increased. As more nursing students became interested in doctoral programs, more advanced courses in research tools and techniques were added and opportunities provided for participation in ongoing research projects.

Gradually, the graduate curriculum in nursing education took on the characteristics, including the level of quality, of other graduate programs in the college.

Alexander Graham Bell once stated that "great discoveries and improvements invariably involve the cooperation of many minds." The nursing faculty had labored hard and devotedly, and through their participation reached maturity as a graduate faculty.

GS: How did the nursing education fit in with the rest of Teachers College?

RLM: The organization of Teachers College itself and the relationship of its instructional units changed over the years. Considerable freedom and responsibility for developing the plan of organization and programs within the Division of Nursing Education had always been given to the director. In some ways this had prevented full integration of nursing education with the rest of the college. For example, from the beginning, responsibility for handling and evaluating all admission credentials and the placement of graduates had been retained by the division because the problems involved appeared to differ so much for nurses from those in other fields of education. Responsibility for the division's admission and placement functions had been delegated to me from 1925 to 1929 while I was employed part time as a departmental secretary in the division. Perpetuation of this policy appeared to continue the isolation of the division within the college, and transfer of these functions to the general Office of Admission and Office of Placement was soon worked out to the satisfaction and benefit of all.

A change in the statutes of the college provided for setting up a committee composed of the dean, provost, controller, and heads of each of the five instructional divisions to advise the president on matters pertaining to college policy, program, and budget. Dean Caswell called me in to tell me about the new committee. "You are technically a member of the committee as Director of the Division of Nursing Education. However, much of what we will be discussing will be about budget and finances and many things that will not relate to the Nursing Education Division and wouldn't probably interest you. When we do get to matters pertaining to you, such as your divisional budget, we will let you know and you can attend those meetings." Quickly I broke in: "I'd be very happy to be a member of the Committee on Policy, Program, and Budget and will do my best to plan my time so I can attend every meeting that is called. I may not know much about the college budget or understand very much of what is discussed, but I hope by attending I will learn." He looked at me with some surprise and said, "Well, I don't know that you will particularly like it. We may sit with our feet on the table and we're not used to having a woman around. Some of our language—" I said, "I've seen feet on the table before and I've been where men talked, and I don't think it will faze me." I declared myself a full member of the committee and arranged my schedule to attend every meeting I could. Many benefits were to accrue to the division (and to me) from this new plan of organization. The division's budget was no longer distributed ready-made to the director but was initiated, proposed, and defended by her in committee.

GS: *Could you give an example of how you benefited by being on the committee?*

RLM: Yes, I soon discovered what I had surmised, that the salaries at each rank for nursing faculty members were substantially lower than those in other divisions and promotions slower. Justification for correcting this situation was presented, using criteria I discovered were in use in other divisions, and the salaries for the nursing faculty were soon brought into alignment. Opportunities for educational leave for advanced study, writing, or participating in research (often on salary) were made available to nursing staff. Within a decade the nursing faculty had come to be recognized as a graduate faculty in every sense of the word.

Measurement and Guidance

GS: *Dr. McManus, many may not remember, nor today's younger generation know about, your pioneering work in the field of measure-*

ment and guidance. However, under the auspices of the former N.L.N. E., you are acknowledged to be the one person largely responsible for the groundwork which made possible the use of modern testing methods in relation to licensure, selection, and achievement in nursing. Would you please tell about it?

RLM: After my husband's death (1934) I accepted a position offered me by Isabel Stewart as research assistant on the National League of Nursing Education's extensive curriculum study, which she was directing as chairman of the League's Education Committee. My work included assisting in some of the major studies related to special aspects of curriculum research as reported in the *Curriculum Guide*. One of these studies, headed by Dr. Laura Eads, was concerned with evaluation of the outcomes of instruction. The courses proposed in the curriculum had outlined objectives of instruction. Evaluation dealt with identifying the outcomes of instruction in terms of the student's achievement of the objectives. This study renewed my interest in testing, the field in which I had started to work before my marriage. I became enthusiastic about the potentials of objectives testing for the whole field, of expanding the *Curriculum Guide's* proposals for evaluation into a field of achievement testing as a future activity for the League. Isabel Stewart agreed with me and urged the League to appoint a new Committee on Nursing Tests to carry forward the idea. She was appointed the new committee's chairwoman and I served as the committee secretary. I started again on my own doctoral program, which I had put aside when I married, and began exploring more deeply the fields of tests, measurement, and guidance. Dr. Ben Wood and Dr. Flannagan, who were operating the Cooperative Test Service (at that time housed on the campus of Columbia University), were generous of their time and advice concerning objectively scoreable tests, particularly machine-scored tests. We discussed the possibility of adding a "department of nursing tests" as an integral part of the Cooperative Test Service. They told Isabel Stewart that they thought the League might be able to secure funds to initiate the program from the Carnegie Foundation, which had given support to the Cooperative Test Service.

Isabel Stewart enlisted the help of Dean Hawks (of Columbia University and chairman of the American Council on Education's Committee on Tests) to present the Committee on Nursing Tests plan for a Comprehensive Nursing Test Service grant proposal to the Carnegie Foundation. They showed interest in the project but asked for assurance that the tests would be used widely enough and at a charge sufficient to enable the proposed Comprehensive Nursing Test Service ultimately to function without outside support. The committee immediately sought

and obtained by questionnaire substantial evidence of interest and expected use of objectively scoreable tests of nursing achievement, by
schools and college admission departments for employment and by
health agencies and by state boards of nurse examiners for licensing
purposes. Unfortunately, at the time of the next meeting of the Foundation (and when the evidence they had sought was ready for presentation), World War II clouds were so heavy that the Foundation decided
not to grant funds to launch any new projects. We were all disappointed, of course. Shortly afterward, Isabel Stewart resigned (1940) from
the Committee on Nursing Tests, and I was appointed its new chairman.[9] Although the hopes of the committee were shattered, we decided to try to find at least one phase of the comprehensive plan as a
starting point, even without funding. A growing number of schools of
nursing were beginning to require all applicants to take the Psychological Test Services battery of tests prior to admission at a cost of $5 per
student. We believed that our committee could offer a Prenursing and
Guidance Test Service to nursing schools at that price, which would
provide, in addition to test scores, assistance to the school's committee
on admissions and to those responsible for the guidance of the students upon admission. If so, while waiting for the hoped-for grant to
come to us in the future, and counting upon using the income from fees
for operating expenses and volunteer workers for the service, we could
get started. Dr. Flannagan arranged for us to be licensed to use (for a
fee per test paper) the American Council on Education Psychological
Test and several other standardized tests of academic achievement
which provided norms based on applicants to college. These norms
permitted meaningful comparisons with norms we assembled for nurse
applicants. Arrangements were also made for our test papers to be
machine-scored and reports prepared by the Cooperative Test Service
on a cost-plus basis. The committee had immediate need of money for
operating expenses, office supplies, printing of tests, and so forth. Although the N.L.N.E. board gave approval to the committee to operate
the N.L.N.E. Prenursing and Guidance Test Service at the $5 fee and
approval to establish its own bank account in that name, it could not
make any money available to the committee to get started. It did, however, give permission for the committee to borrow $1000 toward its
expenses with the understanding that the committee members and not
the League itself would have to assume responsibility for the debt if the

---

[9] The nurse-historian Mary M. Roberts writes: "Mrs. McManus proceeded, against serious odds
reminiscent of those encountered by the founders of the AJN [*American Journal of Nursing*] almost a
half century earlier, to lay sound foundations for one of the profession's most fundamental and useful
services." Roberts, op. cit., p. 421.

committee was unable to pay back the loan. I countered that would be all right; if, on the other hand, we did succeed, the committee could retain any profits for the continued development of its Test Services and for research utilizing the data obtained. I was reminded that since it was a League testing service, the committee should trust the League board to take proper action if profits did accrue. In 1941 the N.L.N.E.'s Prenursing and Guidance Test Service was launched in New Jersey and Connecticut on an experimental basis. Certain committee members administered the tests, and with the cooperation of the state leagues, others arranged testing places and volunteer proctors. Approximately twelve hundred candidates were tested the first year. The Committee on Nursing Tests soon requested a change in name to Committee on Measurement and Guidance to reflect its interest in the use of test results in the guidance of students. After two years, approval was given to the committee to extend the Prenursing and Guidance Test Service to other states wishing to use it. The income was, as had been anticipated, sufficient to repay the amount borrowed and to employ part-time and then full-time staff to operate the ongoing service. Meanwhile the committee turned its attention to a second phase of its comprehensive plan, the development of tests of achievement in clinical nursing. A comprehensive Test of Medical-Surgical Nursing, drafted by Ida Sommer, an early member of the committee staff, had reached the tryout stage and was included as an adjunct to one state's own state board examinations. Soon the committee's help was urgently requested by the American Medical Association (A.M.A.) Committee on State Boards' Problems. World War II was necessitating the rapid enrollment of many nurses in the military nursing services. Newly graduated nurses could not enroll until they were licensed, and the state boards of nurse examiners needed help in speeding up the licensing process. They requested the help of the Committee on Measurement and Guidance in setting up a test service especially for use by the state boards, using machine-scoreable tests and providing prompt issuing of test reports. There were many problems to be solved. State laws and board regulations regarding the subject areas to be tested, the passing score, the person authorized to prepare and give the tests, the licensing fee required, and the amount paid each examiner on the state board varied from state to state. The Committee on Measurement and Guidance could only roughly estimate the costs of preparation, printing, and operation of a test service of the type requested by the state board of nurse examiners. The need was so urgent, however, we decided to try our best. After much discussion, representatives of several state boards said that they hoped to be able to use the tests and would if they could arrange to do so legally. They also agreed to pay to the committee per examinee per test the amount that it had actually cost in the home state in the previous year. The cost estimates turned out to range from a few cents per test to $1 or more, according to the state. To proceed on this inequitable basis was indeed hazardous, but the need was urgent. The income from the Prenursing and Guidance Test Service was by then sufficient to cover its own costs and give us some reserve. We decided we should risk taking on this new venture and hope for the best. In mid-1943 we sought and secured the League board's approval of our plan to assist the state boards as a war effort. The state boards of nurse examiners had also agreed to contribute objective test items for at least one test area. From these we hoped that we could pool sufficient items and that, by adding some to fill in the gaps, we could assemble useful tests in machine-scoreable form. It proved later to be impossible to find suitable test items that related to competence in the practice of nursing in the area of nursing tested. New tests in each area or subject were quickly prepared by the committee staff, using agreed-upon competencies of the professional nurse as a blueprint.

Six months after the request from the state boards of nurse examiners came to us, we had a battery of tests in typed form ready to present to the state boards of nurse examiners at their December meeting. Not all wishing to use them had been able to get authority to do so, or they were not able to pay out-of-state for their use. Still others did not wish to use them. Only three states assured us in mid-December that they could and would use them providing they were ready for use in examination dates already scheduled for January! Perhaps with more courage than common sense, the committee decided to get the material to the printer with a rush order. Just in time for New York State's first testing date in January 1944, the first issue of the State Board Test Pool Examinations was ready and delivered to the examiners, complete with a manual to guide them in the administration of the test and in the safeguarding and returning of the test booklets and the machine-scoreable answer sheets. A few days later the test results were returned to the New York State Board of Nurse Examiners, showing in tabular form for each test area the distribution of all scores mean, and standard deviation for the group as a whole. Also, a breakdown of range and mean scores by schools represented, and an I.B.M. report card for each candidate examined, showing scores in each test area. The committee provided a manual to help the examiners in interpreting the test scores and in determining the lowest passing raw score acceptable in that state for that examination.

Before June of 1944 the State Board Test Pool Examinations had been administered in fifteen states. Two years later the legal and financial problems of other states had been ironed out to the point where every state in the Union made use of the State Board Test Pool service. With the service to state boards under way, a third phase of the committee's Comprehensive Nursing Test Service program was planned.

The development of a series of achievement tests in nursing for use in nursing schools was started and continued concurrently with the operation of the two established services. Norms on achievement tests were developed which enabled any school to compare the level of achievement of its students in each subject with all others tested. Guides for the interpretation of test results helped other individuals, teachers, and faculty appraise individual student and class average achievement in light of the students' learning capacity as reflected in the intelligence test scores recorded on the Prenursing and Guidance Test Service report. In addition to the research needed to develop test norms and to improve the tests themselves, several studies were made based on early test reports. The results of some of the studies posed problems for nursing educators. The American Council on Education Psychological Test scores average for students admitted to schools of nursing, for example, was found to be substantially below the "two years of education beyond high school level" upon which the *Curriculum Guide* had been based. Should admission standards be raised to the desired level, sharply reducing the number of acceptable applicants, or should the instruction level of the schools of nursing be lowered to the learning capacity of students actually admitted to the schools? The need for a research program was pointed out, but plans made for one were not implemented. The League's Test Services were first operated in 1941 from a second desk in a corner of my fifth-floor office at Teachers College, where I was then a part-time instructor. As the service developed, staff were employed. Teachers College gave the committee rent-free the use of two offices in the Lower Annex building. Soon we had five offices! By that time the committee was in a position to offer to pay token rent, an offer which was accepted by the college, of course. Soon the volume of work and the size of the staff needed to carry on the Test Services for both professional and business functions became more than could or should be administered on a volunteer basis by a committee chairman, and I urgently needed to return to earning a living. By common agreement, the committee turned over, for administration by the League at headquarters as a Department of Measurement and Guidance, everything pertaining to the Test Services. This included the employed staff, office equipment and supplies, the committee's historical and current operational files, its audited financial records, and a bank account. The Committee on Measurement and Guidance continued to serve for several years in an advisory capacity on matters referred to it by the Department of Measurement and Guidance. The growth of the League's Test Services, their continued usefulness to the profession, has been a source of personal satisfaction. The extent of financial support that the League has derived from the Test Services over and above cost operations has not been revealed of late, but when last reported, it has certainly been substantial. The committee's dream, that a major portion of the profits of the Test Services could go into organized research in nursing and nursing education, has not yet materialized.

GS: *Did you always have a flair, a talent for mathematics and statistics?*

RLM: I wouldn't consider it a great flair. I was interested in the research procedure and was interested in going along in research design and the use of statistical information.

GS: *Well, you certainly have been a creative—I would say visionary—thinker.*

RLM: Well, while that's visionary, that's me. The development of machine-scored, integrated, and comprehensive examinations—we did that.

Institute of Research and Service in Nursing Education

GS: *You are credited with having established the first organized unit for research in nursing (1953). How did you come to do that?*

RLM: Facilities for educational research programs at Teachers College are organized under the Institute plan for administration, financing, and staffing. Usually the director of the Instructional division most closely related to the area of research is also director of the Institute. When Teachers College closed its experimental school, the Lincoln School of Teachers College, the research funds released became available for educational research to be administered under the institute of organization. An Institute of Educational Research was set up at Teachers College to carry on research programs in conjunction with ongoing educational programs in a variety of educational institutions across the country.

As plans for the new Institute of Educational Research were discussed in the Committee on Policy, Program, and Budget, I asked if the Division of Nursing Education's share of the research funds could be made available for nursing research. It was explained that the money in question had been designated exclusively for research in public school education but that the Division of Nursing Education could set up its own Institute of research if we wished and *if* we could find the funds for its organization and administration. I promptly asked for and was given permission to seek the funds needed.

First, a plan of organization for an Institute of Research and Field Service in Nursing and Nursing Education was drafted along with objectives, proposed program, and budget for a trial five-year period. On the advice of the dean, in support of our grant request, I prepared drafts of several research projects for investigation in a variety of problems in nursing and nursing education. The drafts were to be used as samples to illustrate both the areas of need for research and the scope of research activities we had in mind, for which funds would be sought elsewhere if support for the administrative costs of the Institute could be obtained. With the dean's and the president's approval of the general plan, budget, and sample project proposals, I was authorized to go forth and seek funds—and this I did.

GS: Where did you go?

RLM: With grant request and drafts of sample projects in hand, I approached several foundations, individuals, and government agencies for funds. A professional fund raiser for universities had once told me that a good batting average was one success out of twenty tries and that the seeker had to face refusal nineteen times to earn the right to success once. Encouraged by this thought, I kept on trying and was fortunate in securing the grant from the Rockefeller Foundation (much to the surprise of the dean and the president of Teachers College, I may add). Dr. Helen Bunge, then at Western Reserve University, accepted appointment as the Executive Officer of the Institute and served in this capacity for six years. She was followed by Dr. Leo Simmons.

Funds for individual research projects had to be sought from foundations, government agencies, and elsewhere. My task as Director of the

Institute was ably aided by a project proposal drafted by Helen Bunge and others of the Institute staff. Several members of the nursing education instructional staff availed themselves of the opportunity open to all to submit proposals for research of field service projects. The Institute sought funds for them, and when they were procured, the faculty member was released temporarily from instruction and transferred to the Institute's budget and staff with an appointment as a research worker.

GS: Could you give some examples of some projects?

RLM: For two projects under the Institute's field service category for financial administration, I served as principal investigator. The project initiated under contract to the United States Agency for International Development (A.I.D.) mission in Turkey is discussed with other international nursing activities. The second project involved the development of plans for, and bringing into existence of, the National Fund for Graduate Nurse Education. The project arose from the concern of a group of deans and directors of graduate nursing education programs for increased financial support of their programs. Tuition scholarships and cost-of-living stipends had been made available to many graduate nurses for university study. No additional funds had been made available to the university to expand the programs for the many new nursing students enrolling. The financial plight of the deans endeavoring to protect and improve the quality of the programs on a decreasing per capita budget had become acute. During a meeting of deans and directors, in which their financial and resulting educational problems were discussed, attention was called to the success of the National Fund for Medical Education. This fund had been set up through the efforts of deans of medical schools to raise funds specifically to help their schools and to be used in any way that each dean saw fit to benefit the educational program. The nursing deans decided to organize, to define and make known their common needs, and to take steps toward setting up a new organization to raise funds specifically for graduate nursing education programs. Dr. Marie Farrell and Dr. Ruth Kuehen and I acted as a steering committee for the deans in investigating the various types of fund-raising organizations. The institute secured a small grant for us for the employment of a part-time staff assistant and for travel expenses for the committee. We were fortunate to enlist the interest and help of Josephine E. Nelson, who was well informed about nursing and experienced in the field of public relations.

GS: How did you go about organizing the National Fund for Graduate Nurse Education?

RLM: After investigating many types of fund-raising organizations, the pattern of the National Fund for Medical Education seemed most promising for us. With the advice and counsel of many friends and of the college accountants, and legal assistance from the college lawyers, plans for the National Fund for Graduate Nurse Education were developed. We had been advised everywhere that we should be prepared to provide to those we asked to serve on the proposed National Fund's Board of Trustees and its staff reliable information about the costs of graduate nurse education to the university, over and above the income from tuition fees, from endowment, and from other sources, and the resulting need of the program for funds. With the help of Mary Rockefeller, financial and advisory help on getting cost information was received from the Rockefeller Brothers Fund. They made it possible for the firm of Peat Marwick Mitchell & Co., accountants of Teachers College, to be employed to make a cost study of graduate nurse education programs throughout the United States. With the assistance of the financial office of the university programs, a representative sample of university program data was obtained. It was discovered that the average tuition fees paid by the student covered no more than one-third of the average cost. Endowment and financial resources of the university could not be relied upon for more than another third. One-third of the costs remained to be found from some source if the schools were to continue. Meanwhile the graduate nursing school deans gathered materials that illustrated the public's great need for many nurses qualified to fill the various positions in hospitals, schools, public health, industry, and community health agencies for which graduate education programs offered preparation.

With the cost-study data and statements of need provided by the deans of graduate nursing programs, we began a search for potential members to serve on the Board of Trustees of the proposed National Fund for Graduate Nurse Education. We had been advised that they should include socially prominent people who were informed, or interested in learning, about the needs and willing to help meet them through the Fund. We had been cautioned, too, that while there should be a continuous flow of information from the graduate programs themselves, interpreting their program needs, there should not be lines of control between the professional nursing organizations per se and the Fund. The National Fund for Medical Education, for example, had not wanted the A.M.A. tied in with their fund, whereas the Fund's trustees needed information about the cost of medical schools and the help of the deans in establishing policies for the distribution among them of the money raised by the Fund.

While we searched for potential trustees for the National Fund for Graduate Nurse Education, steps were taken to set up the structure of the Fund's organization and to incorporate it in New York State with tax-free status. Signing the articles of incorporation was a joy indeed. Although quite a number of very able and prominent people had agreed by then to serve on the Fund's board of trustees (including two former Surgeon Generals of the United States, Helen Hayes, Mary Rockefeller, and other socially minded individuals), no one able or willing to serve in the leadership role as board chairman had been found. About that time George Smith, who had recently retired as president of Johnson & Johnson Company, became a trustee of Teachers College. I arranged a meeting with him and explained what we were trying to do and our urgent need for a chairman. He expressed much interest, thought we had made remarkable progress, and agreed to do his best to get one of the several suitable people he had in mind to accept the chairmanship. Further he said, "I can assure you that if I can not get one of them to do it, I will take on the chairmanship myself because this is too important to be left undone." Soon, as Chairman of the board of trustees, he took over responsibility for the Fund's further organization and directed its activities.

It had been the dream of the steering committee that Josephine E. Nelson would be the one to continue with the project as a staff member of the Fund. The Fund's officers, however, feared that the big business organizations to which they were going for money would be unlikely to respond as generously to a woman as they would to a man fund raiser. It was a disappointment to us all, but we felt we were in no position to insist upon having our way.

GS: *What was the Fund's growth?*

RLM: The Fund started operation in 1961 and is still a going concern, raising money for graduate nurse education programs. A report released over a year ago indicated that by that time the Fund had turned over to universities offering accredited graduate nursing education programs over $1.5 million, to be used exclusively to augment the regular budget for the graduate nursing program at the discretion of the dean or directors of the program. That's a lot of money made available for graduate nursing education that might never have become available to the schools if no organized effort had been made to inform many organizations and individuals across the country of the need to contribute to the preparation of leaders of nursing. The small project developed under the Institute's administration, with the cooperation of the deans and directors of graduate programs in nursing, has provided and continues to yield rich dividends for all concerned.

GS: Was a goal of the Institute to train nurses in research?

RLM: Yes. We of the Institute of Research and Service in Nursing Education from the first had been able to provide a laboratory setting for training nurses in research. An organized research training program was set up for graduate students with lectures, seminars, and participation in aspects of ongoing research projects. Students employed as part-time research assistants could better decide whether or not to embark upon a career as a nursing research worker. The Institute's facilities were used as a laboratory in which many doctoral students in nursing had valuable experience under the tutelage of the Institute's staff.

By the time the initial grant for the administrative expenses of the Institute terminated, the income derived from the proportional administrative costs built into each project proposal budget was not sufficient to maintain as full and active a program.

The Institute's records attest to the extent of success in research fund procurement, the volume and scope of research activities, and the findings reported. Within Teachers College, and perhaps among all professions, the establishment of the first facility specifically organized for conducting a research program in nursing and nursing education marked the start of the year for the coming of age of nursing as a profession with its practice based upon findings that stemmed from systematic research.

The Junior and Community College Program in Nursing

GS: I would now like to turn to your leadership role in the development of the associate degree program. Where did you get the idea? How did it evolve?

RLM: One of the research drafts I had prepared, for inclusion with other samples to support the request for funds to set up the Institute of Research and Service in Nursing Education, was a proposal for research in cooperation with selected junior or community colleges across the country in the adaptation of preparation for registered nurse licensure in programs leading to associate degrees. The President's

Commission on Higher Education had earlier strongly recommended that two years of education beyond high school be made available in many communities, and more new junior and community colleges were being established. Nursing as a career field had not been able for some time to attract the numbers of high school graduates needed to fill their programs and to meet health needs. The work-oriented training program and nursing home residence requirements of most hospital schools of nursing made competition for applicants less favorable than in schools preparing for other occupations, and the shortage of nurses became continuously more acute. The concept of the spectrum range of nursing functions had placed the functions of the registered nurse who worked under supervision routinely in the category of technical function. Among the studies undertaken earlier during the division's curriculum study, practical nurse education had been investigated. Mildred Montag had been employed to study vocational and technical education relating to spectrum-range functions of nursing. She extended her study to make application specifically to vocational and technical education in her doctoral project. In her published report she proposed preparation for nursing technicians.

As the junior and community college movement expanded, the system of education they developed was geared by design especially to prepare for technical functions. Could preparation for registered nurses for practice under supervision be adapted to fit into the patterns of the technical programs of junior and community colleges? If so, nursing might successfully compete for students desiring junior college study. By qualifying for the registered nurse licensure in two academic years rather than three calendar years, the nurse would start earning a whole year earlier, and the community's supply of nurses would be built up more quickly. It seemed worthy of experimentation.

While waiting for the decision of the Rockefeller Foundation, which had under consideration our request for a grant to enable Teachers College to set up the administrative machinery for the Institute of Research and Service in Nursing Education, the draft I had prepared proposing a five-year Cooperative Research Project in Junior and Community College Education for Nursing remained for some time with the other sample projects in the bottom drawer of my desk.

One day a representative of the board of managers of a well-known school of nursing in New York City came to request help in locating a new director for the school. In the discussion that followed, she bemoaned the acute shortage of nurses in the hospital, particularly on the wards at night. "What can be done about the shortage?" she asked.

"What are you doing at Teachers College to help the communities get more nurses?" Taken back a bit, I reached in my bottom drawer, took out the research proposal involving associate degree programs in nursing, and said, "Here is one plan we have been thinking about. I think registered nurses can be prepared in two rather than three years and thus can be ready to work earlier; and the cost of the two-year education programs could be paid for as for other educational fields, taking the financial burden off the hospital and ultimately off the patient."

After many questions she asked, "How much will this research cost and may I have a copy of the proposal? Perhaps money can be found for it. It seems such a good idea."

As soon as she left, I dashed to the controller for help in setting up a budget for the five-year project and obtained official approval for submitting the grant request; within ten days the check for the full amount arrived from a donor who wished to remain anonymous. Thus, funds became available for one of the projects proposed to be carried out under the Institute's administration before the Institute itself was funded and established.

Had we been certain we could succeed in securing support for the Institute, we might have waited to initiate the Junior College Cooperative Research Project. We were only certain that we had money for one important project in hand and decided to start it as soon as possible.

As soon as word got about that Teachers College was about to start experimentation in registered nurse preparation in two years, protests poured in from nurse educators in diploma schools and baccalaureate programs alike and from nursing leaders at the League headquarters. Proceeding with our plan would "sell nursing down the river," we were told. I defended both the need and the university's right and responsibility to carry on research, turned deaf ears to their protests, and continued plans to get under way.

GS: Mildred Montag is usually given the credit for the associate degree program concept. What was her role exactly?

RLM: Mildred Montag was interested in serving as director of the project and was soon released from her instructional responsibilty to start it. Together we visited junior and community colleges across the country that had indicated interest in participating in the research as pilot schools and the state boards of nurse examiners in those states to secure approval for the experimental programs in nursing. An advisory committee representing nurses, physicians, educators, hospital administrators, and consumers of the services of nurses was set up and met frequently throughout the research project. The nature of the cooperative research (in which many people participated), the types of experimental programs developed, and the evaluation of the competence of the graduates of the new-type program are all fully described in the several published reports of phases of the project.

Three years later, well before the five-year research program was completed, some of the former doubters had changed their minds, and the League appointed to its own staff a consultant in junior and community college education in nursing to give advice and help to those considering the development of the new-type two-year program.

One of the answers to the question raised two decades ago about what Teachers College was doing to help communities get more nurses is reflected in the following facts. There has been a great increase in the number of junior and community college programs in nursing and in the proportion of today's registered nurses being prepared in them. Many diploma schools of nursing across the country have been closed down, thereby relieving the hospitals of the cost of their operations.

The time needed to qualify as registered nurse has been reduced by at least one year to the advantage of the nurse who can start earning a year earlier and to the community that benefits from the nurse's services.

Education for nursing at long last is now firmly established as an integral part of the system of higher education of the country.

International

GS: When did you begin to get interested and involved in nursing on the international level?

RLM: Early in my career I became keenly interested in nursing internationally through attending the 1925 International Council of Nurses (I.C.N.) conference in Helsinki, Finland. At the I.C.N. meeting in Stockholm, Sweden, in 1949, I was appointed a member of the Florence Nightingale International Foundation (F.N.I.F.) Council. The Council's task was to plan and carry out a program of research in relation to nursing significance internationally. Income from the invested funds of the F.N.I.F. would supply the budget for the Council's activities. At the first meeting in London early the next year, I reluctantly became chairperson of the Council (1950–1956). For the next five or six years the Council struggled with getting a program under way.

GS: *What were some of the obstacles?*

RLM: Concepts of research varied among the Council members almost as much as opinions about the relative importance for nursing, internationally, of some of the projects proposed. The Council was further hampered by the I.C.N.'s policies regarding advertising internationally all positions vacant and selecting for appointment only from those applying by mail for the position advertised. Relatively few nurses with research experience or training applied for the staff position open. Much time was lost and money spent before work on any of the studies projected was under way. The level and type of research to be undertaken had to be in balance with research competence of the staff available. Travel costs prohibited holding Council meetings often enough to reconcile differences of opinion among Council members and to give the staff the help and supervision needed with the research undertaken. In spite of all these problems, two descriptive studies were eventually completed.

GS: *Could you amplify?*

RLM: One was a study listing and describing all post basic nursing programs offered in all countries; the other was a study of a selected sample of programs in basic nursing offered in selected countries. The Council arranged with the Welcome Historical Library to have a qualified historical researcher compile for the F.N.I.F. information that still remained in the many boxes and cartons in the basement of St. Thomas's Hospital.

From the start the Council tried to work with and through national nursing organizations to enlist the help of their members knowledgeable about research in nursing. Their interest was often much greater than their competence in research. If we could get them all together for instruction in research methods and training in planning studies, they could be of much more help to the council and in their own countries.

A proposal for a conference or seminar on international nursing research to be sponsored by the Council was drafted and permission of the I.C.N. board sought for it. Each country would be invited to send one or more nurses with some experience in research or study making, and to pay travel expenses for their representative. The Council's budget could not be stretched to cover the administrative expenses of the seminar. The I.C.N. board gave approval for holding the conference, providing the Council itself could raise the funds for it. So once again I found myself asking here and there for money. It was not easy to find, but eventually the Rockefeller Foundation gave me $10,000, a bit over half the amount needed. The conference planning went ahead while I was still seeking to obtain the amount needed. At the last moment a good friend of nurses gave the remaining amount of money required to get under way.

At the Council's request the U.S. Public Health Service (U.S.P.H.S.) released Margaret Arnstein on leave to chair the conference. Many others contributed their time and services to make it a success. The securing of funds and the planning for the conference had taken so long, my term of office on the Council had already terminated by the time the conference met. However, I was invited to attend and to participate in the first International Conference of Nursing Research, sponsored by the F.N.I.F. Council. The conference was held in a delightful spot in Sèvres, France, in 1956. A few years later the I.C.N. arranged with the F.N.I.F. for a new use of its income, the support of the I.C.N.'s Department of Nursing Education. The F.N.I.F. Council was thus disbanded, and the research program was discontinued.

GS: You were a consultant in Turkey on the project on the University of Istanbul–Florence Nightingale College of Nursing from 1956 to 1961. Would you elaborate upon this, please?

RLM: From Sèvres I journeyed to Istanbul, Turkey, in response to a request from the United States A.I.D. mission in Turkey and the F.N.I.F. of Istanbul for Teachers College help in developing a university school of nursing at the University of Istanbul. Plans were developed for what became one of the first field service projects of the Institute of Research and Service in Nursing Education at Teachers College, similar in pattern to field service projects carried on by other institutes of the college to aid in education internationally. At the initial meeting with the administrative officers and faculty at the University of Istanbul, the foundation's board, leaders in medicine and nursing in Turkey, and the United States A.I.D. staff, a proposal project was drafted. In a visit to Beirut, Lebanon, a year earlier, I had been distressed to find that after fifty years the American University School of Nursing there was still staffed by Americans. Local leadership had not been developed or employed as faculty by the American University School of Nursing. Remembering this, I said, "If you wish the new-type university program to be instrumental in improving nursing in Turkey, the system of nursing education started in the university here must be one that will be acceptable to the Turkish people. Therefore it should be under Turkish leadership and staffed by Turkish nurse faculty from the beginning. That will mean arranging for some of your best, experienced Turkish nurses to qualify for university appointment as teachers in the new program." United States A.I.D. agreed to finance teacher preparation for ten Turkish nurses to be se-

lected by the F.N.I.F. of Istanbul. Teachers College agreed to accept
the nurses as Turkish faculty trainees, assisting them first to qualify for
Columbia University admission, then to complete the requirements of
the baccalaureate program for registered nurses at Teachers College.
Eight of the nurses chosen were also able to complete the requirements
of the master's degree and prepared as teachers of nursing. A special
aspect of the program was a faculty training seminar each week to
discuss step by step the organization and function of the faculty as a
group and the responsibilities of individual faculty members. Together
we went through each step in the process of formulating aims and
devising a plan of organization for the proposed University of Istanbul–
Florence Nightingale College of Nursing. For this, information was obtained from Turkey such as the university organization and regulations,
the Ministry of Health reports about major health problems of Turkey,
and so on. A sample curriculum thought suitable for Turkey was drafted
with suggested sequence and length of courses including class, laboratory, and clinical practice hours, which together would fit into the pattern established for other programs in the University of Istanbul.

On completion of the program at Teachers College, each nurse returned to Turkey and together they began to work in earnest as the
faculty-elect of the new school. Teachers College arranged for Eugenia
Spalding to go with the first of the returning students to guide them in
making a survey of nursing education in Turkey as a research experience from which they and the school profited. Teachers College appointed Dr. Katherine Sehl as its representative in Turkey and as a
continuing consultant to the new faculty on matters pertaining to the
establishment of the new program.

All went well until the time came for the final action to be taken on
the administrative relationships previously agreed upon, in discussion,
between the new College of Nursing, the F.N.I.F. board, and the University of Istanbul. The Foundation insisted upon retaining control of the
nursing curriculum, lest it be interfered with by some of the medical
faculty. The nursing faculty-elect protested, but to no avail. After much
discussion the university representative said, "If the Foundation wishes
to control the nursing curriculum, as is its prerogative, the university will
withdraw from the project entirely. There can be no official tie with the
university of any program if the university does not control the curriculum."

This action by the Foundation necessitated my presence in Turkey
for an immediate review by Teachers College of its contract with the
United States A.I.D. mission, to assist the University of Istanbul and the
Foundation in the development of a university program in nursing. If the
Foundation's change of mind made it impossible for the University of

Istanbul to continue with the project, Teachers College was not willing to continue. It was obvious that without the participation of the University of Istanbul, our objective, to assist in developing university education for nursing there, could not be attained. I arrived in Turkey on the very eve of the overthrow of the Turkish government by the military coup. A wild drive from the airport got me to the hotel just at curfew. During that night soldiers marched in the streets and surrounded nearby government buildings. Sherman tanks ground up and down the streets, all traffic stopped. Dr. Sehl and I were stranded in the hotel for some time, for martial law kept civilians off the streets and hotel employees couldn't get in to work. Eventually the new government announced that the public could go about ordinary business. Hotel food, elevators, and telephone service resumed. Within a few days a meeting with the A.I.D. mission staff and the Foundation board was arranged. In spite of the fact that the Foundation had inadequate funds to continue the development of their plans for the school or to support it once established, the board was still adamant about controlling it. The Foundation insisted that they would operate their own school with no university tie. Teachers College therefore withdrew and the contract with A.I.D. was terminated.

GS: *What were some of the direct implications?*

RLM: The effect upon the ten nurses whom Teachers College had prepared for university faculty positions was my most serious concern. They were ready for work in a university-level program and unhappy with the Foundation board decision. Two of the nurses found employment in Ankara. The thought of leaving the others stranded was hard to bear. I arranged a meeting with the Minister of Health in Ankara and told him of the ready-made nursing faculty without a school. Could the Ministry of Health possibly arrange with the Foundation to take over the organization and financing of the proposed Florence Nightingale College of Nursing, and could a higher-level nursing program be offered there under the joint auspices of the Ministry of Health and the Ministry of Higher Education in Turkey, and could the Ministry employ the ten qualified nurses as faculty of its new school? It took some time, but much of my proposal did finally come about. The Minister of Health did employ the prepared faculty who remained in Istanbul and gave them freedom to continue to develop the higher-level nursing program. Since 1961 the Ministry of Health has operated the Florence Nightingale College of Nursing. Only lycée graduates are admitted to the program. Within a short time the program was recognized by the Ministry of

Higher Education as a higher-level program, and the school's diploma—as are all other Turkish higher-level programs outside of the university—is recognized as the equivalent of a Turkish university degree.

Recently there have been new plans discussed for the absorption of the Florence Nightingale College of Nursing program into the University of Istanbul, a long-hoped-for goal!

The two faculty trainees who found employment in Ankara when the Teachers College A.I.D. project came to a halt in Istanbul were employed by Dr. Dogramaci, head of the department of pediatrics at Ankara University and the Ankara Children's Hospital. A program for aide training had been set up there, but a university-level program in nursing was wanted. With a few changes, the sample curriculum which had been developed in the Teachers College faculty training seminar was placed before the Ankara University Senate and favorably acted upon in May 1961, the evening before I arrived in Ankara for a visit. Dr. Dogramaci urged me, as I was about to retire from Teachers College, to take the position of Acting Dean of the Ankara University School of Nursing. I insisted that qualified Turkish nurses should be appointed to the university faculty from the state. Would I at least be a consultant to the university and help them? I agreed to help, but only as a volunteer. He had funds for travel for consultants. I was made welcome in the residence that had been built by the United States A.I.D. mission for nursing staff and students. In October of 1961, the first students in nursing were admitted to Ankara University. That same month the Turkish Ministry of Health opened its Florence Nightingale College of Nursing in Istanbul, and both schools have continued and flourished ever since. For several years I continued to serve on a volunteer basis as consultant to the Ankara program and as Visiting Professor of Nursing on the medical faculty of the university (on the same honorary basis). I attended meetings of the medical faculty. Since I understood little Turkish, a "whisperer" was assigned to me to interpret matters under discussion. The need for the establishment of a new university was under discussion, and particularly a new medical school, to be organized on the lines of American universities in contrast with older European universities. Ultimately, parliament did act favorably upon the proposal and set up a second university in Ankara, the Hacettepe University. The Ankara University School of Nursing and the medical faculty that staffed the Children's Hospital became the nucleus around which the new Hacettepe University was built.

The nursing program has continued to grow and improve. Ten of the early graduates of the university school were given scholarships for advanced study of nursing in the United States to prepare for teaching nursing in Turkey. After earning their master's degrees here, they returned to Turkey and are serving on the university faculty. A graduate program in nursing has been developed under the graduate faculty of the university, and several of the faculty and graduates of the new school of nursing now have doctoral degrees. While in Turkey I had the opportunity to take part in several conferences of significance in nursing, notably the conference on nursing and nursing education held in Tehran, Iran, which brought together representatives of nursing from all the Central Treaty Organization (CENTO) member countries—Pakistan, Iran, Turkey, England, and the United States—under the leadership of health personnel from each country. Firsthand contact with nurses coping with problems unknown to us in the United States, under conditions which would baffle registered nurses in this country, I found most educative and humbling.

A Summing Up

GS: In looking back over your productive and distinguished career, what would you say have been one or two—meaning one or two only— of your greatest satisfactions?

RLM: Well, one is really getting the League testing program on the road. I think the organized program for research in nursing—the initiation of that—because that was the first organized program financed and set up especially for research. Not that research wasn't *done* other places, but this was purposely set up for research and research training, a combination. And I think the clarification of the distinctive role of the master's-level program in comparison with the baccalaureate program, and the role of graduate study in nursing, in general, which includes the doctoral program. It's very interesting that the first university program in 1899 for graduate nurses was established in a teacher-training institution. That was the only place that would admit them. The original idea was to put nurses in the classes for teachers, and that way they would get enough help to become good teachers of nursing. Then it was decided that it wasn't enough, and they have to have more and different instruction. At least nurses had a toehold in a university, but the role of *that* particular college was to prepare teachers. We came to see that it wasn't enough to teach about *methods* of teaching; teachers also had to have more content. This is one of the things we defined through our curriculum study: that it was essential for teachers to have advanced study of the content relating to the subjects which they were going to teach. If they were going to teach nursing, they needed opportunity for the advanced study of that subject. And, therefore, the university had to prepare to offer such instruction. When other universities first started programs for graduate nurses, they failed to set up a new pattern that would be more appropriate to focus on adding to the body of knowledge relating to practice of the profession in their universities. Yale didn't attempt graduate education for some time; its program was to prepare people to *become* nurses. But many of the universities—the University of Chicago, Catholic University, New York University, and many others—had programs for graduate nurses before they had preservice or general programs to prepare for the practice of nursing. They tended to copy the program that was suited for a teacher-education school. They didn't set up programs that were clearly for advanced study in many clinical nursing fields. It took a long time for that. And, interestingly enough, when they first got the idea about the proper role for graduate study in nursing, they turned around and blamed Teachers College for preparing teachers rather than practitioners—which wasn't the point. And neither did they recognize that by that time Teachers College was in the business of offering advanced study of nursing practice in specialized clinical fields. One of the first studies we did at the Institute of Research was in surgical nursing per se. It's been interesting to see the shift of emphasis in many of the programs. Rightfully so. It's been a long time coming.

GS: Could you please say something about combining marriage and a career? You married, at the age of 33, a widower who had six children, and you subsequently had one child. You were happily married for four years; then your husband died suddenly. Could you please comment on your own experience?

RLM: Well, I certainly had a very happy and fortunate marriage: fortunate in my children, unfortunate in losing my husband so early. I don't see any reason why marriage and a career can't function if both are willing. I think I felt very much that I had neglected my daughter, particularly when I was working on my dissertation. But I was not only working on my dissertation; I was also teaching extramural classes and at the same time developing the test service—running out here, there, and everywhere. I think I felt that I was doing a less satisfactory job in my family situation than I would have like to have because I was doing it *alone*.

GS: How would you describe yourself? Your personality?

RLM: Very disorganized, very disorganized. I find it hard to do things I don't like to do. If I have a job to do, I put it off. Then I can find a *dozen* things to do that interest me more than what I have to do.

GS: What do you consider to be some of your strategies in terms of working with people? You have been very successful with the faculty, the administration, the president of Teachers College, and in Turkey, to cite only a few examples. What is your secret?

RLM: I don't have any secret. I think you just have to study the particular situation and do what seems the most important, yet practical, thing at the time. Sometimes it does take planning to think ahead of what the interest of that person is. It's silly to go to a person who doesn't have any interest. But to create the interest, you can plan the gradual involvement of that person. But I have had some very lucky streaks, like . . . I was trying to help the anonymous friend of nursing by telling her I saw at least *one* way of helping relieve the nursing situation which she was interested in, and boy! Did she help me! Later, she said that the success of the two-year (junior or community) college research project had given her more satisfaction than any other project she had helped with or experienced. She liked particularly the fact that she had been instrumental in helping make it possible for this new area of nursing education to be opened.

GS: Is there anything you wish to add?

RLM: There are certainly two mistakes that I made, or perhaps it's the same mistake made twice. When I turned over to the League the work of the Committee on Measurement and Guidance, I turned over *all* the records—the official records of the committee, minutes, and progress reports from the beginning of the Committee on Nursing Tests— everything went to the League. Also, all the data we had collected from nursing applicants tested in the first two or three years of our activities, priceless materials in relation to test scores and the experimental data forms and the like, on which I hoped we or they would proceed with research. The League, of course, had not enough storage room for everything, all the data, we and they had accumulated all these years, but much of the material has not been found. It was evidently *not* kept. They'd been housekeeping. Everybody new coming in cleans house. So whether any of that material exists or not, I don't know. I think, however, that for my own personal satisfaction I should have kept more of my own materials than I did. What I have here represents duplicates that I gleaned to use as illustrative material in my courses on nursing tests, and so on. Again, when I turned over the National Fund for Graduate Nurse Education project to the staff of the new organization, I turned over all the files from the beginning, all the historical material, committee minutes, study reports, correspondence, and so on, especially all of the letters I wrote to prospective trustee board members. I have no idea whether any of that historical material exists. Nowadays, I think that the thing to have done was to have had it all microfilmed. In those days we didn't use microfilming of records that way. But after all, it's far less important that I have it in my files than it is for them to have it. But I just wish that they had kept it.

Activities before and after Retirement

While serving as Director of the Division of Nursing Education at Teachers College, opportunities to serve informally on advisory committees or as consultant to a variety of agencies came to me, as they did to many professional associates in similar positions. These included serving as a civilian consultant to the U.S. Navy Bureau of Medicine and Surgery; consultant to the Department of Nursing, Walter Reed Army Institute of Research; on the Dean's Committee of the Veterans Administration Bronx Hospital; consultant to the U.S. Veterans Administration's Nursing Service in Washington. I held appointment as a member of the National Health Council Advisory to the United States Surgeon General. I was invited by General Marshall to be a member of the Defense Advisory Committee on Women in the Services when it was first founded, and served on the committee for a six-year period.

Some of these activities continued for a time after my retirement, and a few new ones were inititated. One assignment took me to Kenya, East Africa, to help a mission board determine how best to prepare for African nurse leadership in the mission's hospital and training program for enrolled nurses. With Kenya's new policy of denying permits for non-Kenyans to hold paying positions there, the mission's hospital could no longer look forward to being permanently staffed by British and American nurses. It was urgent to start planning for Kenyans to prepare themselves academically and professionally for positions as teachers, supervisors, and administrators of nursing in the hospitals. It was a challenging and interesting assignment for me. Upon completion of my duties, I visited several of the East African game reserves on safari with my camera.

For the New England Yearly Meeting of Friends (Quakers) I have served ten years as a Trustee of the Lincoln School of Providence, as a member of the board of the New England Yearly Meeting of Friends Home for the Elderly, and on the permanent board of the Yearly Meeting itself.

When plans were initiated for the Cape Cod Community College to be established, I called on the newly appointed president-elect to suggest the inclusion of an associate degree program in nursing. In due time an advisory committee was appointed to help with plans for the program, particularly with recruiting applicants, interpreting the program's purposes and needs in the community, and encouraging the support of community health agencies. Acting on advice, the president arranged for the nurse-director of the program to be on campus a year before the students were to be admitted so she could work with the faculty and community health agency personnel in planning the nursing curriculum, including nursing practice fields. After the first year, recruitment was no problem; applicants poured in and continued to exceed class openings five to one. It was satisfying to the nursing faculty, to the college administration, and to the advisory committee for the program to become fully accredited just after the first class graduated. As in many seemingly isolated, quiet communities, there abound on Cape Cod many opportunities for participation in community health, social welfare, and educational activities. After helping initiate the Falmouth Family Planning Service, I have continued on its board. As they first organized, I participated in the activities, often serving as an officer, of such organizations as the Cape Cod chapter of the American Association of University Women, the Cape Cod Community Health Council, the Cape Cod Islands World Federalists Association, and the Cape Cod United Fund.

Believing in continuing my schooling, I enrolled in several courses offered by the Falmouth Adult Education program in the evenings, seeking more skill in tailoring, furniture refinishing, and cake decoration.

The Barnstable County Extension Service program has provided opportunities to explore a variety of crafts and to discuss ways of improving the quality of home and family life, under the leadership of home

economists on the staff of the University of Massachusetts Extension
Service. As Barnstable County Extension Service Council Scholarship
Committee chairman, it has been satisfying to have helped raise the
funds to grant full-tuition scholarships for two Cape Cod young women
each year to enroll in programs planned for careers in the field of home
economics.

The best way of continuing my education after retirement that I have
found to date has been to travel. After four times around the world and
many shorter excursions by air, I tried by cargo liner twice and then by
the still slower twelve-passenger freighters. I've traveled abroad alone
and with friends and relatives. Few invitations to travel abroad with me
have been turned down by my granddaughters, ten of whom accepted
and now are traveling enthusiasts. With twenty-three grandchildren and
eleven great-grandchildren to date and much more of the world to visit
or revisit, the future looks promising.

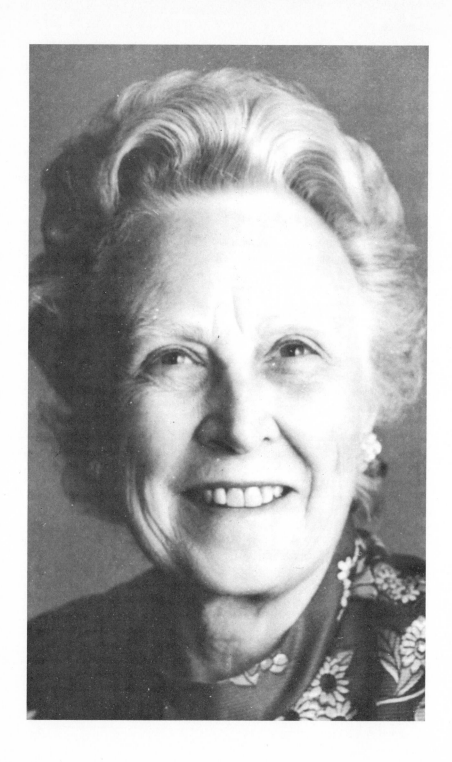

9

"Regents of the University of Minnesota
As a Token of High Esteem
In Recognition of Noted Professional Attainment by

MILDRED MONTAG

Distinguished Graduate of the University of Minnesota
Professor of Nursing Education at Teachers College, Columbia University
Enthusiastic Researcher in Diverse Areas of Nursing Education
Creative Leader in Developing Effective Nursing Curricula
Skillful Author of Valuable Manuals on Nursing Care and Education
Deem Her to be Worthy of Special Commendations for
Outstanding Achievement
Conferred on May Seventh, Nineteen Hundred and Fifty Nine"

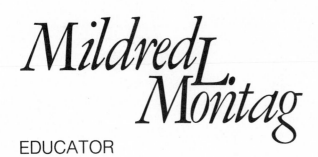

EDUCATOR

Mildred L. Montag is known as a foremost nursing educator. She is credited with implementing the junior and community college education for nursing in the 1950s. She was born August 10, 1908, in Struble, Iowa. Her father died when she was quite young, and her mother died when she was sixteen. Dr. Montag, the eldest of three children, had a brother four years younger and a sister six years younger than she. They were all adopted by an uncle who was in the real estate business and later in the restaurant business, so that financially there was no hardship.

Dr. Montag was brought up in a somewhat strict Protestant religious environment. She received her B.A. from Hamline University in St. Paul, Minnesota, in 1930. She received a B.S. degree from the University of Minnesota in 1933 and an M.A. and Ed.D.[1] from Teachers College, Columbia University.

Her numerous professional experiences include starting the nursing program at Adelphi College in Garden City, New York, in 1943, and serving as its director. She was a member of the faculty of nursing education at Teachers College and was the Director of the Cooperative Research Project in Junior and Community College Education for Nursing, 1952–1957. She was also the Director of the Teachers College section of a five-year project, involving four states, for implementation of the associate degree programs in nursing.[2]

Dr. Montag has published extensively.[3] In addition to being very active professionally, she has been the recipient of awards, such as the Outstanding Achievement Award from the University of Minnesota, and of several honorary degrees.

Entering Nursing

GS: *Where did you get the idea to go into nursing?*

MM: I suppose from friends of the family. A friendship had begun because the oldest member of that family had been a nurse and had taken care of my mother when I was about two. Her youngest sister

---

[1] The title of her published doctoral dissertation was *The Education of Nursing Technicians*, G. P. Putnam's Sons, New York, 1951.

[2] Published as Mildred L. Montag and Bernice E. Anderson, *Nursing Education in Community Junior Colleges*, J. B. Lippincott Company, Philadelphia, 1966.

[3] Among her key publications are *The Community College Education for Nursing*, McGraw-Hill Book Company, New York, 1959; and *The Evaluation of Graduates of Associate Degree Programs*, Teachers College Press, Columbia University, New York, 1972.

also became a nurse. I've had that kind of contact through the years with nurses, and I suppose that may have contributed.

GS: *Did you like nursing?*

MM: Yes.

GS: *Had you ever thought of quitting once you were in?*

MM: The only time I thought of quitting was when my uncle died, and that wasn't because of nursing. It was because I felt that I'd had five years of education and that there ought to be a little less spent on me at that point.

GS: *Did you ever feel a stigma attached to it?*

MM: No, not after I got into it. Oh, I do think there are times when people still look at nursing as a very menial thing.

At Adelphi

GS: *Dr. Montag, could you please talk about your starting the nursing program at Adelphi?*

MM: It was called the School of Nursing at Adelphi because at the time I went there it was a college; it's now a university. It was, if you recall the date (1943), wartime. It was a time of a shortage of nurses and a time when hospitals were short-staffed. Some of the hospitals that had closed their schools in the thirties, following the Grading Committee study, were beginning to talk about reopening them. When those requests went in to Albany, as they would have to do in New York State, it was noted that several of them seemed to cluster around the place where there was a college. So at that time Adelphi, Keuka College, Wagner College, Alfred University, the Manhattanville College of the Sacred Heart, and the College of Mount St. Vincent all opened schools of nursing. Now how this came about I really do not know, but Adelphi got a grant from the U.S. Public Health Service (U.S.P.H.S.) to do a survey—I suppose now you'd call it a feasibility study—to see if there were hospitals in the area that would cooperate in such a venture; and I was asked to make the survey. Usually the person who made the survey was likely to be the person appointed to the chair of the department or the head of the school, and I was. So we began a School of Nursing at Adelphi in January 1943, to which we admitted about twenty-five students. The base of the program was at the college, and we used the hospitals in the area for clinical experience for the students. In the time I was there, we graduated over 500 students. Financing of the program was almost exclusively through the U.S. Cadet Nurse Corps. Because Adelphi had a fairly large program, the college was able to get, for the first time, dormitories on campus through government construction grants. As a result we had two dormitories and a dining hall. The nursing program also accounted for the first minority students on that campus. We took the first black students. Through the War Relocation Authority, we got several Japanese students. They were charming young women, excellent students. That really opened the door at Adelphi to three new things: first, dormitory availability, which meant that they could become a residential college as well as a commuting college; second, it introduced minority groups; and third, because of the residential facilities, students could be recruited from a wide geographic area. We had nursing students from Alaska, Ohio, Washington, Massachusetts, to name a few areas represented. This was one of the benefits to the college for having the nursing school.

GS: Do you care to add anything else about your leadership role there?

MM: I'm trying to think what that might be; one thing, I had an excellent faculty. I had a small faculty but a very good faculty. I made a choice at that point that I would rather have a well-qualified baccalaureate graduate than a poorly qualified or unqualified master's degree holder. I took two young women who were graduates of Skidmore and one who was a graduate of New York–Cornell, all of whom had bachelor's degrees. They turned out to be excellent people; one of them went on for her master's and later went into health education and made quite a contribution in health education in teaching. I think that was a wise choice of faculty. I think we did some things in reducing the work week of students, and another thing we did was to make the nursing program an integral part of the college and the students bona fide students of the college. They came back every week for their classes. We had no classes in the hospitals. They did not go to school there. The program had some characteristics of the hospital school, but it also broke with many of the old traditions. One cannot look at a 1943 activity in the light of 1975. We've come a long, long way. I feel what we did there was as significant as some of the things that are being done now, because we made a great break with the past, a great break. We admitted students through the college admission procedures, held them to college requirements, and opened college activities to them. They were college students, and I think that was significant. We worked hard at that, and as I say, it was not always easy. Many of those graduates have gone for further education. It seemed to me that an unusual number did graduate study, and I think this is a result of what they got at Adelphi. I think the fact that a large percentage of them continued in nursing—even if it's part time—is also significant.

At Teachers College

GS: What brought about your going to Teachers College and getting involved with the junior college program?

MM: I went to Teachers College in 1948 to pursue my doctoral study, and was quickly pushed into full-time teaching. I was going to teach two courses to finance my tuition, but I became a full-time instructor at the end of the first semester. Thus my doctoral study was slowed.

GS: What stimulated you to take the initiative to go to college for further education?

MM: First of all, Katharine Densford. Oh, Katharine Densford used to say to me daily, "When are you going on?" Finally, I said I would. Lucile Petry (Leone) advised me to apply for an Isabel Hampton Robb Scholarship, which I did. I was third in a line of sixty-five applicants and received a scholarship of $300. So I was again a full-time student, this time at Teachers College. I've only been a part-time student a very small part of my educational career, and, even then, being on the grounds at Teachers College through part of it made me seem not quite as much a part-time student as if I had had another job. I did, however, continue my graduate work while I was at St. Luke's and Adelphi, again at the insistence of Isabel Stewart. I had thought that the master's was enough, but Isabel Stewart told me when I was leaving that I ought to go directly on for my doctorate. There was a course being offered the following semester that she advised me to take. It was by an Englishman—Laski—on American democracy. I registered for that course, and thereby hangs the rest of the tale; I kept on. When I returned to Teachers College in 1948, I was well along in my doctoral study and had to begin to think about my dissertation. This period was the beginning of auxiliary help in hopsitals; it was a beginning of vocational education and adult schoolwork in practical nursing; and I took courses in vocational education, trying to see if there was something relevant for nursing. And, incidentally, those courses proved most useful.

GS: How did you get interested in the junior college programs?

MM: Precisely, vocational education; but also because of the philosophy of the man who was head of the department, Dr. Forkner, under whose auspices I took the courses and who ultimately was on my doctoral committee. He left before I finished but was very influential in the early philosophical approach to vocational education. I had felt from the beginning that we would rue the day when we permitted nursing to be taken over by practical nurses or allowed it to go increasingly into their hands. At this time practical nurses were virtually unprepared. The more I read about practical nursing and how it was changing and how they were adding to it, the more convinced I became this was not the way nursing ought to go. I began, again as a result of vocational education courses, to read in the area of community colleges and technical education. There was a kind of merging and emerging of the notion that we already had this technical worker in the diploma school. What we didn't yet have was what we would call professionalism, except as people became professionals through their own efforts. We really didn't have professional education. I got part of this idea from Louise Mc-Manus, who first introduced the notion that you could differentiate the functions of nursing, that nursing had too broad a range of functions to be encompassed in a single individual.

GS: Was this before the Brown Report?

MM: At about the same time. The book written by the Committee on the Function of Nursing, titled *A Program for the Nursing Profession,* came out about the same time as the Brown Report. They were not connected in any way, and I'm not sure that Esther Brown even knew that this committee, which had been brought together by Louise Mc-Manus, existed. This group did not do research in the technical use of the term but used armchair strategy. Then Louise McManus enunciated rather specifically the differentiation of function. As a result of many ideas about professional and technical education, my doctoral dissertation was concerned with the introduction of a new worker in nursing, a technician. The dissertation also proposed where these new workers would be prepared (the community college) and a curriculum for their preparation.

GS: Was this project published?

MM: Yes, it was published in 1951 under the title *The Education of Nursing Technicians.* Later, Louise McManus wrote up a project proposal based on this proposed program. One individual gave $110,000 to finance a five-year project to test and develop the new program. The project took the form of a cooperative, which meant that we would not set up what you might call an ideal exhibit kind of program, but rather we would follow the pattern that had been introduced at Teachers College of cooperating with existing and ongoing educational institutions if they worked with the ongoing school system. We chose seven colleges with which we would work, with the understanding that each of these colleges would develop a program according to certain criteria, operate it themselves as they would any other program, and work with us then in the curriculum development and the sharing of data. We would offer consultation services to those programs. The $110,000 we got, which was $22,000 a year, financed consultation visits, workshops for the faculty, and the collection of data, with the colleges financing the operation of the program itself. I think the single biggest contribution of the associate degree program was to show that it was possible for colleges to assume the responsibility for a nursing program. This meant total responsibility for the nursing program: They admitted the students; they set standards for graduation; the students were held to the same requirements as all other students. The college employed the faculty and paid the total faculty on the same basis as all faculty members. In other words, the nursing program became an integral part of the college. That was not true in the fifties in baccalaureate education, and I think that, really, the financing was the most important achievement.

GS: *Your ideas seem to fit in with those of Martha Rogers?*

MM: Well, I think Martha Rogers and I are in agreement the greater part of the time. She feels very definitely that we should have professional education, that we should have baccalaureate education which is truly professional education; and she makes the comment often that many a person has a degree without professional education, has a baccalaureate degree but without having had professional education. And I agree with that. She also feels very strongly that there is a role for the technical practitioner; in that we are in agreement. She really comes out strongly for this separation of the professional and the technical functions and hence the professional and the technical workers.

The Professional Practitioner

GS: *How do you define the professional nurse, and where should she get her education:*

MM: Well, I think the professional practitioner—and I'm indebted to Louise McManus for this—is one who has functions (I'm almost quoting this from Louise McManus) comparable with those of a physician. In other words, in looking at the patient, the professional practitioner would identify the diagnosis, if you want to use that word, that demands nursing intervention. I hate that word; it conveys a meaning which I don't like. I would identify the task of the professional practitioner as that of identifying the diagnosis, the gathering of such data as are essential with respect to identifying the diagnosis; making a nursing care plan which would implement, which would put into action that which the patient needs to have from the nurse; delegating to those working with the nurse those tasks or activities or aspects of the function that do not require the nurses's knowledge and skill; evaluating the plan, and replanning. This, then, would require a kind of education which would be geared to producing this kind of person from the beginning rather than starting with the technical skill and forcing the person into the technician role first, before going into the professional. I would see the professional skills as, for example, taking the nursing history, interviewing. I think this is a highly developed skill which requires a kind of expertise the technician does not have and does not need and should not attempt. This is a kind of in-depth probing (and I don't mean in the negative sense) to get the information the professional needs, then interpret that information in a way that lends credence to the nursing care which that patient will receive. I would stress the role of the professional and the skills of the professional from the very beginning. Now if they need technical skills of some sort—manual skills—I would tack them on at the end or make them electives or something, but put them out of the mainstream. What I've said many times—and this gives me some worry with respect to the associate degree or technical program—is that many an associate degree graduate goes into a baccalaureate program and comes out a technician with a baccalaureate degree; and many a practical nurse goes into an A.D. program and comes out with an associate degree, but with no change in either abilities or concepts, and is still a practical nurse. I think to do this does grave injustice to both kinds of education. Now I've been thinking for a long time that we should develop, experimentally at first, a one-year nursing program which would be based on a liberal arts degree, making the grand total for nursing preparation five years. In that, then, you could develop a program quite different from what we have now. If all of the groundwork is laid, one wouldn't have to worry about communication skills. Students would have had a background in the general biological and physical sciences; a background in the general sociological, anthropological, and political science aspect. They would have had logic, philosophy, and history, all of the latter now missing in baccalaureate nursing programs. It would be a foundation upon which to build. You would have a more mature student, and you certainly would have a motivated student. If someone with a four-year college degree chose nursing, one could assume considerable motivation. It would then, I think, make us more comparable with some of the other professions: law, medicine, social work, engineering. I think that might establish a little more purity, if you will, which is now kind of missing in the baccalaureate education. We try to do a little bit of everything in the four years. I think that may be what I would like to see happen in the future rather than the development of four-year programs.

The Birth and Growth of the Associate Degree Programs

GS: Could you comment on the first associate degree program?

MM: We had seven programs at the beginning, and those seven programs developed: two in 1952, three in 1953, one in 1954, and one in 1955. We chose those first for a variety of reasons; first, location, so that we would cover the United States; second, under different administrative structures; third, there was one school for the black nurses because blacks were then not readily admitted to nursing school. All of these programs remain except Virginia Intermont. Virginia Intermont closed, not because it wasn't successful, but because it's a very small, church-related school that did not wish to get large. Had it developed a nursing program, which would be financially feasible, it would have had to outweigh the other students in the college. Also, we had to go into states where the state boards of nursing would permit a two-year program. Many states at that time had laws, or regulations, which required thirty-six months and specified the actual number of days, the number of courses, the sequence of courses, and all that type of thing. We had to go into states in which the state board was willing to do as we requested, which was to waive all existing requirements and let this program develop as outlined, with the guarantee that the graduates would be qualified to take the licensing examination at the end of the program. That meant that the faculties themselves could develop their own curriculum. California had very much more rigid regulations but gave us permission for the program in Pasadena, *with* restrictions. We have been asked recently why we didn't request a change in the law before the programs began. We had no basis for asking for a change in the law; thus we had to work within the framework of the law or the regulations of the state. The requirements or restrictions which California placed upon these programs meant that the first programs there tended to be very much more traditional than those in the other states because they had to provide certain courses in certain sequences for certain lengths, which we did not have in any other state. Almost imme-

diately upon the completion of the five-year period, laws—or regulations, as the case might be—began to change in other states, until
today there are no longer any regulations in any of the jurisdictions that
prohibit the two-year program from developing. We had a very rapid
change of law and regulation once the project was over. I think in the
mid-fifties, somewhere around 1957 or so, there were about thirteen
states that would permit these programs, and now we have fifty states
and three jurisdictions. In California, an amendment to the law eliminat-
ing the internship was introduced because they found the internship
absolutely unnecessary. It was found that within a matter of days to
weeks, the graduate was doing the work of the registered nurse. The
amendment was in effect for five years, and at the end of that time the
amendment became part of the law. Since the law was changed, the
programs in California have developed along very much less traditional
lines. I think the one at San Jose, with which Verle Waters was associated, was one of the first developed according to other than the old
traditional sequence of courses. Then the one at Marin was developed
along markedly different lines. That began a whole trend of changes.

GS: How was the project evaluated?

MM: We carried on two evaluation studies. One was toward the end
of the project itself, during the last two years. Lassar Gotkin was the
one who did that part of the study which evaluated the graduates at
work. The evaluation study was carried on in two ways, partly by questionnaire and partly by interview. Lassar Gotkin interviewed a sample of
the graduates of all of the original programs that had graduated a class
at the time of the study. He interviewed graduates working in some
twenty-five hospitals. He interviewed the head nurses and the directors
of nursing service. The result of that study, to put it very briefly, was that
something like three out of four of those graduates being evaluated
were rated as good as, or better than, their counterparts who were of
the same experience working in the same unit, under the same head
nurse, for the same length of time. We didn't have quite a matched
sample in that study because the non-associate degree graduates were
not in sufficient number in all situations to have a completely matched
sample. Now, a word about that. We were forced in this evaluation into
comparing them with graduates of other programs, not against determined criteria. There were no qualitative standards then identified by
which you could objectively evaluate the graduates. Therefore, we had
to take what was the current norm—the existing graduate—which,
while it was not the way it should have been done, was the only way it
could have been done. We were specific in the characteristics which
we used for comparison. The forms we used in this study are in the

published report, *The Community College Education for Nursing;* unfortunately that is now out of print but should be in many libraries. When we finished our project in 1957, we had about $10,000 left and we asked the donor if we could keep it for a second evaluation study which would be done somewhat later. The second study included a much larger sample. We included the original seven programs and added to it about 50 percent of all those programs that had developed since. We took a sample of the graduates from these several programs. This study was done entirely by mailed questionnaires instead of interviews as in the first study. We used essentially the same questionnaires; this will be found in the report of that study.[4] We found virtually the same results; about 75 percent of the graduates were rated as functioning as well as, or better than, their counterparts with similar experience. We also had another part in both of those studies, the state board test results. In the first evaluation we found that the graduates were able to pass at about the same rate as all others taking the same examination. There was less than a percentage point difference. In the second study, the percentage passing the first time had gone down, but so had it for all graduates. That aspect is developed quite extensively in the report. Why the state board test scores or the passing rate had gone down in all programs I don't know. It has been speculated that associate degree graduates have more difficulty because the state board test examinations are set up in the traditional lines: medicine, surgery, pediatrics, obstetrics, and psychiatry, whereas that is not the way the typical A.D. program is organized. These, then, are the main points in the evaluation of the graduates undertaken in our project. There have been many other evaluation studies, but I haven't been involved in those.

Leadership

GS: Could we talk a little bit more about your leadership role at Teachers College? We have discussed it here and there, but I think there's more to say.

MM: I suppose chairmanships represent some evidence of leadership. We had at the time, right after the Brown Report, what we called the prespecialization program. We changed our program from specialization on the baccalaureate to making the baccalaureate at least approximate that which we now call a generic program. I was chairwoman of that program and was largely influential in the plans that went into it

---

[4] Published as *The Evaluation of Graduates of Associate Degree Programs,* Teachers College Press, Columbia University, New York, 1972.

and its implementation, and I advised students. As a part of this program we developed several nursing courses, one of which was Leadership and Team Nursing. I was the first to teach that course and taught it several semesters.

GS: Is that right? Was the concept yours?

MM: The concept comes out of *A Program for the Nursing Profession* and Louise McManus. You have to kind of read between the lines, but you see the team concept coming out. If you do not divide people's work by what the procedure is—for example, all temperatures can be taken by practical nurses, all enemas can be given by practical nurses—and if you don't divide nurses' assignments according to categories of illness, what do you have? Well, the *Program for the Nursing Profession* report says you take what the patient needs as your clue and you have a team approach, you see; rather than identifying a task you take "what does the patient need?" Eli Ginzberg was really the one who wrote the report *A Program for the Nursing Profession.* He was secretary of that group to which I referred, which Louise McManus initiated. One of the things we said needed to be taught to the professional practitioners in the prespecialization program was leadership skills: how to be a team leader now. If you look back at the catalogue of Teachers College, Nursing 150P, I was its instructor. We started out at Morrisania Hospital. We went then to Woman's Hospital and about that time, or thereafter, Delafield, and that's when Eleanor Lambertsen came into the picture. I decreased my activities in that area when the project came into being; I was the chief administrator of the Cooperative Research Project, which took from 1952 to 1957. Then we were engaged in another project from 1959 to 1964, which was financed by the Kellogg Foundation. That was a four-state project in which Texas, California, New York, and Florida participated. Each state had three parts to its project. One was a demonstration center where an ongoing program could be used for visitors; second, a teacher training institution, which was Teachers College (we had a special program set up for the preparation of teachers); and third, providing some financial aid in the planning year to institutions instituting a two-year program. I was responsible for the part of the project at Teachers College, and I also cooperated with the other two parts of the project, the demonstration center and the conference group, which helped to determine which program should get the planning money. So, from 1959 to 1964 that was my major responsibility along with teaching.

GS: What did you focus upon before your retirement?

MM: In the later years from, I would say, the early sixties to the time of my retirement, my chief leadership role was with the doctoral students. I chaired the Doctoral Committee of the department for about ten years. That committee was responsible for all of the policies, the procedures, and the activities with respect to the doctoral program of the department; those all were, of course, consonant with those of the college. I was on the Doctor of Education Committee for the college for two different terms of three years. I was also on the Faculty Executive Committee for two different terms. The Faculty Executive Committee was elected to office by the entire faculty of the college. Membership on the Doctor of Education Committee is an appointed office. The work with the Doctoral Committee in our own department had to do with the development of what we call certification examination, the review of candidates, the admission of candidates. Any problem, issue, question, plan, and procedure that had to do with doctoral candidates came into the Doctoral Committee, of which I was chairperson. So that meant I had to work very closely with faculty members and with students. I advised a large number of doctoral candidates, and I suspect that's as much leadership as anything, helping them with their dissertations. I am still doing it in an informal way with several doctoral candidates.

GS: Do you care to add to your feelings about nursing education?

MM: Let me say I have one general feeling about nursing education at this moment. I think we're making too many compromises. I think professional education—or baccalaureate education—is not doing what it should. I think associate degree education is doing more than it should. I believe we should straighten this out pretty soon. I do not believe we can go on without greater distinction between the programs in nursing. We have arrived at a point where there are more than half of the students today in some kind of collegiate nursing education program. The diploma schools are declining. I believe we must have a greater difference in the nursing care that patients get pretty soon, or we can't justify prolonged educational programs. I'm not sure that we are yet making the impact on nursing care that we should be making. I would blame nursing service in part for this, but I would also put some of that blame at the feet of the educators. I think until we get professional practitioners honestly prepared and equipped to practice in no other way, we will not get professional practice in the hospitals accepted or permitted or required.

GS: What is your opinion on preparing teachers for nursing schools?

MM: Of course, coming from a teachers' college I probably have some bias. I do not believe that simply knowing one's subject makes one a teacher. I believe that the arguments between ''should you know *what"* or "should you know *how"* are all spurious arguments. I think you need to know both and that there are techniques and skills of teaching just as there are skills and techniques of surgery; and the greatest physiologist in the world, or anatomist in the world, does not become a surgeon. He or she has to know how to do surgery. So, I don't believe the clinical specialist is prepared to teach unless skills in teaching and curriculum development are included in the preparation. I have no qualms about people being qualified in the practice of nursing, but they need something else if they are to become teachers. I think we gave them both of those things at Teachers College. We are credited with giving only the how-to's, the how-to-do-it; but we also have clinical courses, and they are as vital in our curriculum as are the curriculum skills. But teachers need to know how to develop a curriculum, how to implement a curriculum.

Opinions on What the Big Issues Are in Nursing Today

GS: What do you see, then, as some of the main or major issues in nursing today, and the trend?

MM: Well, I think one of the issues in nursing—not precisely in education—is, what is the American Nurses' Association (A.N.A.) doing and going to do? I have some qualms about the emphasis upon collective bargaining and the economics side of it. I feel very strongly about the strikes. That's one issue, I think. What the role of A.N.A. is in the education of nurses is, I think, another issue. I had great hopes for the Commission on Education, the whole commission structure when it went in a few years ago. I think the Commission on Education has been absolutely dormant until very recently. They showed more vitality at the last meeting. I think they should have taken a very much more active role than they have. They should have set the stage in leadership. I think what the A.N.A. has done about the Position Paper is incredible. I think their statement in 1973 relative to diploma programs was unbelievable, *unbelievable!* The A.N.A. has done nothing since 1965 but to dilute the Position Paper, which has been the official position of the association since 1965. Another issue might be which organization should be responsible for accreditation of nursing programs. I happen to believe that accreditation belongs in the A.N.A. or under its general auspices. I do not believe it belongs in a nonnursing organization.

GS: Why do you believe it should be under the A.N.A.?

MM: Because I believe a profession controls its own education, its own entrance into the profession. I think we ought to be responsible for the kind of programs we develop and what kind of products we produce. As far as I know, all other professions do that. Perhaps the new organization, the American Association of Colleges of Nursing (A.A.C.N.), will fill this role.

GS: *What do you think is going to happen? What do you predict?*

MM: At this moment I would hate to predict who will win; it will depend a lot on the leadership of A.N.A. I think the role of A.N.A., with all of its activities, is one of the great issues of the day.

I think the number and kind of nursing programs we have is another issue. We have about 1300 schools of nursing today, and I don't think we need 1300 schools. There are too many master's programs to staff properly. I think we cannot dilute the quality of education by having so many programs which we cannot staff with qualified faculty. Most master's programs today have unqualified faculty in large measure. And then we talk about promoting doctoral programs. Where are we going to get faculty for those programs? I think we need to come soon to some decisions about the number and kind of programs. I think we need to come to some kind of decision with respect to how many nurses we need. How many can we support? How many can the economy support?

GS: *When you talk about nursing, are you talking about the professional nurse?*

MM: I'm talking about *all* nurses. I think we need to determine how many nurses we need in total, then what proportion would be from baccalaureate and what proportion from associate degree programs. My own feeling is that the number of associate degree graduates will greatly exceed the number of professional graduates, if you go by what's happened in other professions, in other occupations, where a commonly cited ratio is 1 professional to 8 or 10 technical workers. I think we ought to discontinue practical nurse programs as soon as possible. Instead of declining, they seem to be proliferating.

GS: *You mentioned quite a few key issues. Do you see any more?*

MM: I think the whole question of how nurses are used is certainly a problem. I think if we employ professional practitioners, we ought to permit—to demand—that they practice in a professional way. So, too, the technical. I don't think there is any such thing as an interchangeable nurse.

GS: What is your view on the concept of the so-called extended role of the nurse–nurse-practitioner–clinical specialist?

MM: I do not believe in the extended role. I don't think you extend a role. I think, rather, you fulfill it. And if we were really fulfilling the role of nurse, many of the things they're talking about we should have been doing, for they are clearly within the responsibility of a professionally prepared person. Now, when you say extended role and mean physical examination and physical diagnosis, then I think we're into difficulty. There is a very good article by Barbara Bates et al., cautioning against preparing for physical diagnosis skills on the part of every nurse. Many schools have introduced courses in physical diagnosis, and so forth, without having people qualified to teach them and, also, without questioning whether or not they should be taught. And I think we've got plenty in nursing without getting into medical diagnosis. So, if this is what is meant by extended role, I find this hard to accept. I also find this label ''nurse-practitioner'' hard to accept. What else is a nurse but a practitioner?

GS: What, briefly, are your views on the ''ladder'' concept?

MM: Well, if all that can be conceived as baccalaureate education is putting a layer on top of a technical education, then baccalaureate nursing education is bankrupt. A professional program is not layers on layers of rather discrete things, in my opinion; I think the ladder, and its popularity under some guise of democracy or social mobility, leads to much confusion as to goals.

GS: Do you have any other issues you'd like to mention?

MM: Licensure of individual nurses versus institutional licensure is one. I have moved very definitely toward belief in two licensures: one for the professional nurses and one for the technical nurses, with different labels. We get into all kinds of emotional feelings when we talk about labels. So I think we must move to a clarification of the licensure issue. I think there's much to be done in the area of nursing service. We have a paucity of prepared nursing service directors, and the need in that area is tremendous because so many nursing services are being run on antiquated bases and with procedures popular, but not necessarily good, thirty or forty years ago. I think one of our great lacks is qualified nursing service personnel. I think the move which was made a couple of years ago to designate a clinical major for a nursing service administrator is wrong, too. They're not doing clinical work; they are administering a nursing service, and it runs a gamut of the clinical areas of practice. I think continuing education—whether it should be mandatory or voluntary—is another major issue, and I would vote for mandatory.

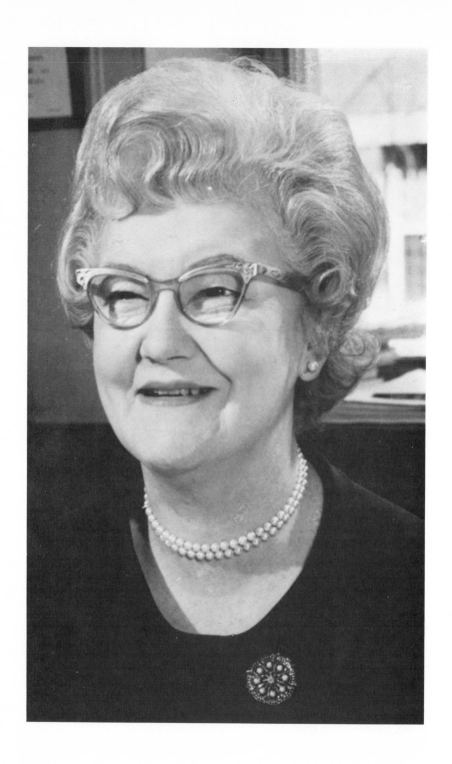

10

. . . for her keen vision and her appreciation of the contributions that nursing can make have led her to promote excellence in nursing, with the knowledge that nursing must expand to meet the needs of a changing society. The example she has set in her own career will serve to remind others that the pursuit of excellence is in the true service of a profession[1]

. . . pleased to acknowledge her monumental contributions to the profession of nursing and to the improvement of the health care delivery system to the People of Illinois . . . [2]

[1]From American Nurses' Association's Honorary Recognition to M. K. Mullane, May 3, 1972, Detroit, Michigan.
[2]State of Illinois Seventy-seventh General Assembly, House of Representatives, House Resolution 760, June 22, 1972.

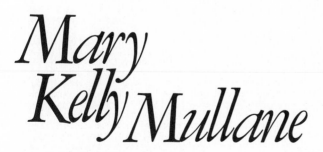

Mary Kelly Mullane

ADMINISTRATOR

*M*ary Kelly Mullane[3] was born September 15, 1909, the eldest of three children. Her background is Irish Catholic. Her father and grandfather, both native New Yorkers, were businessmen in New York City and were active in local politics.

Her mother and father had been volunteers in a new hospital opened in New Jersey in 1925. Mary Kelly Mullane decided to apply to the School of Nursing. She liked nursing and, although several times she had the opportunity to take up something else, realized that she had found her "niche in nursing."

She received her registered nurse diploma in 1931 from Holy Name Hospital School of Nursing, Teaneck, New Jersey; B.S. (1936) and M.A. (1942) degrees in nursing from Teachers College, Columbia University, New York; and a Ph.D. degree from the University of Chicago in March 1957 with a major in administration in higher education.[4]

Among Dr. Mullane's professional positions are her administrative leadership as assistant to Dean Katherine E. Faville at Wayne State University (1944–1952); Dean of the College of Nursing at the State University of Iowa (1959–1962); and Dean of the College of Nursing at the University of Illinois (1962–1971). Dr. Mullane has received numerous awards and honors, among them two honorary doctoral degrees. She has been active in professional organizations and has served as a consultant to many groups. She has written numerous articles.[5]

Dr. Mullane is recognized for her leadership particularly in the following areas:

1 As a member of the Board of Directors, Association of Collegiate Schools of Nursing (A.C.S.N.)

2 As a participant in the Structure Study of the six national nursing organizations

3 For her role at Wayne State University, where she helped Dean Faville build one of the strongest collegiate schools of nursing

---

[3] She married John Thompson Mullane in 1951; her husband was an accountant until his retirement in 1967.

[4] The title of her Ph.D. dissertation was "Identification and Validation of Criteria of Excellence for Nursing Service Administrators."

[5] Among her writings are "Improvement of Nursing Service," *News and Views*, pp. 1–4, August 1957; "What Is Administration?" *Michigan Nurse*, pp. 1965–67, December 1957; "Has Nursing Changed?", *Nursing Outlook*, p. 323, June 1958; "Validation of Criteria for Nursing Service Administration: Report of a Study," *Proceedings of the Forty-first Convention of the American Nurses' Association*, June 1958; *Education for Nursing Service Administration: An Experience in Program Development by Fourteen Universities*, W. K. Kellogg Foundation, Battle Creek, Mich., Dec. 1, 1958; "Nursing Faculty Roles and Functions in the Large University Setting," *Memo to Members, Council of Baccalaureate and Higher Degree Programs*, pp. 1–4, National League of Nursing Education, New York, 1939; "Women and Their Role in Shaping Society," *Occupational Health Nursing*, pp. 7–9, June 1970; and "Summary, Synthesis, and Future Directions," *Research on Nursing Staffing in Hospitals*, Report of the Conference, May 1972, Division of Nursing, H.E.W., Washington, D.C., Government Printing Office, March 1973.

4   As dean of the College of Nursing, where she developed the University of Illinois College of Nursing into one of the leading nursing programs in the United States

5   For her role in faculty development at the University of Illinois

6   For advancing better administration of nursing services

Contributions to Nursing

GS: *What do you consider your main contributions to nursing?*

MM: I've helped organize, and pushed forward, college education for nursing. I don't feel I played any particularly distinguished role in curriculum specifically. I felt I was more effective in enlarging enrollment, developing sophisticated faculty, and obtaining resources of space and equipment. I consider those my principal contributions. I'm sure that we'd both agree there are a few people in this world, and I certainly am not one of them, who have really achieved significant, demonstrable progress all alone. This year I've been a university professor for thirty years. I became associate professor of nursing in 1944 at Wayne under Katherine Faville, and I've been involved, except for seven years, ever since. I was to some degree an instrument of major changes in education for nursing at Wayne from 1944 to 1952. When I left there, I came here to Illinois. I suppose I've been a kind of builder, modernizer of curriculum, developer of faculty, and provider of space. I suppose another facet in my career is that I'm often said to be a politician.

GS: *What is meant by that?*

MM: Well, I'm not sure I know, but I've always been rather sensitive to the fact that most progress is made as a result of getting people to acquiesce in support of what needs to be done. For example, Rita Kelleher[6] and I [we were then the principal officers of the Council of Baccalaureate and Higher Degree Programs of the National League of Nursing Education (N.L.N.E.)] came up with a proposal to have more autonomous functioning of the Council. The proposal, in the form of changed operating rules, was voted by the council and was, in fact, approved by the Board of Directors of the N.L.N.E. The board was willing to try it. Unfortunately the changed operation was not imple-

---

[6] Then Dean, School of Nursing, Boston University.

mented after we went out of office. It is my judgment that if it had been, we might not have had to create again an American Association of Colleges of Nursing (A.A.C.N.). I think there could have been and should have been more autonomy in the operation of those collegiate schools within the League.

I have been active in the legislative planning and program defense for the Nurse Training Act as planner and interpreter. I have to be careful how I say this. I'm a public employee in the state of Illinois, and we have a "Hatch Act."

GS: You have a what?

MM: Hatch, H-a-t-c-h, Hatch Act. Actually, Hatch Act is the name of the federal statute, and I don't know the name of the state statute in Illinois. You don't need to know either, but what it means, of course, is that public employees may not lobby.

I've always been interested in interpretations of that principle because I don't think being public employees necessarily means that we have to be second-class citizens. We are prohibited from partisan political activities and from formal lobbying, but we are not prevented from making our views known or from making explicit the likely consequences of alternative public courses of action or programs.

In 1969–1971, as vice president of the Deans of Collegiate Schools of Nursing, I helped design the deans' action program in support of the Nurse Training Act. That's what I think people mean when they say I'm a politician. I think I do try to persuade people to what I believe to be right. I think that's what people mean when they allude to my political skill. I see political know-how to be necessary to success in building any kind of program, whether legislative or educational. I've made some mistakes, and then I hope I've been big enough to stand up and say I was wrong.

I'll tell you what I don't do very well. I've never been very good at consolidating things, and I do think there's a relationship between the institutional or social needs of the time and the people who filter into leadership positions.

GS: What was your experience in relation to the Structure Study and all six organizations?

MM: Very interesting. You know, that's twenty-four years ago this year. At the time (about 1950) I was a member of the Board of Directors of the A.C.S.N., and as a member of that board I was on the Structure Study.[7] There are other people who can remember it better than I, but

---

[7] See Josephine Nelson, *Horizons in Nursing,* The MacMillan Company, New York, 1950, for a

I remember the great hopes we had for it. I think we really thought that we would be able to get one nursing organization. There were, I suppose, three main reasons that I recall why we had to give up the idea of one organization and create two. One was the tax-exempt position of one organization that would also include a legislative lobbying function. We knew the American Nurses' Association (A.N.A.) had to continue as the profession's lobbyist in the interest of both the public and the profession; yet the lobbying function would affect the A.N.A.'s tax status under the Internal Revenue Code, and would deny to the A.N.A. foundation grants or any other private contributions because donors would have to pay taxes on those grants or gifts. A second reason was that we really did study the social positions of some professional groups who had all of their functions in one organization. We looked especially at the American Medical Association (A.M.A.), including its Council on Medical Education. We didn't see the A.M.A. doing very much in the way of regulation, control, or improvement of organized medical services. I think we did really feel that we ought to separate the welfare of nurses from the public interest so that each might have the best attention we could give it. The welfare of individual nurses, and the advancement of the profession as a profession, was urgent, as it still is. In those days the eight-hour day for nurses was not yet adopted everywhere, and job security was even more tenuous than it is today; so we knew that the individual welfare of nurses had to be looked out for. Nursing has always responded to social need, often giving a higher priority to the public need than to the profession's own welfare. To assure continuance of this dedication we decided to separate organized services and education from the necessary self-development of the profession.

The third reason was that part of the strength in the National Organization for Public Health Nursing (N.O.P.H.N.) and in the N.L.N.E. stemmed from active nonnurse members, and we didn't want to lose that kind of support. Informal inquiry was made of the International Council of Nurses (I.C.N.) about the acceptability of an A.N.A. that in any way, even at the associate level of some kind, would have nonnurse members. The I.C.N. replied that because of then existing political considerations in other countries, an A.N.A. including nonregistered nurse members could not continue membership in the I.C.N. Now the literature may show other reasons, but these are the three that I remember most clearly as preventing a decision for one national nursing organization. As a matter of fact, I suspect that those three reasons would be found as valid in 1974 as they were in 1948. The literature of the period covered the matter thoroughly; for example, annual proceedings

summary of the Structure Study.

of the N.L.N.E. and the *American Journal of Nursing (A.J.N.)* from about 1945 through 1952 carry full reports of this great professional effort.

I lived, too, through the years when the nursing profession, through the A.N.A., was really undertaking the integration of black nurses despite bitter resistance from many state nurses' associations. The National Association of Colored Graduate Nurses (N.A.C.G.N.) was one of the six national nursing associations collaborating in the Structure Study. The education of other members of the Structure Study group by the board of the N.A.C.G.N. was a poignant and exciting, sensitizing experience. It led promptly and directly to the decision to take every step to bring registered nurses who were black into full professional membership. I personally gained much from this leadership experience under impressive professional women such as Mabel K. Staupers and Estelle M. Osborne. Students of interracial relations in any professional group would be enlightened by the strategy and parliamentary processes employed in the A.N.A.'s House of Delegates, which eliminated racial bars to state and national association membership of registered nurses.

Immediately following World War II, as collegiate nursing education matured, sensitivity to the plight of black students increased. Perhaps some review of the development of the programs at Wayne, whose faculty I joined in 1944, would illustrate both the nursing educational developments of the period and the opening study opportunities for black nursing students.

Wayne State University

Katherine E. Faville had become professor and head of the department of nursing in the College of Liberal Arts at Wayne in April 1944. This was her second period of service at Wayne; she had been there from 1929 until 1944, organizing courses through which public health nurses, employed principally at the Detroit Board of Health and the Detroit Visiting Nurse Association, could qualify for the certificate in public health nursing, a thirty-hour program then recognized by civil service commissions and other boards as qualifying registered nurses for specialty practice in public health nursing. Later some courses for head nurses and supervisors were added. At the time, Wayne's nursing program served employed registered nurses who wished to study in the late afternoon and evening. Relatively few registered nurses met the requirements for the bachelor's degree using the public health or supervision courses as the nursing major. As students became interested in university study for beginning nursing, the university offered two years of liberal arts and sciences, in completion of which students sought admission to the hospital school of their choice. When the hospital's nursing diploma had been earned, the university awarded the degree bachelor of science in nursing. This arrangement seems strange now, but in the 1930s and 1940s it was typical of many collegiate nursing programs. By early 1944 it was evident to the nurse leaders of Detroit that the nursing program at Wayne needed major revision, and they joined the university administration in persuading Katherine Faville to return to Wayne. I joined her on the faculty in September 1944.

High on the agenda for reform was the creation of an autonomous school of nursing. Dean Faville convinced the dean of liberal arts and the executive vice president that nursing's full development of undergraduate and graduate programs, as well as its potential enrollment, would require a full-status academic unit. Curriculum revision of the baccalaureate program for beginning students was quickened by finding the files of students whom we could not trace because they were not enrolled in any hospital school program in the Detroit area. The mystery was solved when one young black woman appeared at the university, her transcript from Harlem Hospital, New York, in hand, requesting her bachelor's degree in nursing. At that time, 1945, no hospital school in Detroit admitted black students; therefore Wayne's black students had to seek admission elsewhere. In 1945 no one called this discrimination; few questioned the practice. Dean Faville was one person who did. She sought counsel from black women leaders of Detroit and from distinguished black nurses known nationally. With their advice, especially that of Estelle M. Osborne, then deputy director of the N.L.N.E., strategy was planned both to attract more qualified young women from Detroit's black community and to integrate them into the revised baccalaureate program. Appeal for support and encouragement from the black community was especially necessary because black communities had not yet begun to lay claim to their fair share of our country's opportunities.

Dean Faville in reviewing the several programs she found at Wayne, began by identifying the nature and mission of Wayne as a (then) city university. She taught me clearly that no program like nursing could prosper in a university unless that program was typical of the nature, mission, program form, and quality standards of the university of which it was an integral part. I learned that claims justifying nursing's "difference" in the academic world detracted alarmingly from its acceptance there by other disciplines. We began to lay out the kind of undergraduate curriculum we would have to have if nursing was to be like other university programs. We had two great assets in the university: one was a president who understood and believed in nursing's promise as an academic discipline; the other was an associate dean of the College of Liberal Arts, a chemist, who insisted that our curriculum models should be taken from laboratory sciences and undergraduate university programs, from undergraduate medical education rather than from the internship and residency programs typical of education in hospitals, including the programs of their schools of nursing.

I can remember clearly the day Dean Faville and I went to the President's office with our proposed generic baccalaureate program. We were full of pleas, arguments, justifications, made more urgent by our fears generated by projections of needed faculty and other costs the university would have to meet to implement the program. I learned a priceless lesson that day when, in the midst of a torrent of justification from me, President Henry remarked that I had been giving good arguments but I had not asked the crucial question: "Mr. President, on what grounds does this university give a degree in a major, bachelor of science in nursing, which it does not teach?" He meant, of course, that the major was taught by the hospital schools. He went on to point out that the university was obliged to determine whether nursing was one of the fields within the mission of the university. If so, and if its priority among other demands upon resources available to the university was high, the university was then obliged to search for the resources required. He approved the creation of the generic bachelor's program and agreed to request the board of trustees' approval of Dean Faville's request for phased-in budget for five years' "start-up" costs.

Then we had to make arrangements for teaching privileges for our faculty in nearby hospitals, many of which had, and retained, their own hospital schools. Contracts were worked out under which our faculty were in control of Wayne students' assignments. Black and white students were assigned and accepted equally. Perhaps things went so well because all Wayne students lived either in the university dormitory or at home.

The next phase of development in nursing was the beginning of graduate education for specialty practice in nursing. Much of the impetus for this came from Mildred Tuttle, then director of the Division of

Nursing at the W. K. Kellogg Foundation, and from Ruth Taylor, then Chief of Nursing at the Children's Bureau. In about 1947 they and other nurse leaders began to sense the dramatic changes in technology in medical and nursing care, resulting from efforts required to win a war. If there's any good that comes out of a war, it is, I think, in the advancement of developments in medical science. Antibiotics, new therapy for burns and trauma, and group psychotherapy, which, developed in World War II were, in fact, precursors of more to come from the space program. Revolutionizing medical care, they revolutionized nursing care as well. These women recognized that nursing's response would be crucial to conversion of these medical developments into patient care. W. K. Kellogg Foundation and Children's Bureau grants to Wayne and to other universities made possible the creation of graduate majors in clinical nursing in renovated master's programs in nursing. Soon the National Institute of Mental Health made funds available for graduate programs in psychiatric nursing. Dean Faville used all these funds as "seed" money to revise and strengthen nursing programs, but her budgeting was always based on President Henry's principle that the university is responsible for basic support for its programs. Dean Faville used outside grants to start programs, but her program plans included annual budgets in sequence showing increasing university support and decreasing outside support. Dean Faville and President Henry taught me the advantages and modes of being a "hard money" administrator long before the term was coined.

GS: *What made you decide to go on for a doctorate?*

MM: I'd been at Wayne seven years. We didn't have any kind of sabbatical program there, and I was getting tired, professionally and personally; the only way I could take any time off at all was to go to school. So I decided that I'd start my doctorate. President Henry and Dean Faville weren't happy about it, both feeling that nursing had not yet evolved to the point of needing its academicians to have doctorates. Finally President Henry said that if I could bring him the names of six of my colleagues who were thinking the way I did, he would approve my leave request.

At this time I was a member of the board of the A.C.S.N. and knew most professors of nursing. There was no list of nurses with doctorates; but from my own acquaintances I easily found six who had already earned doctorates and six more of them in doctoral study. Their names satisfied President Henry, who approved my leave. I started that summer (1950) at Teachers College, Columbia University.

While I was there, Mildred Tuttle called me from the Kellogg Foundation to say that the foundation would support a seminar at the University
of Chicago in education for nursing services administration, and wished
to explore my willingness to participate in it. They planned to have three
faculty members: an expert in public administration, one in educational
planning, and one in nursing administration. In exploring the seminar
plans, both at the W. K. Kellogg Foundation and with the project director at the University of Chicago, Dr Ralph Tyler, I learned that I could
combine experience in the seminar (as part-time nurse faculty member)
and study toward the Ph.D. at the University of Chicago. I was committed to return to Wayne with a year's doctoral study completed by September 1951. Combining that commitment with the seminar's work was
a heavy load but was especially attractive, so I transferred to the University of Chicago in September 1950. The challenge examination system
at Chicago was very helpful, and early success in doctoral qualifying
exams helped meet both commitments.

Interest in Administration

GS: What brought about your interest in administration?

MM: My interest in administration goes back more than thirty years.
During World War II, I served as director of the nursing service at Receiving General, Detroit. Though I'd been a teacher most of my life, that
was a very interesting experience.

My interest in the theory and practice of administration began at
Reclining Hospital and was quickened to educational administrative experience at Wayne, but was made more systematic through the Kellogg
seminar. That seminar was, in my view, a milepost of development in
our profession. The fourteen university graduate programs which
stemmed from it offered for the first time preparation for the management of nursing services as distinct from combined management of
schools and services. I wrote the evaluative report of this fourteen-
university program, which the foundation entitled *Education for Nursing
Service Administration.*

GS: Did you go back to Wayne?

MM: Yes, I went home and got married that fall (1951), set up my
new household, went back to full-time teaching at Wayne, organized
the nursing service administration major in the master's program at
Wayne, and again became the Assistant to the Dean.

University of Iowa

GS: *What made you decide to go to the University of Iowa?*

MM: I liked the university. Its College of Nursing was soundly organized as an autonomous college. Myrtle Kitchell Aydelatte had been the
first dean, and her work had led to the college's genuine acceptance in
the university community and in the state. The curriculum still retained
some of the vestiges of a hospital school in that the junior and senior
students at the College of Nursing of the University of Iowa were
housed in the hospital's nurses' home, were not charged tuition, and as
a consequence manned the University Hospital. The next step in matur-
ing the nursing program was to complete the transition of the undergraduate curriculum in nursing to one entirely controlled by its faculty,
and one supported as were other programs at the University of Iowa. I
managed to bring that about in the three and a half years that I was
there.

GS: *What kind of strategy did the change require?*

MM: Even before I was chosen for Iowa and agreed to accept their
offer of appointment, the faculty had made it very clear that the next
step was these curriculum changes. So I committed myself to the faculty, and the university administration committed itself to me for the required changes. In due time the changes were planned and submitted
to the president. Since the college was already staffed for the instructional requirements, the proposed changes carried no increased instructional costs to the university's academic budget. However, re-
placement of student services to the University Hospital would cost
about $500,000 per year. Then the university president said they
couldn't afford it. My position to him was that maybe the hospital
couldn't afford it, but I proposed that the university couldn't afford anything else educationally, pointing out the educational principle that
President Henry had taught me years before. Since the hospital's nursing service administration did, in fact, have the authority "to move our
students because she paid their bills," they could and sometimes did
exercise major control over the heart of the nursing major, clinical
learning experience. The president came to understand that the University Hospital controlled that major; our faculty did not. He saw that as an
educational issue, and agreed that the money would have to be found
for the hospital.

But the administrations of the hospital and the College of Medicine
were reluctant to ask the legislature for this half-million in addition to
other programs they wished to have funded. I learned through conver-

sation with the hospital executive and dean of medicine that they expected me to justify the hospital budget increase required to replace students. I responded that I considered it my business to justify the college budget but not the hospital budget. When told it would be made my responsibility before the legislature's Appropriations Committee, I pointed out that I would reject that responsibility as being outside the function or authority of the dean of the College of Nursing. I pointed out further that if the point of student service requirement to the University Hospital were pushed too hard, the morality of such a requirement as a condition of higher education could also be raised. I thought that might be a very interesting question to have raised, since at least one member of the legislature's Appropriations Committee had a daughter who was then a junior student in the College of Nursing! I don't know whether this was good strategy or not, but there was no challenge thereafter to our curriculum changes or to their cost to the hospital, and the university budget included the increase for the hospital.

GS: Would you say, then, that in your experience most of the leaders have been thrust into positions, or that they have actually sought the leadership position?

MM: I think both occur. I think leadership is a function of time and the required capabilities being joined. No doubt some people could be leaders, but are not in the time or place where their kind of leadership capability is required. I think it is also true that many talented people refuse leadership, being unwilling to commit themselves to the work, worry, and risk that leadership entails.

GS: Do you think that leadership can be taught?

MM: I think some phases of it can be. I keep telling you what I've learned from Katherine Faville and from David Henry. I wasn't born with what I know about planning a course of action; it's steps, and it's strategy at each step. Most things can be taught, but I don't think you can teach all graduate nursing students to become leaders, because I think it's a happy combination of intellectual training and energy and the willingness to commit oneself to the chores and the agony of being a constant student of your field, and being willing to *risk decisions.*

When I was chairwoman of the Council of Baccalaureate and Higher Degree Programs of the N.L.N.E., I really tried to exert constructive leadership. In the short run the efforts succeeded; in the long run they did not. Both before and after I was elected chairperson of the Council, many of the deans hoped I would be willing to help re-create an association of collegiate schools of nursing. It became obvious to me and to Rita Kelleher, who was the Vice Chairman, that some kind of reorganization to free and give greater autonomy to these university programs simply had to be, if the league was going to be kept together. So we gave thought to it and really investigated the matter. Someplace in the Council office there is a tape of analyses and assessments of the structure and functioning—the physiology and anatomy, if you will—of the American Association of Medical Colleges (A.A.M.C.) and other professional groups. I did the basic work on that—dictated tapes for review by officers and staff of the council. We came up with a proposed change in our operating roles that was voted by our own membership unanimously, and finally agreed to with some hesitation by the Board of Directors of the N.L.N.E. But those changes were not implemented.

Now here's an example of a lot of work that went into leadership, and a lot of strategy got it through approved voting channels. One could ask whether or not, had those changes come while Rita Kelleher and I had two more years in office, we might have been able to implement them. I don't know. Here, for me, was an example of something leadership produced that was not vivified, and I can't tell you why. Is leadership still leadership when it doesn't work? I am uneasy about leadership when it's talked about in the abstract. Is it like pudding; the proof thereof lies in its eating?

At the University of Illinois

GS: When did you come to the University of Illinois?

MM: I came here in 1962. This was a relatively new school, inaugurated in 1954. Its first dean, Emily C. Cardew, had succeeded in getting an autonomous school, one organized as one of the constituent colleges of the university. She had laid the structural base for expanding and enlarging the nursing programs. The faculty of the college was ready for it. The president of the university was the same David D. Henry who had helped us do so much at Wayne. The chancellor and other officials at the Medical Center were also ready for the next phase of development of the college.

I came just in time to get ready for national accreditation, due in 1965. As you know, one of the prime requirements for accreditation is a complete self-survey by faculty, staff, and students of the present operation with recommendations for its modification. That self-survey was a superb orientation for a new dean. The University of Illinois is both a state university and a land-grant one. The University of Iowa is a state university but not a land-grant one. While I had learned about the Land-Grant College Act at school, I hadn't really understood what the model was; how being land-grant affects the philosophic operational base of these institutions. I grasped from both literature and my conversation with fellow deans here and in Urbana, our parent campus, just what the philosophic framework of this institution was.

Next I tried to find out what the demography of the state was, the clientele of this institution, not of nursing. All I knew was that nursing here, so new and so small, was not typical of this university; so I had to study the nature of this university before I could begin to help our faculty construct nursing's future directions here. Well, amazingly enough, I got involved in this faster than I expected. I was here just about a month, I guess, when the head of the physical plant came over one day with a document for me to sign, detailing the college's space needs for the coming decade. The document did not contain the kind of planning assumptions the president and the chancellor had explored with me prior to my appointment. We managed to get a postponement that allowed our self-survey and subsequent planning to move forward in an orderly, though accelerated, way. We moved the self-survey along quickly and then undertook to plan programs, student enrollment, faculty head count, space requirements, and budget for the next ten years.

GS: *That must be hard to do.*

MM: Yes, but that's what deans do, what they get paid for.

The enrollment we projected for the college for 1973 was frighteningly large, but we adopted it because its basic assumption came out of the philosophy that guides this university. We assumed that the general proportion of high school graduating seniors enrolling in the University of Illinois at large would be the proportion of the state's nursing students seeking to enroll in the university's College of Nursing. You know, this is a big university; in 1962 we had fifty-five students entering the college, and our projection for 1973 was something like two hundred students. But our reasoning and assumptions proved valid, and in 1973 we had 200 entering nursing students.

We recruited faculty as fast as we could. We also instituted a faculty development program of our own. First we identified qualifications for each faculty rank and for tenure for each faculty rank in the College of Nursing at the University of Illinois. Once that was spelled out, and the faculty adopted it, I implemented it.

In 1962 about half of our faculty had nothing more than a bachelor's degree. Dr. Lohr and I came that year; she and I were the only faculty members with doctorates. The first step was to help those bright young people to select and enroll in accredited master's programs relevant to their future career goals. We also had to urgently recruit nurses with doctorates, since our master's program was inaugurated in 1963. Incidentally, our young faculty members in master's programs in several universities were remarkably successful in identifying among their fellow students nurses in both master's and doctoral study whom they considered possible candidates for our faculty.

The qualifications for rank and tenure were very helpful in encouraging young, master's-prepared faculty to plan for and undertake doctoral study. The qualifications voted by faculty made it clear that any young assistant professor looking forward to promotion or to tenure here had to earn a doctorate in good time. After we made initial appointments to instructorships, we were able to promote to assistant professorships at the end of three years' successful experience. At the end of four years we helped them begin to make doctoral study plans. After five or six years of service here, many began doctoral study; those who chose not to do so moved on elsewhere. We were very fortunate in the availability of federal funds. My service on federal review panels at the National Institutes of Health (N.I.H.) had helped me learn the procedures for application and the criteria for review, and that knowledge helped, of course. Between 1967 and 1971, when I resigned from the deanship, fifteen young assistant professors studied at many universities; about half of them rejoined this faculty on completion of their doctoral programs.

GS: So you would say that in planning the development of this college, recruitment of students and faculty development were part of it? For someone picking up this material and reading it, would you say that your contributions—all of them here at the University of Illinois—are included? Would you care to add anything about curriculum development?

MM: Curriculum development is part of planning. I don't make a special case of curriculum development for the reason that when we talk about program development, I include curriculum development. I really have thought for a long time that in nursing we spend such an inordinate amount of time on the details of curriculum that we avoid badly needed attention to other pressing things. Here we reviewed and updated the baccalaureate program and created and expanded a master's program; and at the present time a program leading to the Ph.D. in nursing is in the process of approval by our State Board of Higher Education. I expect we shall be authorized to admit students to it this fall.

Let me say something else to you, too, in terms of strategy. Hardly ever is a major success a one-person job. One of the reasons, I think, can be illustrated in how we got this building. When I came to Illinois, we didn't have the needs and resources data we needed for planning in the state of Illinois. Our Bureau of Institutional Research in Urbana keeps all school statistics for the whole state. From that source we obtained general data on secondary schools and higher education. What we didn't have were data about nurses. From general data I was able to construct some reasonable, acceptable, general assumptions of need to support our request for this new College of Nursing building. But very soon, working with the Illinois Nurses' Association and the Illinois League for Nursing, through a study commission to get the hard data on nursing needs for planning for nursing in our state, we were able to do this.

Leaves the Deanship

GS: Why did you leave the deanship?

MM: I resigned from the deanship in 1971 because, in the first place, I was tired. Being a dean is a hard job and a constant job.

And second, because there were three things left unfinished from our earlier planning. I knew that with three years I could finish two of them. Though I'd been a university professor for twenty-six years, I had never managed to get a sabbatical. Since one of those unfinished items was graduate work in nursing service administration, I went over to the College of Engineering to investigate systems engineering, to explore advances in the technology of management. When I came back, I reorganized the minor courses in nursing service administration and initiated a new major to prepare nursing service administrators to be more knowledgeable about management science, to be able to understand and apply the newer technologies of systems analysis and operations research.

But the third reason I left was because we were coming up for accreditation. My resignation, effective in 1971, would give a new dean two years for self-survey: a superb orientation for a new dean, a unique opportunity to plan for the next decade and to provide the leadership to implement those plans.

GS: You said there were three things left unfinished from your administration. You have mentioned nursing service administration. What are the other two, and what progress have you made on those?

MM: A second was graduate work in advanced pediatric nursing. I have no competence to help there, but the pediatric nursing faculty are working on that now, I understand.

The third was for doctoral study in nursing. Last year, thanks to a federal planning grant, I was able to inaugurate that effort. Dr. Helen Grace, now assistant dean for graduate study, supported by that grant, served as staff and was principally responsible for the successful completion of the draft of the program. We are all very happy that the program, leading to a Ph.D. with a major in nursing, has cleared all the approval channels of the university and is today being reviewed, and we hope approved, by the Health Education Commission of the Illinois Board of Higher Education. When the entire board approves the program in the spring, my work here will be done. Then I shall retire from the university. Though I shall not have reached the university's mandatory retirement age, I sense that the time is right to close this phase of my career. I feel this college is in very good hands, and I am content to leave it.

Contribution to the Area of Better Administration of Nursing Service

GS: *You are recognized as having made a substantial contribution to the area of better administration of nursing service. Could you say something about your approach?*

MM: I've been interested in nursing service for a long time. I have been an administrator of nursing service and served as head nurse, supervisor, and director of nursing.

Incidentally, I hope some day that we can have real research in the relationship between professional specialties and personality patterns. There's been some work done in medicine, but to my knowledge there isn't any done in nursing. I suspect the demands of a field attract certain personality patterns. I wonder, too, whether demands of the field dictate success for some and no success for others in terms of personality patterns. I feel a great need for nursing service administration to identify what constitutes executive talent for it and then to define and test modes for its search. I think this could be really quite exciting.

I've always been interested in administration and in making things go. I'm interested in the intellectual underpinnings of goal setting and planning to achieve those goals. I'm an activist, but I think I feel very keenly the imperative of the intellectual search which must be basic to the action. I'm also sensitive to the strategies. I suspect you'll find in these tapes the recurring theme that without strategy even the wisest action cannot succeed.

My master's was in the organization and functioning of nursing schools and nursing services; it has always been an interest of mine. Then, too, I was a part-time nurse faculty member in that far-sighted W. K. Kellogg Nursing Service Administration Seminar held at the University of Chicago in 1951. I learned so much through that and the subsequent program that nursing service administration has always been fascinating to me.

All the time I was at Wayne I'd been in educational administration. I've watched our profession espouse fashions, and when we espoused one fashion, we often dropped another. We neglected administration when we turned to training clinical specialists, which I espoused without any hesitation at all. What I'm pointing out is not what we espoused but what we neglected. We neglected the management skills and failed to understand that nursing management must be equally sophisticated or clinical specialization will fail to improve patient care, as we so earnestly hoped. I do believe we made the right choice to separate nursing education and nursing service. Nursing education and justice to students required it. We could not, in fact, control education while it was still inextricably bound to nursing service. Our error was not in what we did for nursing education; our error was in not turning comparable attention to the problem of nursing service, to undertake its analysis and its improvement for its own sake and on its own terms. When we turned our attention to nursing service, we did it because it needed to be better for students. That's the wrong reason. Nursing service elsewhere needs to be better for patients; if it is, then it will be better for students. This conviction turned me back again to reestablish my scholarship in nursing service administration.

Before beginning my sabbatical, I began to review the literature in industrial, governmental, and educational administration, literature with which I had once been thoroughly familiar. I found much refinement in the behavioral science applications, but I thought the ideas not different to the degree that would indicate substantive change in either philosophy or understanding of operations. I was looking for the new ideas—new to me—and I found them in the works on management science, operations research, systems analysis. These concepts were so different, so much more sophisticated than the old time-and-motion studies I used to know as to constitute a major substantive change in administrative theoretical knowledge. So that's what took me over to the department of systems engineering in our College of Engineering. I spent my six-month sabbatical there, trying to learn the modern technological applications of management engineering and management. I became no expert in them, but I became familiar with their terms and their concepts. We have tried to incorporate them into our major courses in nursing service administration here.

Some Strategies and Issues

GS: You have been credited with being a person who works well and effectively with other people. Is there anything that you would care to add to what you have already said in terms of your strategies?

MM: I think I probably have worked well with various people. I don't know that I can conceptualize exactly what brings it about. I am quite sure that one of the reasons is that I always do my homework. I usually try to know what I'm talking about. I try to be prepared when I do something, especially if I'm going to do it outside of my own bailiwick. Another thing that might surprise you: I always try to be well dressed; I try to look the part. I always try to figure out the part I'm going to have to play, and make a conscious effort to look and play that part. My mother used to say, "Stand up straight and stop fidgeting." I've never had a course in speech, but I've been conscious for a long time of the way one can use language, privately and publicly. I try to fit my language as well as my appearance to the task at hand.

Then, too, if I'm going to have to fight, I do fight, but behind closed doors, never in public if I can honestly avoid it. If I make a mistake, I try to admit it and promptly "cut my losses." One can not have the kind of jobs that I have held for years without making mistakes. It isn't just being gracious about mistakes; it's being honest about them.

GS: It seems that you've learned a great deal from whatever mistakes you've made, and that you've really analyzed them and picked them apart. How were you able to work so well and effectively with people with different interests, vested interests?

MM: I did my homework. I tried to know what I was talking about. Second, I knew my field. I knew the people in it, and through them I knew people in lots of other fields. Third, I tried always to meet not just normal expectations for a dean, for example, but to go beyond them. Whatever women do in deanships and such positions, they have to do it this much better than men. I've always known that; any sense of aggrievement about it is only self-defeating.

GS: Looking back over your long and distinguished career, what would you say was one of your big disappointments or big conflicts?

MM: I don't know. I think one tends to—at least I tend to—forget one's frustrations. Maybe that's part of what you call leadership. If you dwell on things, you'll spend energy there rather than on the next step.

I guess I was frustrated lots of times that I didn't make progress faster in this institution. There were a lot of days of frustration here. I really was disappointed at the kinds of things that were natural, that had to happen at Iowa after I had made major changes there. I suppose one of my own disappointments had always been in the large number of fine people who are content with second best, with letting others do the work of progress while they point out all the things wrong with our profession.

GS: What do you see as some of the major issues in nursing today?

MM: I think the biggest issue is how much unanimity of purpose we can hope for in a profession as diverse as our own. Internal warfare in the nursing profession is scandalous. Antagonism between the A.N.A. and the National League for Nursing (N.L.N.) is one case in point. Another is continuing mutual criticism of nursing education and nursing service. A more recent one is the emerging chasm between nursing administrators and nursing staff, precipitated by Taft-Hartley revisions.

Yet, even though these kinds of things come up from time to time, we tend to get them resolved. I'm confident that we shall continue to resolve them, that our professional leadership will be adequate to the task as it always has been in the past.

I often wonder whether young nurses will be astute enough to understand the strength they have in organized nursing—that is, the state and national organizations—and to use that strength. If the Illinois Nurses' Association hadn't helped, I'm not at all sure that we'd have this building. The executive director of the Illinois Nurses' Association went to the Governor about it. I don't have any way of going to the Governor, but she did, and used it for the good of all nurses we could serve through this building.

GS: What is your viewpoint of the "nurse-practitioner" and the "expanded role of the nurse?"

MM: I don't know what we call it. The phenomenon is long overdue. We need to realize that we are kept at the forefront of public confidence only when we serve the public's needs in their terms, not in ours. We did violence to the public's needs by functionalizing nursing. We created the phenomenon and took it to the extreme in functional titles like "med nurse," "stoma nurse." Is that what nursing ought to be? If nurses combine greater clinical knowledge and skill with greater humanization of their application to care of individual patients, perhaps public confidence can be restored. We must also realize that we cannot capitalize on practitioners and expanded roles without changing our organizational structure and philosophy to absorb them into the institutional operation in institutional terms. Young nurses, in zeal and naïveté, have said to me, "Well, I'm not going to take that job; it's too well defined; I want to go and do what I find patients need." My answer to this one is, "If I were director of nursing, I would ask why you think any institution should pay you for such luxury. When we're offered a job, we should expect to be offered a fairly well-defined set of responsibilities for which we will be held accountable and for which we will be paid." Until we really get our structures settled, and until we make a socially defined—not professionally defined—set of tasks and responsibilities for nurse-practitioners, they cannot succeed. To do this we're going to need to train more sophisticated managers. That's one of the reasons why I moved back into nursing service administration. Increasing nursing's response to scientific discovery and technical advance is imperative; it's not a response to professional pretentions. But we have equally urgent need of management that can control the climate, that can define advanced responsibilities in practice and have these accepted and budgeted.

GS: Do you see any other very crucial issues in nursing?

MM: I see another crucial issue to be nursing's tendency to react to changes rather than help design them. If we had less internal dissension, we'd have a lot of political clout, and in our society political clout is the name of the game. We're not yet in a position to play that game as national health insurance, quality controls, PSRO's, and other major developments come tumbling out of Washington. If nursing could get itself together and provide the public with a well-defined redefinition of the role of nursing in modern society—what it ought to be—we couldn't fail, given our large numbers. But we wait to see whether the physicians are going to pay or whether hospital administrators will accept our plans. I hope the next generation of professional nurses will demonstrate their expertise and dedicate their money and energies to speaking with one voice about future goals of Americans' health care. If they can, the public and nursing itself will be better for it.

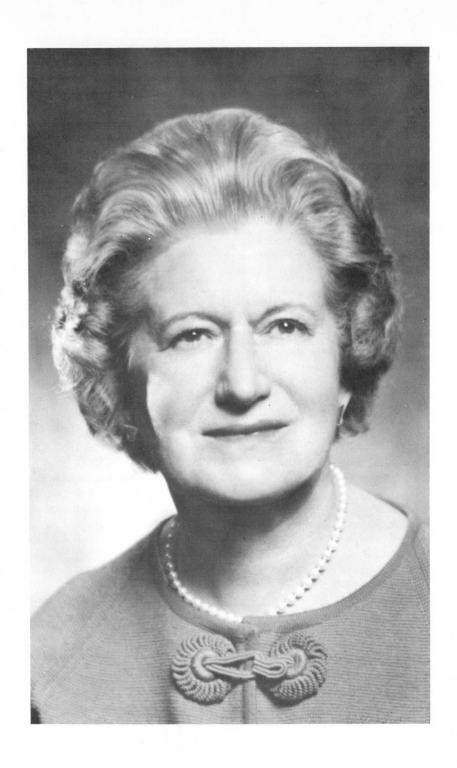

11

Outstanding leader in the world of nursing and nursing education, deeply committed to research as a way to improve nursing care, your intellectual capacity, creative ideas, and firm leadership have been instrumental in shaping the future of nursing education, both in this country and abroad. As Dean of the School of Nursing at the University of California, San Francisco, you have presided over a decade of growth and development which have made that School the equal of any in existence, with a doctoral program dedicated to preparing nurses for clinical research and teaching a highly innovative baccalaureate curriculum, an increasingly well prepared faculty, and a vigorous and growing program of research. For all this and for the decisive and influential imprint of your own scholarship, we salute you—our highest honor.[1]

[1]From honorary doctor of laws, University of California, San Francisco, June 7, 1969.

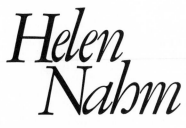

Helen Nahm

EDUCATOR

*H*elen Nahm is considered by her colleagues to be one of the most outstanding nursing leaders in education nationally and internationally. She is described by others as "a lady" first and foremost, but one with an iron fist in a velvet glove.

> *. . . I've seen her (Helen Nahm) irritated and frustrated at NLN (National League for Nursing) Board meetings, and often thought she was at her best in these moments. Her bench marks, however, are that she comes across as a lady and that she is a mediator.*[2]
>
> *She (Helen Nahm) combines an unusually pleasing personality with a clear focus on the work to be done. She is always willing to listen and to modify her approach as long as the main objective is accomplished.*[3]

Helen Nahm was born in a small town, Augusta, Missouri, in August 1901. Her grandfather had emigrated from Germany, and her father was a winemaker. She was the oldest of five children, all girls. When she finished high school, she very much wanted to go to the University of Missouri but did not have any money. After teaching for a year in a country school and saving her money ($200), she was able to enter the University of Missouri at Columbia, where the tuition was then less than $30 for the semester. She had never thought seriously of going into nursing, but when as a freshman she became ill and was sent to the University Hospital, she says, "I was so excited about that experience that I decided to go into nursing."

She graduated from the University of Missouri School of Nursing diploma program in 1924 and went on to obtain a bachelor of arts degree in 1926. She then held teaching and administrative positions in Texas and Missouri. Enrolling at the University of Minnesota in 1938, she was one of the very first nurses to receive a Ph.D. The degree (1946) was in general education and educational psychology. The title of her dissertation was "An Evaluation of Selected Schools of Nursing with Respect to Certain Educational Objectives."[4] The study elicited much response in the academic community.[5]

Dr. Nahm has published extensively—over fifty articles in scholarly journals.[6] Nursing leaders had been writing about the need for greater

---

[2] Letter to author from Lulu K. Wolf Hassenplug, Dec. 27, 1974.
[3] Letter to author from Anna Fillmore, Dec. 6, 1974.
[4] In Boston University's Mugar Memorial Library, Nursing Archives.
[5] Dr. Abraham Maslow, a psychologist, wrote to her commending her on her study.
[6] Some of her bench-mark articles are "Mental Hygiene Knowledge of Senior Students in Schools of Nursing," *Journal of Educational Research*, 41: 193–203, November 1947; "Autocratic versus

democracy in nursing schools and nursing services, but little or no research had been done on what actually took place in relationships among students, teachers, and supervisors. Relationships between physicians and nurses also were authoritarian rather than democratic. Changes in the education of both medical and nursing students were needed.

Dr. Nahm has received numerous awards and citations and four honorary doctoral degrees.[7] . It is difficult to do justice to this outstanding woman and nursing leader in a few pages. Examples of her recognized leadership in the improvement of nursing education are (1) her role in the accreditation of nursing schools and (2) her role as a dean.

Accreditation may be defined as a process whereby an organization recognizes a program of study or university as having met certain predetermined criteria or standards.[8] In 1949 the National Nursing Accrediting Service (N.N.A.S.) came into being, and Dr. Nahm was appointed its first director.[9]

She says, "Except for the job I had later at the University of California, it was by far the most challenging position that I have ever had. I had to develop a whole service from scratch." Up to that time (1949) there were two types of undergraduate educational nursing programs: the three-year hospital diploma program and a small number of college-university baccalaureate programs. Programs for graduate nurses, most of which were also at a baccalaureate level, prepared nurses for public health nursing or for teaching, administration, or supervision. The formulation of specific criteria for the evaluation of each type of

Democratic Beliefs and Practices of Senior Students in Schools of Nursing," *Journal of Social Psychology,* 27: 229–240, May 1948; "An Evaluation of Selected Schools of Nursing," *Applied Psychology Monographs of the American Psychological Association,* Stanford University Press, Stanford, Calif., 1948; "Autocratic versus Democratic Beliefs and Practices in Schools of Nursing," *Trained Nurse and Hospital Review,* pp. 158–161, April 1949; "Planning for the Future of Education in Nursing," *The Canadian Nurse, 56:* 1073–1078, December 1960; with Doris I. Miller, "Relationships between Medical and Nursing Education," *Journal of Medical Education, 36:* 849–856, August 1961; "The Pursuit of Excellence in the West: Five Years of W.C.H.E.N.," *Report of the Fifth Annual Western Conference on Nursing Education,* Denver, Colo., March 22–23, 1962; with Calvin W. Taylor, Mary Harms, Mildred Quinn, Stanley Mulaik, and Jane Mulaik, *Measurement and Prediction of Nursing Performance,* part I, University of Utah, Salt Lake City, 1965; "Nursing Dimensions and Realities," *American Journal of Nursing,* pp. 96–99, June 1965; "Tribute to the Past—Prelude to the Future," *International Nursing Review,* pp. 14–23, July–August 1966.

[7] Some of these are the Distinguished Service Award, University of Minnesota Alumni Association, April 1968; the M. Adelaide Nutting Award, National League for Nursing, May 1967; honorary doctor of laws, University of California, San Francisco, June 1969.

[8] William K. Selden, *Accreditation: A Struggle over Standards in Higher Education,* Harper & Brothers, New York, 1960.

[9] A nurse-historian writes: "Miss Nahm, with experience in both large and small schools, was *temperamentally* as well as academically and professionally unusually well qualified for this *exacting* and influential position." Mary M. Roberts, *American Nursing: History and Interpretation,* The Macmillan Company, New York, 1954, pp. 516–517.

program for accreditation was the first task. In 1949, students were continuing to provide the bulk of nursing care in hospitals. As a consequence, both they and patients were exploited. The rationale behind the accreditation movement was that it was necessary to improve nursing education in order to improve health care.

Dr. Nahm directed the N.N.A.S. between 1950 and 1952. The service was absorbed by the National League for Nursing (N.L.N.) in 1952. As director of the Division of Nursing Education of the N.L.N. from 1953 to 1958, she continued to exert leadership in the accreditation program.

In 1950 there were approximately 1,170 basic programs of which 35 basic collegiate and 113 noncollegiate programs were accredited (total of 148). In 1974 there are approximately 1,492 programs that prepare for licensing as registered nurses. Of these, 433 diploma, 207 associate degree and 234 baccalaureate degree programs are accredited (total of 874).[10]

In addition, 74 master's degree programs are now accredited.

Dr. Nahm became the Dean of the School of Nursing, University of California, San Francisco, in 1958 and remained until she retired in 1969. Her many accomplishments there included improving and revising the curriculum, recruiting highly qualified faculty, getting faculty to conduct and to publish research,[11] and getting a doctor of nursing science (D.N.S.) degree approved.[12] Two of Dr. Nahm's important innovations were to recruit social scientists as regular full-time faculty members in the School of Nursing and to develop an integrated nursing curriculum, building upon the social and physical sciences and the humanities. Dr. Nahm retired February 1, 1969.[13]

The following quotes from former colleagues and students of Dr. Nahm describe what kind of a person she is: "She has idealistic goals." "An important characteristic of her personality is her sensitivity to other people; however, this does not prevent her from making decisions with which other people would disagree." "I admire her intellect." "Helpful to others."

---

[10] Helen Nahm, "The Accrediting Program in Nursing Education," paper presented at the American Nurses' Association Convention, San Francisco, June 1974.

[11] Today this is standard practice, but at the time there were not many nurses in academia.

[12] There are several such programs today in the United States, and others are in various stages of development. Consult the National League for Nursing, Division of Nursing Education, 10 Columbus Circle, New York, N.Y., for the current status of the programs.

[13] Her title: Dean and Professor Emeritus, University of California School of Nursing, San Francisco.

Early Career

GS: *Dr. Nahm, in your early career, first as Director of the University of Missouri School of Nursing in Columbia (1935–1941), and later of Hamline University School of Nursing in St. Paul, Minnesota (1942–1945), what were the main issues and trends in nursing education and your particular role at that time?*

HN: When I was at the University of Missouri, my major concern was the development of a sound baccalaureate nursing program. When I first went to the University of Missouri as Director of the School of Nursing in 1935, the school was still admitting students directly from high schools to a three-year program, and also admitting students who would later go on and complete requirements for the baccalaureate degree. But the degree at that time was not in nursing; students were granted approximately two years of credit for the three years in the School of Nursing; this was done in recognition of the fact that they took a great many regular university courses in English, history, and the social and natural sciences. The nursing courses were set up in such a way that they too merited university credit. However, it still meant that students had to take an additional two years and major in some subject other than nursing to get a bachelor's degree. I entered nursing after a year of college work. After three years in the School of Nursing, I went back for approximately another year and got a bachelor's degree with a major in zoology and a minor in nutrition. After 1935 I succeeded rather quickly in getting approval for a four-calendar-year program which led to a bachelor of science degree in nursing. I think that was one of the things many university schools were striving for at that particular time. One of the other issues at that time was the need to shorten hours of work for students so they could actually be students instead of hospital workers. This had been achieved at the University of Missouri School of Nursing long before I came. When I was a student, we had an eight-hour day, including classes. Many of the graduate nurses who came from other schools were shocked; they didn't think they could possibly learn anything in that period of time. At that time we were also concerned that students have adequate instruction in medical nursing, surgical nursing, maternity nursing, pediatric nursing, and, if possible, some experience in public health nursing. However, with the exception of a few major schools, some of the better hospital schools at that time had their students spend three months with a visiting nurse service, so it wasn't just the university schools that were emphasizing the importance of such experience. Nurse educators were beginning to talk about the need for psychiatric nursing experience. In Missouri, however, emphasis was initially on education of registered nurses in the field of psychiatric nursing. About 1935 or 1936, a six-month course in psychiatric nursing for registered nurses was established in the St. Louis City Sanitarium. The number admitted to this program was never very large, and in a relatively short period of time the program was changed to make it possible for schools of nursing to send their students to affiliate in psychiatric nursing. The University of Missouri School of Nursing was one of the schools that sent its students to the St. Louis City Sanitarium for a three-month experience in psychiatric nursing. Another issue was whether students should have experience in tuberculosis nursing. Since the University Hospital in Columbia, Missouri, was rather small, we sent students for one month of tuberculosis nursing experience to a large TB sanitarium near Minneapolis. They also spent six months (three months in pediatrics and three months in obstetrics) at the University of Minnesota School of Nursing.

Another major concern in 1935 was the need for better preparation of nurse teachers. Most schools at that time were proud of themselves if they could get teachers with bachelor's degrees. There were not many available who had master's degrees. Few of those who held master's degrees had had advanced content in the clinical area of nursing; they had preparation in teaching or in supervision or in administration. In fact, when I went to the University of Missouri as Director, I didn't have a master's degree. I knew I needed to get one; that's why I decided to go to the University of Minnesota in 1938. I completed work for the master's degree in 1939 and then returned to the University of Missouri for two more years. In 1941 I returned to the University of Minnesota to begin work toward the Ph.D. degree. I went to school full time during 1941–1942 and then accepted a position as Director of the School of Nursing at Hamline University in St. Paul, Minnesota.

Duke University[14]

GS: Why did you leave Hamline?

HN: I found out that I simply couldn't complete my doctoral thesis and carry a full-time job, so when I was offered a position at Duke University as Director of the Division of Nursing Education, I resigned and took six months off to complete my dissertation. The position at Duke was one I was very much interested in. It was exactly what I wanted to do. To me it was a new and challenging opportunity. I have

[14] Dr. Nahm was Director of the Division of Nursing Education, Duke University, Durham, N.C., 1946–1950.

always had a quality—I don't know whether it's good or bad—of being excited about things that are new and difficult. When I accept a position and then feel I've gotten the show on the road and things are going well, I begin to look for something new. The school of nursing at Duke was closely associated with the medical school, and that had created difficulties over a long period of time. However, the Division of Nursing Education functioned under the department of education and was responsible for the preparation of nurse teachers. In this position I had a great deal of freedom.

GS: You mentioned the school of medicine's having power over the school of nursing as a big issue. Would you elaborate here, please?

HN: At that time there were a number of nursing schools in the United States that functioned as departments of schools of medicine. As a consequence, nursing school faculty often had only limited control over their own programs. The Duke University school of nursing was struggling for independence.

GS: What do you consider your greatest achievement while you were at Duke—your greatest source of satisfaction or accomplishment?

HN: I worked hard to develop the nursing education program. I worked with the students, with faculty of other departments at Duke, and with faculty of the basic nursing program. One advantage was that the Duke University School of Nursing had perfectly marvelous basic students, some of the finest students I have ever been associated with. During the years 1946–1950 many improvements were made in the basic nursing program. Each year increasing numbers of registered nurses enrolled in the program leading to the B.S. in nursing education. Many of these were enrolled under the G.I. Bill.

Role in the Accreditation of Nursing Schools[15]

GS: What precipitated your going to New York?

HN: Well, I was offered a job as director of the newly established National Nursing Accrediting Service by Adelaide Mayo, who was then Executive Secretary of the old National League of Nursing Education

---

[15] Dr. Nahm was Director, National Nursing Accrediting Service, New York, 1950–1952; Director, Department of Baccalaureate and Higher Degree Programs at the N.L.N., New York, 1952–1953; and Director, Division of Nursing Education at the N.L.N., New York, 1953–1958.

(N.L.N.E.), and Anna Fillmore, who was then Executive Secretary of the National Organization for Public Health Nursing (N.O.P.H.N.).

When the N.N.A.S. was first set up, it was responsible to the Joint Committee on the Unification of Accrediting Activities, which in turn was responsible to the joint board of directors of the six national nursing organizations. That's how complicated it was at that particular time. The N.N.A.S. had come into being in the fall of 1949. When the N.L.N. was organized in 1952, responsibility for accreditation was delegated to this organization.

GS: What were your impressions working in this new job, besides its being complicated? Did you like it?

HN: Except for the job I had at the University of California, it was by far the most challenging and the most difficult position I have ever had. There were many things I liked about it, and I probably would have stayed on in New York if I hadn't been offered the position at the University of California.

GS: What were some of the things you liked about it?

HN: Well, developing a whole service from scratch. When I went to New York, we had one staff member, Hazel Goff (Hazel Goff died in 1973), who had been working with the old N.L.N.E. accrediting program and who, over the years, had done a very meticulous job.

I became Director of the Division of Nursing Education within N.L.N. in 1953, and accrediting continued to be a major means to bring about improvements in all types of educational programs in nursing.

GS: Could you please comment on your role in the restructuring of the national nursing organizations?

HN: In the years preceding 1946–1950, I was aware that a great deal of study was going on at a national level and that this study, it was hoped, would result in the restructuring of the national nursing organizations. At the state level (in North Carolina) I was aware of what was going on, and there were many discussions about the value of one organization versus two organizations. However, I didn't have a vested interest at that particular time in whether we had one or two organizations. I remember going to a national meeting—I think it was the American Nurses' Association (A.N.A.)—about 1948 at which Raymond Rich Associates presented their ideas about the restructuring of the nursing organizations. However, I was *not* directly involved in *any* of the national committees, either of the A.N.A. or of any other nursing organization that debated the merits of one plan or the other at the national level.

GS: Would you please tell about the accreditation movement and your own role in it?

HN: When the N.N.A.S. was first established, it had four boards of review that passed on whether new programs should be accredited, and that evaluated previously accredited programs to determine whether they should automatically be continued on an accredited list or whether a revisit was indicated. The Public Health Board of Review evaluated all specialized programs for registered nurses other than those in public health; the Collegiate Board of Review evaluated diploma programs.

GS: What immediate problems, if any, emerged from these investigations by the boards of review?

HN: The first meetings of the boards of review were held during the fall of 1949. At that time the Noncollegiate Board of Review recommended that 50 of its 113 accredited programs be revisited. Julia Miller, Acting Director of the N.N.A.S. from the fall of 1949 to July 1, 1950, was responsible for seeing that these visits were made. Hazel Goff was the only full-time additional staff member and the only person who had previously been involved in the accrediting program of the N.L.N.E. During 1950 Ms. Goff made as many of the accrediting visits to diploma programs as she could. Each visit covered a period of five days.

GS: Could you amplify on the nature of these visits?

HN: Endless hours of overtime work went into the writing of reports. At that time it was necessary to evaluate not only the educational program but also the quality of nursing service at the institutions in which students had their clinical experiences. (This often included general, pediatric, and psychiatric facilities.) Hazel Goff was always assisted by a representative of a diploma program to fulfill the requirement that at least two persons be responsible for each visit.

GS: At what stage of this evaluative process did you become involved?

HN: Because it was impossible for Ms. Goff to visit fifty schools in one year, Julia Miller recruited a number of representatives of accredited diploma programs to make visits. Needless to say, few of them had had any experience in making accrediting visits or writing reports. When I got to New York in July 1950, I found a drawer full of reports of visits that had been made by many different individuals. The meetings of the four boards of review were scheduled for November 1950.

The procedure that had been agreed upon was that the report of a visit would be sent to the school for corrections, then retyped, then sent to members of the board of review prior to the annual meeting. This meant that reports of fifty diploma programs had to be processed prior to November 1950. In addition, written reports had been requested of all accredited public health nursing programs and basic collegiate nursing programs, as well as of some of the postgraduate nursing programs.

Lillian Gardner, a public health nurse on the staff of the Public Health Service (P.H.S.) in Washington, D.C., came to New York to assist in preparation of reports for the Public Health Board of Review. Except for a few hours of sleep each night, Hazel Goff and I worked during every hour available to prepare for meetings of the other three boards. Somehow or other we got ready. The meetings were held, decisions were made, and a revised list of accredited nursing programs was published in the February 1951 issue of the *American Journal of Nursing (A.J.N.)*.

A beginning had been made. However, in August 1950 we discovered that the N.N.A.S. did not have enough money to survive for the remainder of the year. The A.N.A. came to the rescue with a contribution of $10,000.

During the time that the N.N.A.S. was being established, the Committee to Implement the Brown Report[16] had also come into being. The name of this Committee was subsequently changed to the National Committee for the Improvement of Nursing Services (N.C.I.N.S.). This Committee early agreed that improvement in nursing services would not take place until such time as there had been marked improvements in nursing education. At that time the number of nationally accredited basic programs was so small in proportion to the total number (148 of a total of 1170) that accreditation did not have much of an impact. It was decided, therefore, that a questionnaire study should be made of all basic nursing programs in the United States. Ninety-six percent of the schools responded to the questionnaire.

On the basis of certain predetermined criteria, the schools were classified as Group I (the highest 25 percent), Group II (the middle 50 percent), and Group III (the lowest 25 percent). Lists of Group I and Group II schools were subsequently published. For the first time in history the nursing organizations[17] had had the courage and the strength to make public their knowledge about the status of nursing education programs in the United States.

---

[16] Esther Lucile Brown, *Nursing for the Future*, Russell Sage Foundation, New York, 1948. Dr. Brown conducted a classic and highly influential study of basic nursing programs at the end of World War II.

[17] The National Committee for the Improvement of Nursing Services was responsible to the joint board of directors of five national nursing organizations.

When the first list was published, the N.C.I.N.S. promised the schools that a follow-up study would be made within two years. Responsibility for the follow-up study was taken over by the N.N.A.S.

GS: Dr. Nahm, could you say something about both the nature of your group's follow-up study and its results?

HN: In lieu of a second classification, it was agreed that a program of temporary accreditation should be developed for all programs not then fully accredited. Criteria for temporary accreditation were much less stringent than those for full accreditation. Of a total of 904 basic programs that applied for temporary accreditation during 1951–1952, 624 were approved for a period of five years and 276 were not approved. It was initially hoped that at the end of a five-year period (1952–1957), the majority of temporarily accredited schools would have met criteria for full accreditation. However, this period of time was much too short, and it was not until 1962 that it was possible to discontinue listing, as a separate category, certain developing programs that were not yet ready for full accreditation.

I have certain vivid recollections of the years that I functioned as Director of the N.N.A.S. (1950–1952) and as Director of the Division of Nursing Education of the N.L.N. (1953–1958).[18] These have to do with the continuing need for money and the responsibility for dealing with all of the emotional reactions associated with accreditation. Three times in a period of nine years, Marion Sheahan[19] and I went to foundations to obtain support for what came to be known as a ten-year program of school improvement. These were the Commonwealth Fund, the Rockefeller Foundation, and the National Foundation for Infantile Paralysis. Each time we literally held our breath, wondering whether we would have enough money to continue the program of school improvement. (Funds eventually totaled over $800,000.)

GS: Could you elaborate on some of your extrafinancial problems?

HN: In addition to our worries about money, we had to deal with hospital administrators; college and university presidents; deans, directors, and faculty of nursing schools; boards of trustees of hospitals; and hospital and medical associations (state, regional, and national); all of them had some type of personal or financial investment in one or more nursing education programs. The most difficult problems were those associated with the hospital schools of nursing.

[18] In 1952 responsibility for accreditation was assumed by the N.L.N.
[19] Executive Director of the N.C.I.N.S. and later of the Department of Nursing Services of the N.L.N.

From the time these schools were first established, students had been depended upon to furnish the bulk of hospital nursing service. To say that to be accredited, a school should have a well-prepared faculty, a library, adequate physical facilities, and a budget, and that students should have time for study and recreation, was looked upon by some schools as absolute heresy. Many collegiate schools of nursing were also very poor. College and university, as well as hospital, administrators did not relish being told their programs did not meet agreed-upon national criteria. But somehow or other the accrediting program in nursing survived. It now continues as an established function of the N.L.N.

I was directly involved in questions concerning the restructuring of the nursing organizations during the time I served as Director of the N.N.A.S. However, my primary concern then was the question of which organization would be responsible for the accrediting service.

GS: Were you ever discouraged in your work?

HN: Well, many times, but for the most part the work was endlessly interesting and exciting. I met people from all over the United States, not only people associated with the nursing schools themselves but leaders in education, social sciences, medicine, hospital administration, and other fields. I met national nursing leaders from all over the United States and from other countries of the world. I traveled a great deal during those years, especially with Marion Sheahan, who continued on the N.L.N. staff as Director of the Department of Nursing Services.

GS: On the basis of your experience in accreditation, can you recommend a strategy for leadership which might have wider applicability for others thrust into similar positions of responsibility?

HN: Well, I think one thing that is very important if you're working for a nursing organization is that you be as clear as possible about what is going on and that you make information available to the decision-making groups; in other words, you try to state the issues as clearly as you can. But you accept the fact that when you're working for an organization, the decisions are made by the officers and members of the organization. Now this is very difficult at times, and particularly when you apply it to accrediting of nursing schools. You may have been very much involved with a particular school in consultation to try to help the faculty and perhaps also with the administrators of the institution that conducts the school (hospital, college, or university). You know the faculty members and the director or dean of the school; you have spent a good deal of time with them; you then have a report of their program for accreditation which must be acted upon by a board of review of the accrediting service. You try to state the strengths and weaknesses but then stay in the background while you watch that board of review make a decision. The dilemma arises from the extent to which you can be neutral, or whether it's crucial at a particular point that you step in and make a bit more information available.

GS: *How have you resolved this dilemma? Do you have any concrete suggestions?*

HN: It takes a great deal of judgment not to try to influence the decision that is made. If a decision is made that is unpopular, and many decisions are, again your role is to try to state the issues on both sides. Schools always have the possibility of appealing a decision if they feel they haven't had a square deal. However, the school often needs help in presenting evidence in such a way that it can get a square deal. Your role is not to side with the school or with the board. It's these kinds of things that make being a staff member of an organization difficult, particularly when there are critical issues around very sensitive problems in which human emotions are involved.

GS: *To what extent does the factor of psychology enter leadership strategy? Can you offer any dicta in this regard?*

HN: You must learn to respect the human beings with whom you are dealing, whether you agree with them or not—to listen to people, to treat what they say as important, and to avoid making them feel inadequate (and this, of course, would be easy to do with many weak schools).

GS: *Did you derive any other insights into leadership strategy, from your involvement in the accreditation process, which others might find beneficial?*

HN: Well, one thing I learned had to do with a decision that was made by the deans and directors of baccalaureate and higher degree programs about 1952: that all bachelor's degree programs, including those for both registered nurses and basic students, should be generalized rather than specialized programs and should focus on preparation for nursing practice at a professional level rather than for teaching, supervision, and administration. Now, this represents a decision which was made by leaders in the field of nursing and which was based upon a very sound principle. However, emotional issues were involved. There still was a tremendous shortage of teachers for all types of nursing education programs: collegiate, diploma, and the newly developing associate degree programs. There were tremendous shortages of nurses prepared for supervisory and administrative positions. To say that at a bachelor's level, registered nurses should be prepared in a generalized rather than a specialized program focused on teaching, administration, or supervision seemed very unfair to many people. But from this I learned that if the decision that is made is basically a sound decision, it can be defended. In the defense it is not necessary to antagonize or hurt people who initially do not agree. As a staff member, you can listen and interpret and reinterpret. Gradually, people who have disagreed go through a process of change, and sooner or later you begin to get consensus.

GS: Would you begin to get a little bit angry or frustrated when you would know that it was really the right decision, but the other people were not moving in that direction fast enough? Would it irritate you?

HN: No. I honestly do not remember being irritated, because I think I realized they were not attacking me; they were presenting and discussing their own beliefs. This is a bit different from the situation you are in when you are responsible for a school and you're trying to put your ideas across. It's very difficult then not to feel that you're under attack. If you represent an organization, the decisions around which that organization operates are those of the organization. You did not make them, though you may have contributed information which helped elected members to make decisions. In a service such as accrediting, staff members have to remember that when people are upset, they may need a target. Accept the fact; let them be angry. If that's the way they feel, it's okay. If you can accept that, pretty soon things begin to work out.

Out West—Dean of the School of Nursing, University of California, San Francisco

GS: What was one of your biggest jobs?

HN: One of the biggest jobs was recruitment of faculty. One of the first persons I brought to the University of California Medical Center was Dr. Anselm Strauss. My reason for recruiting him was to try to get social sciences integrated throughout the nursing curriculum. In addition to being concerned about social sciences, I was also much concerned about the fact that many schools of nursing had revised their baccalaureate curricula, and yet seldom had they done anything to try to evaluate outcomes of the changes. I felt it was very important, when a new curriculum was instituted, to try to evaluate what outcomes actually took place.

When the new curriculum was developed, we decided to offer during the first year a two-semester-ten-credit course in human growth and development. Chancellor Saunders was interested and very supportive because he believed firmly that it was important for medical centers to have strong social science departments. He envisioned at the time that eventually a department of social sciences would be created which would be of benefit to all the four schools of the medical center—medicine, nursing, pharmacy, and dentistry.

GS: What about some of your other problems?

HN: When I first came to U.C., I was asked to develop a ten-year plan, and I think that during the years I was on the faculty I developed a ten-year plan every year for eleven years. [*laughter*] I was expected to include in these plans numbers and preparation of faculty, numbers and types of students, curriculum development at undergraduate and graduate levels, the kinds of facilities and resources that would be needed, the research that was projected, the amount of money that could be obtained from other sources for research, and funds for the School of Nursing that must be forthcoming from the state. But it was very good experience to develop ten-year plans because it made you think about where you were going and what you were trying to do. One of the major problems when I came was getting enough space to carry out the program of the School of Nursing. Another major task, when I first went to the University of California, involved strengthening the baccalaureate degree program in nursing so that students could be admitted to the master's degree program in nursing. We did accomplish that in a very short period of time. Changes included reorganization of courses (unification of Maternal-Child Nursing and Medical-Surgical Nursing). Public health nursing and psychiatric nursing were maintained in the basic program. We introduced a number of new courses, including the one-year course in human growth and behavior, plus additional social science and biological science courses that extended through the three-year period.

Gradually, the idea of developing a curriculum around problems that were typical of the problems that a nurse must face at the time of graduation began to evolve. Faculty agreed that the entire approach to the new curriculum would be a problem-solving approach.

We decided to retain the five-academic-year curriculum because the faculty felt that at the time they could not do all of the things they wanted to do or prepare the kind of person they hoped to prepare in four academic years.[20] I had some qualms about it. I felt that, in a way, students were being penalized.

In addition to changes in the baccalaureate program, a great deal was done to strengthen the master's program. After the master's programs were well established and we had sizable enrollments in the program, I felt strongly that we should be one of the schools of nursing to take the initiative and develop doctoral programs in nursing. However, whether or not it would be possible to get a doctoral program in nursing approved at the University of California was something that had to be considered. In retrospect I think I made a good decision at that time. I decided that we needed assistance from other strong schools of the university, and the best way to get such assistance would be to set up an advisory committee made up of representatives of all the schools of the medical center itself: medicine, dentistry, pharmacy, plus hospital administration and nursing service; and also, from Berkeley, public health, education, social welfare, and letters and science. The advisory committee was involved in the development of the doctoral program. It assisted in getting the necessary approval from the university as a whole.

We decided from the beginning that the doctorate would be focused on clinical nursing and nursing research, and would lead to the D.N.S. degree.

Professional Organizations

GS: Dr. Nahm, you have been extremely active in professional organizations. Would you give me, out of your numerous involvements, one or two as illustrative examples?

HN: Yes, I'd like to talk about several activities that had great meaning for me.

I was a member of the Board of Directors of the N.L.N. for ten years and Vice President during four years of that time. One of the major concerns of the League during these years was accreditation of all types of nursing education programs. There were constant arguments about the need to improve baccalaureate and graduate programs in nursing and to strengthen and continue diploma programs. I remember vividly the concern of members who represented hospital associations and hospital schools about preserving and strengthening these schools. The representatives of baccalaureate and higher degree programs were equally concerned, of course, about the very great need to strengthen baccalaureate and graduate programs in nursing. They

[20] The curriculum has been revised, and, in the fall of 1974, a four-year curriculum was started.

were also concerned about employment of larger numbers of baccalaureate graduates by nursing service agencies. Public health nurses who were members of the Board of Directors of the N.L.N. always exhibited a great deal of foresight about health problems of the nation and the role of nurses in the community. It was always difficult, or so it seemed to me, to get representatives of public health nurses to express their opinions about the need to improve nursing services and also to feel that they had the freedom to do something. Their ideas always seemed to be overridden by representatives of the hospital associations. The N.L.N., of course, was set up to have varied membership, not only nurses representing hospital nursing, public health nursing, and nursing education, but also practical nurses and interested citizens of the community. The need to have varied membership was discussed over and over again; the League did have some very prominent and very interested, dynamic lay members. Mary Rockefeller was one of the persons who served on the board for many years and who always brought the point of view of the public to the board.

Though I think the N.L.N. was quite a dynamic organization, its major attention over the years was directed to problems at the national level. My concern was that it was very difficult to strengthen the state and local Leagues sufficiently to make a real impact on the community or to gain enough lay members or members of other professions so their voice could be heard in the improvement of nursing services and nursing education. I think, however, the League performed a very important role, and continues to do so. At times there were real power struggles between the N.L.N. and the A.N.A., but in recent years I think the situation has improved. The two organizations have always cooperated in the matter of legislation, particularly as it related to the strengthening of nursing schools, scholarships and loan funds for students, capitation funds, and funds for construction of nursing school buildings. The N.L.N. provided a great deal of the information that was used in testifying, and certain representatives of the League also testified in Washington about the need for support of nursing education in this country.

Some people were concerned when I accepted the appointment as a member of the A.N.A. Committee on Nursing Education (later the Commission on Nursing Education), but personally I felt no real problem. When I was a member of the Board of Directors of the N.L.N. or working with educational programs under the N.L.N., I felt they had an important mission to perform. The strength of the League came primarily from the fact that it had membership from the schools of nursing themselves. And the representatives who came to meetings represented their schools. This is a different type of representation from that of an individual-membership organization (A.N.A.).

Committees of the A.N.A. to a far greater extent represented individual nurses, and even though there were many factions in the A.N.A., the battles were fought out in committees and in big meetings of the associations at local, state, and national levels. There were times when many people thought that the A.N.A. was very biased toward baccalaureate and higher degree programs. When I was a member of the A.N.A. Committee on Nursing Education, one of the first tasks that this Committee turned its attention to was the preparation of a statement on nursing education. As you know, this statement was finally published.[21] The major recommendations were that all nursing education should eventually be in colleges and universities and that there should be two types of nursing education: baccalaureate education as basic preparation for professional nursing, and associate degree education as basic preparation for technical nursing. This was a statement for the future. It was prepared as a guideline for schools and service agencies and for people in general to use in future planning. The third recommendation, which created a good deal of furor, was that assistants to nurses should be prepared in short, preservice programs. The idea was that the present one-year practical nursing programs would gradually either be strengthened and absorbed into the associate degree nursing programs, or shortened into short, preservice programs to prepare assistants to technical and professional nurses. Personally I still think it's a good idea. Much of the problem would be solved if we simply had nurses prepared for direct service under supervision in associate degree or semiprofessional programs, and nurses prepared for truly professional nursing at baccalaureate and higher degree levels. Personally I hope that eventually preparation for most professional nurses will be beyond the baccalaureate degree level. I think baccalaureate education, for the present, is probably as much as can be achieved, but I do not think that we can include enough preparation in basic sciences— biological, physical, social, and behavioral—and the humanities to really prepare a top-level professional. That's my own bias, but I realize it can't be achieved overnight. Well, as you know, the statement on nursing education created a furor and, to a certain extent, continues to do so. Perhaps the mistake that was made in the statement was to present the ideas as though they should be carried out. It might have been better to present them as recommendations for further study so that, if people could have studied the recommendations and then come forward with plans, we might have ended up with the same recommendations, but many more people might have given thoughtful attention to them instead of reacting emotionally. That's just a matter of strategy, I

---

[21] The American Nurses' Association issued its statement on required educational preparation for nurse-practitioners and assistants to nurses in *A Position Paper*, American Nurses' Association, New York, 1965. Dr. Nahm was on the committee which prepared the recommendation.

think, that organizations need to think about when they publish statements in the future. I was still on the Committee when the statement on continuing education was published. It was well received, and I think has been widely used. Additional statements on continuing education are now being made that relate to the need for continuing education as a basis for continuing licensure.

Retirement

GS: What have you been doing since retirement?

HN: I have been quite active. I serve as a consultant to university schools on nursing in their baccalaureate and graduate education programs. I have also been involved in working on regional surveys, such as for the New England Board of Higher Education (N.E.B.H.E.), and on various projects involving university schools and nursing education services in San Francisco.

GS: In summing up, what is one thing you would like to emphasize?

HN: After years of national experience, I have come to the conclusion that in order to solve problems, one has to do it on the local scene. Nursing leaders must get involved at home and challenge younger nurses to do the same. Younger nurses must get involved to bring about important changes in our community and our society.

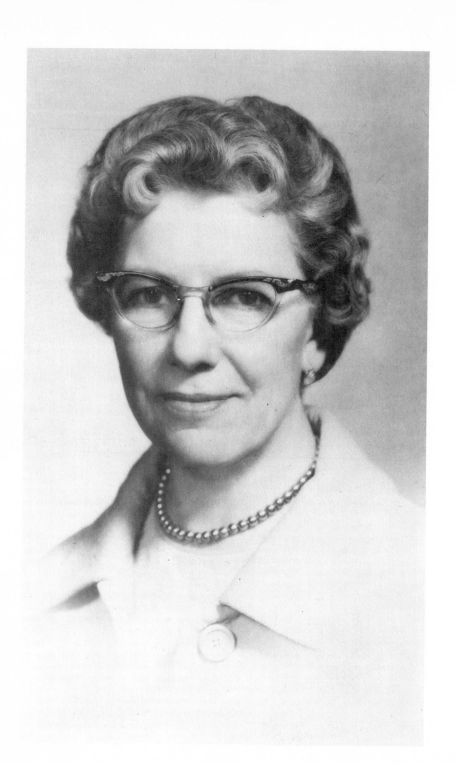

12

Dr. Notter's contribution to nursing research has been that of encourager, stimulator, and enabler—without which much of research would lie fallow . . . As the first full-time editor of *Nursing Research,* she has encouraged nurses to report their research, has given them thoughtful criticism, and through expansion of the magazine's pages and number of issues per year has enabled an ever increasing number of nurse researchers to share their findings with others . . . in 1965 she was influential in launching the *International Nursing Index,* a valuable research tool, and its first editor . . . as project director for the American Nurses' Association's annual nursing research critique conferences. . . . Dr. Notter has been tireless in her efforts to enable established as well as young investigators to present their studies, to stimulate participation in the conferences, and to insure the give and take necessary for inquiry.[1]

[1]From the Citation, Alumni Achievement Award in Nursing Research and Scholarship, Nursing Education Alumni Association of Teachers College, Columbia University, New York, May 9, 1971.

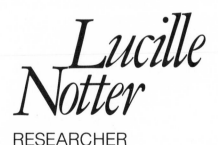

Lucille
Notter

RESEARCHER

*L*ucille Notter's contributions as the editor of the journal *Nursing Research* (1961–1973) go unquestioned. She developed and expanded the publication into a highly respected journal of nursing research. She was the editor of the *International Nursing Index* (1965–1973).

As Project Director of the American Nurses' Association (A.N.A.) Annual Nursing Research Conferences (1965–1973), she brought nurse-researchers together to present a superior level of research papers and critiques. The 15 highly stimulating series of conferences served as a catalyst for regional nursing groups to institute similar conferences.

Among her past positions are Head Nurse, Supervisor, and Instructor, Michael Reese Hospital School of Nursing (1932–1940); staff nurse, supervisor, administrative assistant, and Educational Director of the Visiting Nurse Service of New York (1941–1950); Director, Joint Education Program, Visiting Nurse Service of New York and Visiting Nurse Association of Brooklyn (1950–1954); Assistant Executive Director, Visiting Nurse Association of Brooklyn (1956–1960); Adjunct Assistant Professor, Hunter College of the City University of New York (1960–1963); and faculty member, Writers' Workshops, Boston University School of Nursing (1963–1966). She is currently (1975) coeditor of *Cardiovascular Nursing* and Director of a National League for Nursing (N.L.N.) project, "An Evaluation of Open Curriculum Projects and Open Curriculum Students in Nursing Education."

Lucille E. Notter was born in Frankfort, Kentucky, on Friday the thirteenth, 1907. She was the eldest of five children. She came from what she describes as a "modest lower-middle-class" background. Her father was a salesman with a public utilities company, well known and respected in the community. Her grandfather had immigrated to the United States about six years before her father's birth. Her mother was a "very warm, spontaneous, artistic personality."

Lucille Notter was reared as a Catholic and attended Catholic parochial schools. Because there wasn't much money in the family, especially with five children, there was some question whether she could go to college. She worked for about two years as a record-room clerk in a local hospital, where she bacame acquainted with nursing and with Mabel McCracken, a graduate of Saints Mary and Elizabeth Hospital School of Nursing in Louisville, Kentucky, who influenced her to enter nurses' training there. Lucille Notter "loved" nursing and says, "I never planned on nursing when I was in high school. It was the last thing I had on my mind. I don't know what I thought I was going to be, but I certainly hadn't thought I was going to be a nurse, and I didn't know very much about it. However, my family encouraged and helped me with my plans to become a nurse."

She graduated from Saints Mary and Elizabeth Hospital School of Nursing in 1931. She received her B.S. in nursing education in 1941, an M.A. in supervision in public health nursing in 1946, and an Ed.D. in administration of educational programs in 1956, all from Teachers College, Columbia University.

Among her honors are an Award for Distinguished Service to Public Health Nursing from the Public Health Nursing Section of the American Public Health Association (A.P.H.A.) in 1974; an Alumni Achievement Award in Nursing Research and Scholarship from Teachers College, Columbia University, in 1971; and a Citation for Outstanding Achievement from Wagner College in 1958.

Her membership and participation in many professional organizations have been considerable.[2] Her editorial page of *Nursing Research* was eagerly awaited by the readers of the journal. The topics were always timely, relevant, and well written.

Dr. Notter is the author of several books.[3] She has published numerous articles throughout the years on research and other topics. One of her key articles is "The Vital Significance of Clinical Nursing Research," which demonstrates how the end result can be improved patient care.[4]

Editor of Nursing Research

GS: You have been saluted by other nursing leaders as an outstanding leader in research. Could you discuss your position as editor of Nursing Research? How did you get into it, what is your definition of research, and what have been your major contributions?

LN: Lucy Germain, who was at that time (1961) Executive Director of

[2] To mention only a few: chairman, Governing Council of the Society of Distinguished Practitioners, New York State Nurses' Association; former member, Board of Directors, N.Y.S. Nurses' Association; past President and former Secretary, N.Y.S. Nurses' Association; Executive Editor's Board, *International Journal of the Addictions;* Treasurer, Board of Trustees, Institute for the Study of Drug Misuse; member, Nursing Advisory Committee to the Director of Nursing of the New York City Prison System; and member and former consultant, Nursing Archives, Mugar Memorial Library, Boston University.

[3] *The Essentials of Nursing Research,* Springer Publishing Co., Inc., New York, 1974; with Eugenia K. Spalding, *Professional Nursing: Foundations, Perspectives, and Relationships,* J. B. Lippincott Company, Philadelphia, 1976; and, with Audrey F. Spector, *Nursing Research in the South: A Survey,* Southern Regional Education Board, Atlanta, May 1974.

[4] *Cardiovascular Nursing,* 8:19–22, September–October 1972.

the American Journal of Nursing Company, talked me into taking the position as Editor of *Nursing Research*. I was interested in the journal for the simple reason that I had been on the Editorial Board of *Nursing Research* for several years (1957–1961). During part of that time, several of us on the Board who lived in or near New York City used to go into the office periodically to handle correspondence and to decide on the disposition of manuscripts, based on reviewers' comments. Edith P. Lewis, the present Editor of *Nursing Outlook,* was Managing Editor and did the actual preparation of manuscripts for the printer.

I must admit that I had been interested in *Nursing Research* from the time the Association of Collegiate Schools of Nursing (A.C.S.N.) began planning for it. I recall one meeting of the A.S.C.N. I attended, at which Helen Bunge and the Committee to plan the journal discussed *Nursing Research* and solicited subscriptions and contributions for the new journal. I was heart and soul behind it. I felt that this was an important step in the development of scientific inquiry in nursing and that the new journal would make a very important contribution to our profession. I became a charter subscriber and continued to take the journal throughout the years, using it in my teaching. So when Lucy Germain asked me to become the Editor, I already had a great interest in the journal and an appreciation of the kind of contribution it had made under Helen Bunge's leadership and through the work of Barbara Tate, part-time Editor from 1959 to 1961.

I went on the staff of the American Journal of Nursing Company as Editor of *Nursing Research* in the fall of 1961. At that time there weren't too many nurses with doctorates and not too many doing research. The increase in research has paralleled the increase in nurses prepared at the graduate level—especially at the doctoral level, that is—to do research. In this, I think nursing has taken the same route other professions have, and particularly the professions in which women are involved. For example, in the early 1900s a college education was not as readily available as it is now, and especially not for most women. However, as opportunities arose in higher education for women generally, and for nurses particularly, the possibilities for nursing research also arose. As the master's degree programs flourished in the 1940s and the 1950s and the doctoral degree programs in the 1960s, we began to have more research by nurses.

The first issue of *Nursing Research* in 1952 carried one major research report in nursing, Dr. Marjory Mack's report of her doctoral dissertation. Much of the research reported in later issues during the 1950s was not about nursing practice; the research was more likely to be about nurses or about nursing education or nursing service administration. This reflected the kind of research in nursing that was being done during that time.

By 1961 there were more articles reporting research, but the journal was still a relatively slim one, published four times a year. It had become a quarterly in 1959, and it became a bimonthly in 1968 as a result of the gradual increase in the number of publishable manuscripts that became available.

My philosophy was always to produce the very best, that is, to publish reports that represented the best research being done. Although much of this research was often doctoral research by nurses or research by nonnurse scientists, some of it represented master's work by nurses. I felt strongly that young nurses coming along with good master's studies should be encouraged by seeing themselves in print. These master's studies were often published in the "Briefs" section. They were usually small but carefully done studies, often in clinical areas and indicating areas in need of further research. I was hopeful that reporting them would encourage more research in nursing practice and would also give these nurses the push they needed to go ahead with doctoral study and to continue their interest in research.

I always saw the purpose of *Nursing Research* as carrying reports of a variety of kinds of research in nursing (clinical research, research in nursing education or administration, and historical research) as well as general articles about research. The term "nursing research" may imply nursing practice or clinical research; however, the journal *Nursing Research* has always carried articles that are broadly representative of the various types of research in nursing, and I believe this policy is a good one.

Views on Nursing Research

GS: Is this, then, how you would define nursing research?

LN: I would define nursing research as that research which aims to improve clinical practice, that is, is relevant to nursing practice. Much of it will probably be research which is based in the behavioral or biological sciences, as these are related to nursing practice. I also see the need to continue to have studies of nursing education and studies of nursing service administration. Studies in these areas will also eventually improve nursing practice. However, I believe that eventually more nurses will be working more directly to improve nursing practice through research. Perhaps with the development of doctorates in nursing, our research will become more practice-oriented.

GS: Is this the direction you think nursing research is taking?

LN: Yes, I believe that there is an increasing focus on clinical nursing research. I have the feeling that this focus will continue. The movement toward clinical specialism in nursing may help in this respect. Clinical specialists may be in the best position to identify problems in nursing and to help with, or carry out, the needed research. The growing practice of giving baccalaureate students in nursing an introduction to nursing research may also be influential in interesting young nurses in using the findings of research and participating in research to the extent possible.

GS: Do you prefer a quantitative type of research orientation in teaching?

LN: Over the qualitative type? I think that it's very difficult in a practice profession not to be also interested in qualitative research. I don't have a preference, but I have a feeling that we need to emphasize both. Overemphasis on quantitative measurement may possibly hinder the development of some kinds of clinical research, such as case studies or field observations. Much can be learned by carefully done qualitative research. Of course we also need good experimental research, even though collecting data and controlling the intervening variables are difficult in the practice setting. There are many problems in doing experimental research in the clinical setting; for example, there are some variables which one may not be able to control. However, we need to go ahead and do the research even though we cannot control all of the variables or quantify all of the kinds of data observed. Applied research, that is, research for the purpose of discovering ways to improve patient care, can be as important as basic research, which has as its aim discovering new knowledge.

GS: Yes. And there are fashions in research, too. The experimental models are considered technically sophisticated, but do you think that many times they may have meaningless goals?

LN: I wouldn't say many times, but now and then one gets the impression that in some experimental research, the design used may have assumed more importance than the purpose of the research.

To go back to the purpose of clinical nursing research: to improve patient care, I hope that all nurses as they graduate and go into practice will have inquiring minds and that they will begin to keep records of what they observe in order to eventually study the problems they identify. If one keeps good records, data can be collected that in the long run may prove more valuable than an experimental study of a handful of patients that has perhaps little or no relevance to patient care.

Trends in Nursing Research

GS: *What have you noticed as major trends in nursing research?*

LN: In the 1950s the studies funded by the A.N.A., their five-year study of nurses, influenced greatly what happened during that period. Nurses seemed to be the most studied group of people in the country during that time. Psychologists and sociologists were looking at nurses—what they were like, what their attitudes were, what their roles were, and how they differed from other people. At the same time there were some excellent studies in nursing education as well as studies in clinical nursing and some historical research. But the studies of nurses monopolized the scene. During the 1960s, research in nursing education assumed more importance, and there was a gradually growing interest in clinical research. Today, the emphasis appears to be definitely on clinical research. There is also a growing interest in historical research.

GS: *What, do you think, has brought about this latter interest? What has acted as a catalyst for this interest in historical research in nursing?*

LN: There probably have been several things operating. It became possible for nurses to get their doctorates in history. Also, the interest in the development of nursing archives may have been an additional influence. We began to note a rising interest in nursing history and an increasing realization of its importance to present-day nursing. Because a few nurses have had more than a passing interest in historical research, their influence has been felt. There were always some nurses interested in history, for example, Adelaide Nutting, Lavinia Dock, Isabel Stewart, and Anne Austin, to name but a few of those who have made a contribution to this field. However, the current interest in historical research will, I believe, significantly increase the numbers of nurses who will study our heritage and its contribution to the present and future of nursing.

I am happy to see the growing interest of nurses like yourself in historical research and to see the results of their work as it appears in print. I am impressed with the zeal these nurses show in promoting careful historical studies and reports. Their growing interest in oral history is also an important trend of great significance to future nurses. In the Winter 1965 issue of *Nursing Research,* I commented in an editorial on the urgency of the need for historical research.[5] As a result of a suggestion by the A.N.A. Research Committee, I had encouraged an

---

[5] "The Urgency of the Case for Historical Research," *Nursing Research,* 14:3, Winter 1965.

article by Mildred Newton on "The Case for Historical Research." My editorial pointed up the need for historical research as did Dr. Newton's article, which appeared in the same issue of *Nursing Research*. At that time, as Dr. Newton pointed out, "historical research in nursing [was] . . . pitifully meager."[6] I used Dr. Newton's title seven years later as the title of another editorial to highlight the continuing need to place emphasis on historical research in nursing.[7] By that time I was able to note some increasing interest in this form of research.

Major Contributions

GS: What would you say you feel would be your major contribution with respect to leadership in nursing research?

LN: I would like to think that I made some contribution to nursing research. As Editor of *Nursing Research,* I was in a unique position to know the field—to know about ongoing and completed research and to know many of the nurses and others who were involved in the field. Also, I became further involved in the nursing research field when I assumed the responsibility of project director of the A.N.A. Nursing Research Conferences. The A.N.A. Research Committee and, later, the A.N.A. Commission on Research served as the advisory committee to these annual conferences, nine of which were held between the years 1965 and 1973. The conferences, which provided a forum for scientific interchange among nurse-researchers over the nine years, brought together a large number of nurses interested in research and did much to promote an interest in scholarly research. I believe that both the journal *Nursing Research* and the A.N.A. Nursing Research Conferences made significant contributions to nursing during a very important period in the development of research in nursing.

Involved as I was in the above activities, I had the opportunity to stimulate research activity among nurses and to encourage nurse investigators to communicate their research and its findings to others. It is a truism that a piece of research is not complete until it is communicated to other interested researchers and to those who can implement the findings in the practice field. The early nurse-investigators often needed encouragement to report their research in scientific journals like *Nursing Research*. I never missed an opportunity to speak to nursing faculty, particularly those in graduate programs where students and

---

[6] Mildred E. Newton, "The Case for Historical Research," *Nursing Research,* 14:20–26, Winter 1965.

[7] "The Case for Historical Research in Nursing," *Nursing Research,* 21:483, November–December 1972.

faculty were doing research or wanted to start a research program. These occasions, I hope, served to stimulate both research and writing about what they were doing for the various journals, including *Nursing Research*.

If I did make a major contribution to the field of nursing research, I believe that it was through the stimulation of research and the encouragement of communication of the findings of research. In addition to meeting with faculty, this was accomplished through my personal contacts with many nurses and through the selection and presentation of the best of the current studies in nursing in *Nursing Research*. I had a lot of faith in the ability of the nurses I met and talked with as well as faith in the future of nursing research. It was a wonderful experience to be a part of the development of research in nursing during the years that I was the editor of *Nursing Research*.

The publication of the new *International Nursing Index*, beginning in 1965, was also an important event in helping to promote research by improved communication. Guiding this important bibliographic tool during its early years was an exciting experience. The *Index* made, and continues to make, a significant contribution to nursing research by providing researchers with easy access to the wealth of nursing literature in nursing journals and related health journals.

GS: What would you say was your biggest point of frustration in your work?

LN: Having enough time, I guess, to do all of the things I wanted to do. When I first came as editor of *Nursing Research,* I did all of the editorial work with the help of a part-time secretary. This was all that was needed. As the journal grew in size, a full-time secretary was employed and later a part-time assistant editor. As I said earlier, I was also involved in other activities that helped promote the journal, such as visiting faculty in universities, attending research meetings, and serving as director of the A.N.A. Research Conferences. However, I guess that I would have liked to be able to see even more of the people interested in research and to keep even more in touch with ongoing research because, as time went on, the field of nursing research grew. It became increasingly difficult to know all that was going on, not only in universities but also in the nursing service agencies. For example, nursing service in Veterans Administration hospitals and in a few large medical centers and health agencies began to employ nurse-researchers to head their research programs.

Today it is increasingly difficult to keep abreast of all of the research in nursing. Although *Nursing Research* has done most in terms of influencing research and communicating research in this country because it is the one journal devoted exclusively to reporting research, I suspect that, as time goes by, more of the research will be reported in other journals.

GS: You mean nursing journals or other journals?

LN: I really mean other journals as well as nursing journals. I think, for example, that some of the nurse physiologists, nurse-anthropologists, and those in other fields will continue to report their research in other journals related to their specialties. Some researchers will report their work in health-related journals. But I would like also to see reports of clinical research, written in a simple, clearly understandable but scholarly manner, in other nursing journals. Nursing research should be reported broadly so that all nurses have access to its findings. As research becomes a way of life in nursing rather than something esoteric, I think we will see it reported in many more nursing journals. I believe there are many nursing journals in the field today that have an interest in communicating the findings of research to nurses in the practice field, in education, and in nursing service administration.

Future Directions in Nursing Research

GS: To recapitulate, would you define nursing research, or research in nursing, and, then, where you think it is going?

LN: I believe that nursing research can be defined as systematic, scientific investigation of problems related to nursing with the ultimate purpose being improved patient or health care. It encompasses both basic and applied research and includes studies in search of theories of nursing, methodological studies to develop needed research tools, clinical practice studies, studies of patterns of patient or health care, nursing education studies, and studies of the historical roots of nursing. All of these investigative areas—and perhaps more could be added—are necessary as we strive to improve the nursing care of people.

The emphasis at the moment appears to be on clinical investigations. Both basic and applied research are encouraged. Some are investigating the quality of care given by nurses; others are attempting to study the effect of nursing care on the patient. The latter kind of research is admittedly more difficult because of the problems involved in the control of intervening variables. Still others are carrying out basic research related to patient care, studies based in the biological and psychosocial sciences. All are important to the improvement of nursing practice.

The emphasis on clinically oriented research has been needed in order to interest more nurse-researchers to work on nursing problems. The trend toward offering doctorates in nursing should, I believe, promote research in nursing practice.

The next decade or so should see the expansion of clinical research in nursing, both by large-scale investigations in nursing research centers or by collaboration of investigators from various university centers, and by smaller-scale research by individuals, including doctoral students. Promising efforts at comprehensive studies have started, for example, in the studies of pain, rest, and fatigue. In the past there have been too many small, uncoordinated studies. The trend toward collaborative studies and toward the coordination of research efforts of faculty and graduate students in university centers will do more to help us accumulate useful scientific knowledge in nursing.

As stated earlier, there will continue to be a very real need for educational research, particularly for evaluative research. Both traditional and the newer nontraditional programs need to be examined. For this purpose, better evaluation tools are required for the study of new curriculum approaches and new teaching methods, as, for example, the use of multiple media.

GS: *Are you talking about things like videotape?*

LN: Yes, videotape is one of the methods needing study. Others include modular learning, programmed instruction, self-pacing, and other methods not yet invented.

Lately there has been increasing criticism of the product of nursing education by employers and consumers. Perhaps we need more studies to determine wherein the problem lies. Here we need studies which will help us determine whether the criticism is valid and, if so, whether the problem lies in education or in nursing service, or in both.

But, to go back a bit to the subject of the future of nursing research. I would really like to see progress made on all fronts—clinical, patterns of delivery of care, education, administration, historical, and philosophical, both basic and applied—with emphasis on the goal of improved practice. My point of view has been, and continues to be, that we need practice-oriented research and research-oriented practice, that every nurse should be helped to make use of the results of research. I am afraid that the climate in many institutions or agencies where nurses work is not conducive to changes in nursing based on the findings of research; however, I am hopeful that the use of research-minded clinical specialists and nurse-practitioners will help change this.

Of course, the introduction of research and research-oriented teaching in the basic baccalaureate program and in in-service and continuing education will also help. It is hard to know how much journals, such as *Nursing Research,* are used by nurses and by educators. Publication of the results of research is important, but avails little if it is not read, evaluated, and implemented when indicated. Nurses, like other professionals, must keep abreast of the knowledge in their field. Keeping up with the research literature in their specialty and in general is one way of keeping abreast.

It is perhaps important to remember that initial evaluation of the research reported in a scientific journal like *Nursing Research* has already been made by a review panel of experts in the field before it is accepted for publication. This review or referee system ensures that the studies reported make a contribution to the literature.

Perhaps *Nursing Research* is used more by graduate faculty and their students who are learning to do research. In this case, the journal is used for both its archival and its current value—to know what has gone on before and what is currently being reported. But the future should see all educators, both those in educational institutions and those in service agencies, making use of journals that report research, particularly clinical research. And, as noted earlier, as the volume of clinical research increases, more will be reported in a variety of journals.

GS: When you retired, what would you say were the approximate number of manuscripts you were receiving for publication?

LN: Roughly, in the neighborhood of 200 a year. We published about sixty-two.

GS: Would you ever solicit manuscripts?

LN: Oh, yes. Most commonly, when I met nurses who were doing interesting research, I would indicate an interest in receiving a manuscript reporting their research when it was completed. Later, of course, the prospective author might need a reminder. Also, articles of general interest on research methods or theories basic to research were frequently solicited or encouraged from experts in the field. Then, too, research conferences were often a good source of authors of prospective manuscripts.

GS: You said that you received 200 manuscripts. Was this a gradual increase?

LN: Yes, it was a gradual increase. *Nursing Research* was initiated in 1952. At that time it consisted of a forty-eight-page journal issued three times a year. When I became Editor in 1961, it was a sixty-four-page quarterly publishing in each issue around seven to eight articles and fourteen to sixteen pages of abstracts of studies in nursing which had appeared in other journals. With the growth in research at the master's, doctoral, and postdoctoral levels, there was a corresponding growth in the number of manuscripts to be considered. The number of submitted manuscripts which were published began to approximate one out of every three received.

GS: Would you agree or disagree with the statement that the recent increase in the number of manuscripts is due to pressure for people in academic life to publish?

LN: I would say that the statement is partly true. There are at least two things operating here. First, and most important, more research is being done and more nurses are writing for publication. Second, there is a push for publication. It is true that nurse faculty, like other faculty, are now more often required to show evidence of their contribution to the literature.

GS: About what proportion—just a rough estimate—of the articles would you say are sincere, valid attempts to communicate research findings important in improving patient care?

LN: That's a very difficult question to answer. I would estimate that at the time I retired in 1973, roughly a third of the articles reported were about research specifically related to patient care. I could not say that any of these articles were not sincere, valid attempts to report research in the interest of improved care. It is possible that some individuals just like to get what they've done in print; however, I believe that the nurses who sent in manuscripts were really more interested in making a contribution to nursing. A few nonnurses did occasionally submit a manuscript that was obviously not related to nursing; in this instance, the interest in contributing to nursing might be hard to establish.

Working with Prospective Authors

GS: To what extent were you able to encourage or assist authors?

LN: There were three major ways in which I, as Editor, could be helpful to authors: (1) by encouraging nurses to write, (2) by meeting with groups of nurses, usually faculty groups, to discuss writing and especially writing for *Nursing Research,* and (3) by helping prospective authors who were asked to revise their manuscripts.

Despite the "publish or perish" syndrome, many nurses still need to be encouraged to write articles reporting the studies they have done. Every effort was made through personal contact with nurses to encourage them to commit themselves to writing. There is no better way to learn how to write than by starting to write. A letter to the editor inquiring about interest in an article reporting one's research and then a specific commitment to deliver the article help one get started.

Meeting with groups to discuss writing for *Nursing Research* was, I found, most helpful because individual questions about writing could be answered. Also, individual conferences could be held with those persons who were ready to start, or had started, an article.

Because the volume of manuscripts was not too great, individual letters briefly indicating the reasons for rejection could be sent, in which an attempt could be made not to discourage the writer. In the case where revisions were indicated before acceptance could be considered, suggestions were made to help the author with rewriting. Also, in any meetings with nurses, I found it important to stress that a rejection should never keep one from trying again and that good writing is a matter of rewriting. Suggestions for revision are almost always made to improve the presentation of the research report—perhaps a matter of reorganizing the content and sometimes a matter of adding details not included because the author knew them so well they were simply forgotten.

GS: Did you take any special courses or classes in editing or writing?

LN: No, I learned on the job, I guess, and by talking with the other editors at the American Journal of Nursing Company. I did do one thing; a couple of years after I went with the journal, I went to a Bread Loaf Writers Workshop for two weeks. I also occasionally attended meetings of medical writers, but I never really took a course in editing or writing. I am sure it would have been helpful had I done so. I might say I learned a lot from working with authors and with the members of the review panel and the editorial advisory committee.

GS: What did you like most in your job?

LN: I liked meeting the people, getting to know the people in nursing research. And I really liked working on manuscripts; this was something that I hadn't known would be true when I accepted the position as editor. Sometimes a manuscript that sounded as if it were going to be easy turned out to be the hardest to edit. But a really tough manuscript that turned out to be good was always a pleasure.

I don't know what I liked most about my job. I didn't mind rewriting or working on a manuscript; I rather liked it. Then, as I say, I thoroughly enjoyed meeting the people, some of whom I knew through correspondence only but many of whom I later met personally and got to know quite well. You may think that being an editor is being closed up in an office with nothing but paper and pencils around. Actually, that's not true at all. One does do a lot of pencil work, but it's more than that.

I liked my work as editor very much, as you can see, and I still liked it when I retired. In fact, I can't think of anything else I would rather have done during the years I spent as Editor of *Nursing Research.*

Some Issues and Problems in Nursing Research

GS: What are some of the issues in nursing research as you see them?

LN: I think one of the issues is whether we should be doing basic research or applied research, whether the person who is doing the research should be concerned about whether it is going to influence practice. I believe there is beginning to be a swing, if I read correctly what people are saying, toward accepting the idea that scientists may have some responsibility for promoting the implementation of the results of their research. Now, I know that in basic research the investigator pursues the research with the idea of learning new knowledge, and has traditionally not been concerned with the use to which that knowledge will be put. However, with the tightening of funds available for research, including nursing research, the question about the usefulness of the expected findings will more often be asked. The investigator may need to show that the research is going to have some impact on the improvement of patient or health care. As a result, I think that more nurses will be investigating nursing problems and will be taking responsibility for seeing that their research results are communicated not only to other researchers but also to nurses generally. They will write not only for scientific journals but also for journals read more frequently by the practicing nurse.

Today, because of the demands for faculty with doctoral degrees, not enough of those prepared to do research are actually engaged in it. Perhaps at issue is the problem of time for faculty to do research. Often, teaching loads are heavy and time for research is at a premium. On the other hand, even when there is a philosophy which would permit time for research, it may not always be done. I think that it is possible that some nurse faculty would really rather teach.

Another issue or problem is related to funds for postdoctoral fellowships. A doctoral degree prepares the nurse to do research but does not necessarily make the nurse an expert researcher. There is a need for more attention to be focused on this problem. Of course, to get funding for research and for postdoctoral fellowships one must be able to sell the need for this. Society as a whole may not as yet see nurses as scientific researchers. There is a job still to be done here, but a good start has been made with the funding of research projects in nursing and of such programs as those preparing nurse-scientists.

Another issue faces nurses interested in doing clinical research. Patients have traditionally been readily available for medical research, but not always as available for nursing research if objections are raised by the medical or nursing staff. The issue of patients' rights further complicates the picture, and institutions are increasingly cautious about granting permission for research to be carried out using their patients. It is possible that nurses wanting to do patient care research will find themselves in competition with physicians for the available patients. This issue must be faced when it is encountered. However, a number of nurses have been able to do clinical research without the issue being raised. Much depends on the quality and type of research planned and the relationships established. If the research is well designed, the patients' rights are respected, and the goal of improvement of patient care is demonstrated, there should, as a rule, be no difficulty.

GS: *What about funds for research?*

LN: Right now funding agencies seem to be tightening their belts. Nobody really has the money to spend that they did in the 1950s and the 1960s. During that time nurses grew accustomed to looking to the Public Health Service Division of Nursing and to the research grants program in nursing for support of research and for fellowships and traineeships; they did not always look beyond that to other sources of research funds. They now are beginning to look at many more sources, both public and private. Nurses will increasingly have to look for research support in the marketplace, just as everyone else does. This may not be as hard as it sounds, but it means doing a bit of searching for the available funds in a variety of places. The kind of research that some of our nurse investigators are doing can stand up very well in competition with others.

Generally speaking, hospitals and health agencies have not been accustomed to supporting research in nursing. I think they might be willing to support studies if they could be convinced that care would be improved. As stated earlier, some hospitals and public health agencies have employed a nursing research director. If this trend were actively promoted by nursing, it could go far to increase the amount of clinical research in nursing.

Also, I believe nurses can be much more of a force in society as a political action group to promote better nursing care through both education and research. The idea that research is as much a part of nursing as it is of medicine and the other professions must be accepted by nurses and by society. Acceptance of this idea may not always be easy to effect, but it can be done. Perhaps the reason so many do not understand why nurses should be doing research is that so few nurses in the past were doing research that made a difference in patient care. Nurses are going to be assuming greater responsibility and accountability for patient care than they have in the past, and for broader areas of patient care. This responsibility will entail improving this care and adapting care to new conditions as these arise. Research to validate changes will become increasingly important and, I believe, more acceptable to the public as an inherent function of nurses.

Present Interests

GS: What have you been doing since you've retired?

LN: I have been busy doing some writing and some consultation on both writing and research. However, I also have taken on two part-time jobs. I am working half time in the Division of Research of the N.L.N. on their open curriculum project. My original responsibility was for the Open Curriculum Conferences held as part of the project. I am currently serving as director of the project, "An Evaluation of Open Curriculum Projects and Open Curriculum Students in Nursing Education." Objectives of the project, which grew out of the N.L.N. Board of Directors' approved statement on "The Open Curriculum in Nursing Education," include dissemination of information about open curriculum programs and opportunities for career mobility in nursing education, as well as the development of guidelines basic to the development of sound open curriculum systems.

I am also serving as coeditor of *Cardiovascular Nursing.* This is a three-year appointment that will terminate at the end of December 1976. *Cardiovascular Nursing* is a bimonthly publication of the American Heart Association. It is distributed to interested nurses and institutions through the association's local affiliates, and serves to provide nurses with up-to-date scientific information about cardiovascular diseases and the care of patients with these conditions.

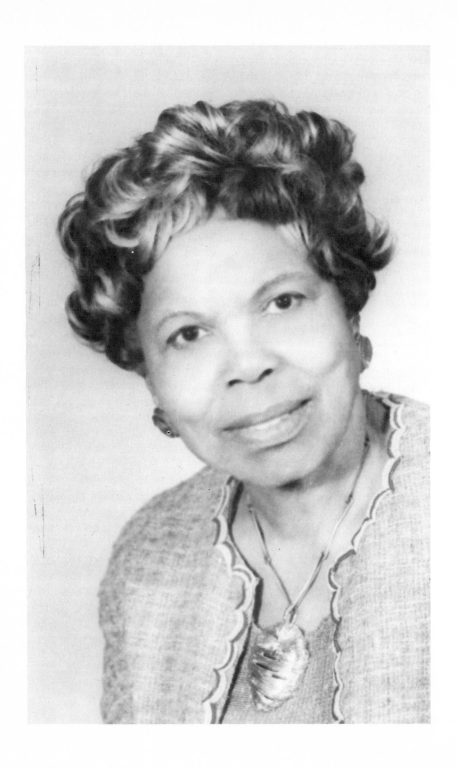

13

Democracy is emerging to a point that we of the nursing profession embrace all nurses. We are allying ourselves with world brotherhood and with more consecrated effort and sympathetic understanding. We work together with an enhanced spiritual desire to love, help and hope that peace passing all understanding will come throughout the world.[1]

[1]Estelle M. Osborne at the National League for Nursing Convention, 1967.

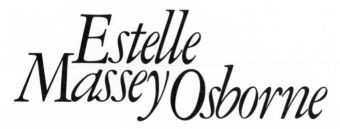

Estelle Massey Osborne

EDUCATOR

*E*stelle Massey Osborne was a pioneer in creating opportunities for the black nurse. She is a warm, gracious person who suffered humiliation and prejudice. She has had to have tremendous courage and determination to successfully fight racial discrimination.

She has lived to prove herself primarily bigger rather than primarily bitter. She should be an inspiration to all young women, of no matter what race, creed or color. Because of her victory as a Negro woman in a predominantly white nation as well as of her contributions to nursing, the next generation of Negroes already have better opportunity for jobs on those levels.

She struck hard for principle and conviction when fighting for minority groups was neither popular nor easily won. Mrs. Osborne must stand tall as one of the leaders in Nursing who contributed substantially to the improved public image and the advancement of educational and economic opportunities for Negro nurses. That she was needed for this task in nursing is disgraceful, but that she was present and answered the need is a bright chapter in nursing history.[2]

Estelle Massey Osborne was born Estelle Massey in Palestine, Texas, on May 3, 1901. She was the eighth child of eleven children. Her father was a janitor and her mother a housewife. She looks back on a childhood full of laughter, fun, and warmth.[3]

Estelle Osborne went to segregated public schools. After she finished high school, she entered teacher training college. She started to teach school in a rural community but, she says:

I didn't find it too inspiring. I taught for two years, and on Sunday night I'd start crying because it was close to Monday morning and I'd have to go to school. The classes were too large; the load was pretty heavy; and some of the boys in the higher grades were older than I was. They didn't know my age, but I knew. When they said twenty-four and I thought sixteen, that was the difference.

After two years I decided that I just couldn't come back to a rural community. There were many social factors, too, that affected my decision: first of all, this limited outlook in terms of opportunity to do something different. Second, my mother had experienced—had at least lived through— things that affected an older sister teaching in a rural community down in Slocum, Texas. Just as her school was about to close, some whites in that

[2] Edna Yost, *American Women of Nursing,* J. B. Lippincott Company, Philadelphia, 1955, p. 98.
[3] For more details of her childhood, see ibid.; Sylvia G. L. Dannett (ed.), *Profiles of Negro Womanhood,* vol. 2, Educational Heritage, Inc., Yonkers, N.Y., 1966; and *Nursing Science,* April 1964.

community rode through and shot up some of the best of the Negro people. Many of those people came to our house seeking refuge. That made my mother very cautious about wanting us in rurals. Then, at the closing of my school the second year, one black killed another.

When she went to visit her brother, who was a dentist in St. Louis, Missouri, he encouraged her to become a nurse because he thought that nursing was going to be a career of the future. She went to City Hospital No. 2 (No. 1 was for whites) in St. Louis and received her registered nurse diploma in 1923. After graduating, she worked at the same hospital but quit because she faced racial prejudice and discrimination. She then worked for the Visiting Nurse Service of St. Louis, but she could never advance in her position because of the color barrier. She was black, and only the whites got the promotions and moved upward. She found this extremely frustrating because, while quite bright and competent, she could not "move ahead." She resigned, and then she thought quite seriously of leaving the nursing profession completely.

A friend helped her obtain a nursing instructor's position in the Central Nursing School in Kansas City in 1927. Knowing that she had to get more education, she borrowed money and in 1927 went to Teachers College, Columbia University, New York, to begin study for her baccalaureate degree. To complete her studies, she was given a scholarship from the Julius Rosenwald Fund, and was the *first* black nurse to be a recipient. She received her B.S. in nursing in 1930 and her M.S. in nursing in 1931, both from Columbia University.

It was now that Estelle Osborne knew in her heart that her role would be to help create social equality for other black nurses, and not just in the South but also in the North. To her, there was overt and subtle discrimination in the national nursing professional organizations and against black nurses in general.

She became the first Educational Director of Nursing at Freedman's Hospital (primarily a black institution) in Washington, D. C., in 1931. In 1932 she and Mabel Staupers were the first black nurses appointed to the committees of the National Organization for Public Health Nursing (N.O.P.H.N.). In 1934 she became the eleventh President of the National Association of Colored Graduate Nurses (N.A.C.G.N.), and for five years as President "worked tirelessly to enhance and strengthen the organization's programs" and "established a sound foundation from which (the program) could be carried forward."[4]

In 1940 she returned to St. Louis to become the first black Director of the Homer G. Phillips Hospital School of Nursing and Nursing Service. In 1943 she went to New York City to serve as a consultant with the National Nursing Council for War Service.[5] There was a known shortage of nurses in the Armed Forces, but black nurses had great difficulty getting into the service. The National Nursing Council for War Service set up a unit for black nurses on an experimental basis, the purpose of which was:

. . . to provide a better and wider use of the Negro nurse by integrating the activities of this group into the total war program. The preliminary work done by the unit was so excellent and so promising that the work was integrated in the overall council program.[6]

The work of the National Nursing Council for War Service and the N.A.C.G.N.,

(with Estelle Osborne) as a spearhead, made a genuine contribution to the upgrading of Negro nurses' qualifications and opportunities—consequently a genuine contribution to the improvement of nursing care for all patients.[7]

In 1948 Estelle Osborne was elected (the first black) for a four-year term to the Board of Directors of the American Nurses' Association (A.N.A.). In 1949 the A.N.A. board elected her as one of four United States representatives to the meeting of the International Council of Nurses (I.C.N.) in Stockholm, Sweden.

In 1946 she accepted the position of Assistant Professor at New York University, and in 1954 she left N.Y.U. to become the Assistant Director of the National League for Nursing (N.L.N.).[8] On July 1, 1959, she became the Director of Services for all state branches of the league, and was advanced to the position of Associate General Director of the N.L.N.

She has received numerous awards and citations. Among these are the Nurse of the Year Award in 1959 from New York University and the

---

[4] Mabel Staupers, *No Time For Prejudice,* The Macmillan Company, New York, 1961, p. 16.

[5] She was recommended by Congresswoman Frances Bolton from Ohio, with whom she maintained a close, warm friendship for many years.

[6] *Nursing Science,* April 1964.

[7] Ibid.

[8] The three organizations—National League of Nursing Education, National Organization for Public Health Nursing, and Association of Collegiate Schools of Nursing—merged to form the N.L.N. in 1952.

Mary Mahoney Award for her contribution to nursing and the opening of professional opportunities to minority groups. She was a member of the Health and Welfare Committee of the National Urban League. She served as a member of the Federal Citizens Committee to the U.S. Office of Education, and was on the Advisory Committee to the Surgeon General, U.S. Public Health Service. (U.S.P.H.S.). She has been Vice President of the National Council of Negro Women; a member of the A.N.A. Board of Directors; and a member of the Alpha Kappa Alpha Sorority, where she served as chairman of their National Health Project. She has written numerous articles in a wide variety of journals.[9]

Estelle Osborne's struggles and accomplishments led to the improvement of the black nurse's status, and her own life in itself is an inspiration to all, not only in nursing but in any profession. She resigned from the N.L.N. in 1967 because, she said, "I was tired," and "I have no leisure time."

Since her retirement, however, she has been on numerous committees and has traveled frequently. Her travels have included Mexico, several islands in the West Indies, the Virgin Islands, Hawaii, Bermuda, a trip around the world, Africa, the Scandinavian countries, and nine other countries in Europe.

Going into Nursing

GS: In looking back over your long, productive lifetime, what things come right to your mind?

EO: Let's start with how I happened to be a nurse. I grew up in a southern community, a member of a very large family. It was a family in which there was a lot of cooperation and shared ambitions, but not too much of the world's goods to help us realize our ambitions.

My older sisters were schoolteachers because that was just about the biggest area of employment for women of the black race; you'd have to be a schoolteacher or just a laborer. My sisters were schoolteachers and wanted me to be a schoolteacher; and so, when I finished high school, I went to Prairie View, the state teacher training college in Texas, and took the two-year teacher training course. I finished high school at fourteen, so I was sixteen when I finished at Prairie View.

I didn't find it too inspiring, teaching school in the rural community. There were many things I tried to do with the people; I've always had a

---

[9] American Journal of Nursing, Journal of Negro Education, and Public Health Nursing Magazine.

community approach to anything I've worked in. In this community the school carried seven grades. Many of the girls dropped out; their education ended there because their parents didn't have either the wisdom or the means to send them to the town 18 miles away to high school.

My mother was taut with fear after my older sister experienced an assault in Slocum, Texas, where she taught. Whites had ridden through the small community and killed many of the well-known black landowners and injured others. Some of them sought refuge in our home. So my mother was supportive of my desire to leave rural areas.

I've told you about one black killing another at the closing of my school. It was an old, old grudge from way back. The victim was a very handsome young man. After the murder, people remembered that they had had a feud over a girl years before, and this guy had just carried that grudge all those years. Well, I went to some of the trials at the courthouse in the town, and I heard truth twisted in such ways as to . . . to free this young guy, that I thought: There just is no justice; you can't expect it.

So naturally I wanted to leave, and I was determined to leave. I didn't know what I was going to do, but I have a brother who is a dentist, and I had worked in his office a little, and I had said I wanted to be a dentist. He said, "Oh, that'll be fine" at one point. Then later he'd say, "It's not a profession for women, just not what you want. You should think of nursing."

GS: Did you feel that there was discrimination at the school?

EO: Yes. Rather, it was in my favor. Remember that this was an all-black institution, except the directors, who were white. When we affiliated for communicable diseases and dietetics at the sister institutions, which were white, a screen was placed in the dining area to separate our table from the others.

I liked the content of the courses. In fact, when I was given my textbook on obstetrics, I just sat and read it one night, like you would a novel. That's an indication of the cloistered kind of background I had. I was very curious about birth and other aspects of living.

GS: What would you consider your first leadership position in nursing, and how did you get into it?

EO: I sort of got into it really as I was a senior student and was told that black nurses were having a state meeting in St. Louis and some of us could go. I went, and I was surprised that so few nurses were there. I was next surprised that it wasn't stimulating.

In my class was a girl, Juanita Caston, who had an excellent family background, and she and I used to get together and gripe and complain and take our complaints to administration. We were usually the ones who went. She and I talked about this so-called state meeting and what ought to be done. So we began organizing little discussion groups. As we were the second class, there was no alumni association. We organized it, and I was its first President.

Then I left and went to Kansas City to teach in what was, so-called, a central school of nursing. The white hospitals in Kansas City had this central program. There were only two schools for black nurses in Kansas City, and so the nearest thing to centralizing was to have the students in these two schools come to the junior college, where the junior college had a person on the staff to teach them. But that person had to be qualified also to teach hygiene to junior college students. In other words, it was an exchange plan. That was the first time *I really felt the opportunity*, that I was capable of providing some real leadership over and beyond just the classroom.

So it was when I was in that position that I started coming East to Columbia to go to summer school. My second summer, someone wisely told me to apply to the Rosenwald Fund for a scholarship in 1929; it was granted, and I stayed and attended Columbia for my bachelor's. Now that again showed me how wasteful nursing education was. I'd had two years of college before nursing and three years of nursing; that was five; and I still had to put in two more years at Columbia to get a bachelor's degree. The Rosenwald Fund saw me through. I had some real problems at Columbia at that time.

Facing Discrimination

GS: How did you find Columbia?

EO: There were attempts at discriminating in terms of my program content. When I was working on the bachelor's level, I did teaching—practice teaching—and a white nurse was my critic-teacher. We got along just beautifully together. When I was ready for graduate work, the head of the department said to this adviser, whose office was next to hers, "Miss Massey's going to stay. She's going to do graduate work. I want her to have the course in critic teaching because I think wherever she goes, she's going to have to do a lot to help the head nurses and supervisors, and this course she should have." That person said to her nonchalantly, "She can't take those courses; there are no colored girls teaching." Right in my presence! Well, the department head was greatly embarrassed and said, "Well, we'll work it out. We'll work it out." Well, I heard it!

GS: *What was your reaction?*

EO: I said nothing at the time. My reaction was to get all of my required courses and then insist upon getting that one. "She doesn't recognize your need for it; I recognize my need for it; I'm going to have it," were my thoughts. Columbia's not supposed to do that. So I went ahead and planned it on the registration day. I had it on the program. You move from chair to chair to get up to the adviser. I got the same adviser who had made the comment, and who knew me very well. She said, "I told you, you can't take the course." I said, "The department head says I can." "Well then, you go back to her again," she said.

GS: *Was the reason because you were black?*

EO: Yes, I'm black, and I can't criticize a white nurse—so she thought.

GS: *Wouldn't this make you mad—angry?*

EO: Of course it does.

GS: *How did you hold it in?*

EO: Well, you don't gain by just exploding. You think through what's the best strategy. I thought the best strategy for me was to get all my required courses so they couldn't hold me for anything, and in the last semester insist upon this.

I'd get faculty support other than in that department because I did have good faculty relationships at Columbia, in the sociology department especially. When the spring semester came, that's when the test was coming, because I was determined I was going to have the course, and I had talked it over with several outstanding faculty people who knew me.

At registration I was told to take Dr. Strattemeyer's course; I was told to take several substitutes; but no, I wanted the critic teaching. This was in nursing, and this was the way I needed it. "Well, you just can't have it."

So then I went to the dean, Dean Russel, and I told him the situation. "Oh," he said, "they can't do that here." He called the head of the nursing department, Isabel Stewart. She was out. He left the message, and he assured me he would explore and notify me. "I'll work on it and I'll let you know tomorrow."

We used to get early mail deliveries in New York then. Before I was up the next morning, my landlady pushed a note under my door, and it was from Dean Russel. "I talked with Miss Stewart about your problem.

I find that she has no prejudice and none has been exhibited toward you. In fact, Miss Stewart says she knows of no student who's had more personal attention than you. In fact, the department helped you get a Rosenwald scholarship. So take this to Miss Stewart and she will work out your problem."

I got dressed in a jiffy. Not to go to Isabel Stewart, but to go to the Dean. And I said to him, "Apparently I didn't make the matter clear to you yesterday. I have no problem: I have the money, the ability, the time, and the desire to take this course, and it's listed in the Teachers College catalogue. So I don't have a problem. And if you think my grades are not adequate for me to be advanced, then you have access to all of the grades here." So, to make a long story short, the dean had to agree with me. He called the department head and we made an appointment to meet her at four that afternoon.

I was there ahead of time. The dean arrived on time. When the conference began, she said, "Miss Massey, what makes you think we are discriminating against you? Why, Dr. Carney and Dr. Kulp have made inquiries about some problems you have." These were good allies I had in other departments. "What makes you think this?" So I repeated exactly what happened, with the dean sitting there. "Miss Muse said to you I could not take the course in critic teaching because there are no Negro girls teaching, implying that I could not be a critic teacher for a white." "Oh," she said, "I should never have done that to Miss Muse. It was just snap judgment." I said, "But you see, if you hadn't done it that way, I would never have known the real reason for being barred from the course. But she came right out and said it." The dean spoke: "Well, we have a problem, and Miss Massey cannot be the victim." And so of course they had to give the course to me.

I taught all the way on the east side of Manhattan, at Lincoln School for Nurses. Columbia is on the west side. I was the most expensive pupil there because Maude Muse used to go all the way to Lincoln. She'd sit in the back of the class so this practice teacher wouldn't get the impression I was the critic teacher. We had conferences to plan each week's work and to discuss her teaching. When we'd have these conferences, usually Maude Muse would try to take the lead, to shut out criticisms I would project. I would just insist on talking. Now the practice teacher herself, who was a victim, displayed no resentment to me. She and I had no conflict at all. She would call and visit me at home.

GS: *Do you think opportunities for black nurses have improved?*

EO: Of course they have.

GS: In what way? Also, what was your role in bringing about some of these changes?

EO: Certainly the opportunities for inclusion have increased. There was a time when there were twenty-seven separate nursing schools for blacks in this country. All of them were diploma schools except two. And those diploma schools varied in their content and status, and so forth, as far as from A to Z. Of the twenty-seven schools, I think twenty-five of them had white directors. These white directors were supposed to be in charge because there were no black nurses qualified. So we would ask: "If you've been a director for ten years, how many of your girls have you helped qualify? What's wrong, then, with your *schools* if none of them can qualify?"

After I received the M.A., the Rosenwald people kept close to me, and those that are living still do. As they would come from Chicago to Washington for various kinds of conferences, they would take me to meet key people and discuss the status of the black nurse and general nursing problems and needs. Dr. Michael Davis was the Rosenwald executive I knew best; I used to call him my fairy godfather. Dr. Davis was an outstanding social worker and one of the directors of the Rosenwald Fund. All through my schooling, all my correspondence was with him.

After I received my M.A., I went to Freedman's Hospital School of Nursing as their first Educational Director. I was working with the N.A.C. G.N. as a volunteer, and many doctors and nurses wanted me to go South. "If you're so well prepared, go South and do so-and-so," they would say. I soon saw that the kind of discrimination that was so overt in the South was just as prevalent in the North. (Look at Boston today. Who would have thought. . . ?) I was teaching over at Harlem (New York) and they neither housed nor fed me with the white instructors. In the dining room the whites sat apart. This was up in Harlem! The whites sat at a table, and if a black sat there, the waitresses would not serve her. So naturally I didn't feel I had to go anywhere in the South to do anything to fight racial discrimination. I wanted to stay close to the national organizations, and I felt that our own national was weak financially.

I went to the annual meeting of the N.A.C.G.N. down in Greensboro, North Carolina, in 1931. The program had been planned by a local group with very limited experience. Also, the program was not sufficiently dynamic for a national group, and quite a few of the people listed as program participants did not come. I wrote the board, and several of us sat down and drafted some recommendations for the next convention: first of all, that a national committee be appointed to plan national meetings. It was also recommended that at the next convention we have two days for an institute which this national committee would plan the program and the participants for. Then there would be two days for the business of the association.

In the meantime, Dr. Davis came into Washington, and he came to see me. He talked very straight and analytically; you could almost see Roman numeral one, a, b, c. He was a man of action. I told him I'd like him to be on our program. He was going to Russia that summer. So he said, "No, I'll tell you who I'd like for you to put on: Alma Haupt, Associate Director of the National Organization for Public Health Nursing." I said to him, "We're a little bit tired of representatives of the national nursing organizations coming to our conventions. They come to sell subscriptions to the magazines (that's really what they used to do) and tell us how wonderful nursing is, and then leave." I said, "We're a little tired of it." So he said to me, "I wish you'd go along with me. I'm doing a little experiment. I want you to come to New York to a luncheon I'm going to sponsor." And at that luncheon Alma Haupt was one of the people who sat very near me. (Rosenwald used to do these things. Oh, they were clever!) Dr. Davis began to talk about a profession and its idealism and obligations to all in a democracy. Then he got right to the point. He said, "I can't get over nursing discriminating in its highest places." So he put Alma Haupt on the spot. She wasn't a defensive person. (She was one of the best friends I've had.) She pointed out things they'd do and some of their problems. Afterwards he asked me, "What do you think of Miss Haupt?" I said, "Well, if she comes I think she's the kind that will be helpful."

When we had the meeting down in Nashville and she was called upon early to bring greetings from the N.O.P.H.N., her first announcement was that the N.O.P.H.N. had just appointed two black nurses: Mabel Staupers to N.O.P.H.N. Organization Committee and Estelle Massey to N.O.P.H.N. Education Committee. Okay, that was fine. But the thing to watch, if you're the one who's been protesting and you get appointed, could be just to shut your mouth.

So okay, we accepted that, and would continue to recommend competent black nurses. Some more needed to be there, and that was the way we began working. Then, you see, it was easy to make it clear to Dr. Davis that we didn't have enough money to get our office together: to do this, that, and the other. So then the Rosenwald Fund gave us the money to implement some national activities, and I wrote all the letters, even though I wasn't the president. They gave us our first grant to set up headquarters. Where we going to have headquarters? Next door to the N.O.P.H.N. and so on. They were at West 50th Street, and our office was at 50 West 50th Street, New York. So this interflow could go on.

As we were trying to build the N.A.C.G.N., we needed money for regional conferences. It makes me sound conceited, but you just didn't have many people to do these things, and I was fortunate that there was the Rosenwald Fund. Most any idea that I had, I could get support financially, and that was important.

I planned and conducted the first regional conference we had right here in New York. One of the purposes of that conference was to bring all the white directors of the black schools together with us because customarily they would go to the A.N.A. and League meetings; we would go to the black nurses; never the twain was meeting. So we invited all of them to this meeting. Then, in addition, for luncheon guests I had outsiders and blacks: Elmer Carter and Jesse Fauset, both of them writers, both of them scholars. Elmer Carter was a Harvard graduate and a most interesting speaker.

Isabel Stewart had said to me once that I talked above my people. She said I was going to run into stone walls. I said, "Miss Stewart, you just don't know my people; there are Negro people who are so profound I don't open my mouth in their presence." So I was trying to give them a sampling of the black intellectual. Just because they saw us in an isolated way over at Teachers College! Maybe we were doing a little more than the average black nurse was doing, but we were certainly not the tops in the black group. But that we had access to the tops was very helpful, because many of our black people who had achieved in other ways really got in and helped us with nursing.

The night that the N.A.C.G.N. went into its formal dissolution at a big banquet at Essex House, the boards of the (then) five other organizations and several hundred other guests were present. I always remember that I sat between Langston Hughes, the writer, the poet, and Adam Clayton Powell, who at that time was a congressman. The person who gave the talk was Governor Hastie, ex-Governor of the Virgin Islands. His speech was broadcast that night over the Voice of America. It's published in one of the early issues (1951) of the *American Journal of Nursing,* and has been referred to by many other groups. This is the first of the voluntary black organizations to work itself out of existence; and it worked it out through the channels of the existing organizations. In other words, we had a contract with A.N.A.; we had to fight for the membership opportunities in seventeen southern states. Not until these things were assured did the N.A.C.G.N. say, "Now the way is open." We knew it wasn't going to mean that every black nurse was going to see it that way. A group met in Miami (in October 1974) to form another black nurses' organization.

It's one thing to say, "Yes, you can come; you can join." But when you get there, nobody sits beside you; nobody says hello. I've been in meetings where, when I have spoken, they would look at me with the amazement that you would get if you bought a dog and he suddenly spoke.

The freeze-out is a very difficult thing to take. I was at a League meeting once in Boston, of all places. Everything was open so far. Only two of us were there, and the other one said, "No indeed, I'm not going to the banquet. I would choke if I tried to eat food there. I know they don't want me there." I said, "Well, I can't go by what they want; I'm going to the banquet." So I dressed up and went into the dining room. Well, you yourself know it isn't the easiest thing to walk in alone, facing a whole crowd of people. You don't know whether you have a friend in the whole setup. But you go on in, acting like you belong. The head-waiter tried to seat me at one table. "All the seats are taken," he was told. He took me to another one. After about three tables of "That's been taken," the headwaiter said, "She's paid her money like everybody else; and she's going to sit here. Have a seat, madam." I sat down. Then, where do you look after you sit down? You feel you've been placed in the middle of a hostile situation, so you . . . Maybe that's why I started smoking; you've got to do something. As a rule there would be one soul who didn't have the courage to say, "Let her sit here," but once you're there would say, "Are you enjoying the meeting? Where are you from?" Just anything to get something going.

Once I went to a luncheon in Cleveland. This is another story. The kinds of people that supported public health nursing, like Congresswoman Frances Bolton, were there. Frances Bolton was up at the dais and saw me come in, and she saw a runaround about seating me. She jumped up from that table, came down, and kissed and greeted me. You almost heard the people gasp.

Along the way I developed many friends. One may develop some enemies in any kind of crusade, and that's true in any area of life. And so we learned to work with our friends, and when our friends understood many of our problems, they were willing to act.

I want to come to my election to the A.N.A. board. We had to fight for membership opportunities. Seventeen states did not admit black nurses, no matter how well qualified they were; if you were black, you couldn't join. That was an issue that had to be decided by the House of Delegates nationally. You can imagine that for several years we were making these recommendations. There would be some reason they didn't get on the agenda: the agenda would be too full, so that would be the thing left out.

So at one convention in Chicago—we'd start a year ahead—we'd go right down and ask Ms. Best and whoever was there as the president,

"What is it now that has to be done a year from now to get this into the right committee?" So we would do all this groundwork and this spade-work. We lost by about five votes in Chicago at one biennial. So then we'd work on the techniques for getting this on the agenda for the Atlantic City convention which was in 1946. Often it is on the agenda. You've got to work to get it at a place on the agenda so that other important things will not crowd it out. And so it was supposed to come at the A.M. session of the A.N.A., and it didn't.

Well, by this time we had some key people around in different places, so we'd alert them as to what was happening. A motion was made that the motion re membership for black nurses be the first item on the agenda of the reconvened session. The first person to speak to it was from Virginia. She said, "The 'Nigra' (that's a compromise between "nigger" and "Negro") . . . The Nigra nurses are working so hard to be in our organization; they would do much better to strengthen their own. And the A.N.A. has already spent about $3000 in looking at the Nigra situation." So she didn't want it to come up. Fortunately we had good people, you see, who would rise at the mikes out in the aisle and say, "No, no; this is our business of the morning and we must attend to it." So they did. The discussions from the floor . . . Many of them were quite negative. Some would say, "We would have them as members, but the law's against it." *There was no law against membership privileges* in those states. And every state didn't even have a law against mixed schools at that time. It was really the custom, more or less, that they were talking about. I was making notes because I planned to get to a floor mike and refute some things that were being said. But as I got to the mike, I stood back and let one or two other people precede me because I wanted to hear what they were saying so that my refuting would include it if necessary. I stood back for a white nurse, and she said, "I'm Pauline Cox of Georgia, and all you-all that want your Nigra nurses in can go ahead and have them. But we in Georgia know our darkies, and we know their place." Well, my dear, believe it or not, she helped the cause. A wave of surprise and disgust went over that whole auditorium! People who hadn't planned to speak were jumping to the mikes, because here was spoken the disdain, the . . . Everything was there! She was followed by another nurse from Georgia whose voice was trembling, and tears were in her eyes. She said she was from Georgia, "and Pauline Cox cannot speak for Georgia nurses," she said. And there were Georgia nurses who wanted to recognize any qualified nurse, the way we needed them, and so on. So we won! The vote was in favor of admitting all qualified nurses as individual members.

Elected to the A.N.A. Board

Katherine Faville, who is one of the strongest people in nursing, in my estimation, asked how individual members would vote and run for office, and so forth. Since the method required some study, the House of Delegates voted to have the A.N.A. board devise a method within the next six months. It was fine that now black nurses could join as individual members, but where would they vote? Could they hold office? So then she made a motion that the A.N.A. board, within a six-month period, work out a plan by which individual members could vote or be elected to office, and so on.

So the A.N.A. board held a special session to do just that. That was very significant.

A lot of correspondence has come through the years to show the different kinds of people who responded and who helped us work on this. Then, you see, we had no black representation on the A.N.A. board. The N.L.N. came into existence at a higher level of racial participation; so there never had to be this race struggle there. The National League of Nursing Education (N.L.N.E.) membership was through schools, and some schools for black nurses had qualified. In 1948 the A.N.A. was meeting in Chicago, and nominees had to be submitted through the state associations. The State Nurses' Association of Oregon submitted my name; they wrote and asked me if they could. I said yes, with no feeling that I'd ever be elected; however, I was elected.

I was a candidate for membership on the A.N.A. board. The afternoon that the election results were announced, I went to visit friends; I felt sure I wouldn't be elected. I was elected, however. There were candidates for two years; there were candidates for four years. I was a four-year candidate, and I was elected with the third highest vote. But I wasn't there to hear it. One of my friends heard it, and she came rushing to where I was to say, "You were elected!" She brought me flowers. It meant that in all of the history of the A.N.A. I was the *first black* to be on the board! (I flinch because I don't want to get too involved in what happened on the negative side.)

The convention was in May; the first postconvention board meeting was to be in Kansas City in September. I received, as did all board members, a notice of this meeting and the information that the A.N.A. was getting a block of rooms for board members, and you were to indicate whether you wished to be included in that or whether you were making your own reservation. I checked the box indicating I wished to be included with the board at the Muehlbach Hotel. A few days after my card was received, I was called by Ms. Best and a member from Missouri who was on a committee at A.N.A., to tell me that I could not stay at the Muehlbach in Kansas City. They understood, and they knew that I had worked in Kansas City. They asked if I would stay with some of my friends; I could stay anywhere and they would take care of all of my expenses; but I just couldn't stay at the Muehlbach. So I said, "No. It's true that I do have many friends in Kansas City. I have friends that I'm so close to that I wouldn't have to write them that I was coming: just get there. But that's beside the issue. I was elected by the national body, and I am sure that they intend that I be treated as any other board member. Even if they don't, I do!" That's when they had Edward Bernays working at A.N.A. there, paying him a terrific salary for public relations. They kept talking, and the Missouri woman got on the line: "Now, Miss Massey. You know Missouri's got to have a little time to come along. It's moved a long way." I said, "You know, I know the history of Missouri too well but I also know the history of people. I think if an organization with the prestige of the American Nurses' Association is going to let a hotel decide what happens to one of its elected officers, that the prestige of the organization drops." "Well, it takes time." "Yes, it does take time. And we waited a long time. But this is the time to be active—be positive, I think. What about Edward Bernays that we've engaged for public relations for A.N.A.? What does he say?" They hadn't even thought of discussing it with Edward Bernays. When we wound up I said, "I'm sorry you can't make the change, but I will. I will see to it that something happens." The assurance that I had about the issue was gained because we kept up with what other organizations were doing along racial lines. Anywhere the social workers had met, we knew we could meet there interracially too. Anywhere the Y.W.C.A. had met, we found public accommodations generally open. I knew that some of my best friends had stayed at the Muehlbach when they attended the social workers' conference.

I finally said, "Well, if you can't, I can take the necessary steps to have the Muehlbach open its doors to me." They gasped. "Well, we hope you don't embarrass the A.N.A." I said, "Well, the A.N.A. is really embarrassed if the hotel doesn't take me in." But I knew that all I had to do was rely upon what had happened with the social workers and just request a reservation directly. A few days later they called me from A.N.A. They were so pleased; the Muehlbach was going to accept me!

I was teaching at N.Y.U. at the time. I had an evening class I couldn't get excused from. So I could not get to Kansas City before the 9 A.M. session opened. So I expressed the hope of joining the board on arrival about eleven o'clock that morning. The limousine went to the side entrance of the hotel, and all the passengers got out and walked into the lobby this way. So I walked over to the desk. The clerk was talking to someone; he just nonchalantly pushed the registration pad out to me, reached up and got a key, and waved to a redcap who came speedily to take me to my room. I signed the register, and the redcap picked up my things. We started across the lobby from the side. The main entrance was to my left. I looked up and saw one of the A.N.A. professional staff running across the lobby and waving at me. She was at the front door waiting for me because they were thinking that I should have an escort through this "hostile" territory.

I went to the board meeting, and they were very gracious. They went through all the formalities of introductions. At lunchtime one of the board members from Oregon said, "We want you to eat lunch with us today. We're going to celebrate. You're our victory." I accepted. We went up to their room and toasted each other before lunch. After the afternoon session another board member said, "I want you to come up to my room and have dinner." By this time I'd told some of my friends in Kansas City I'd see them so I said, "Oh, I'm sorry. Knowing there was no program tonight I just made a social engagement, and I can't." When I came in that night, there was a note under my door from a staff member inviting me to have breakfast with her in her room the next morning. I began to wonder why each invitation specified "in my room." So I just wrote a note: "Thanks. Sorry, have made other plans," and pushed it back.

So at lunchtime, when Lucy Germain, whom I'd known from Teachers College days, said, "Estelle, come up to my room for lunch," I said, "What is all this about? I'm just catching on. Everybody's saying: 'Come to my room.'" I said, "Lucy, I'd be glad to have lunch with you. But I'm going to have it in the dining room. Are you game?" She said, "Well, you know I am. But they discussed it in the board meeting, that you couldn't eat in the dining room here." So I said, "I am going in that dining room. If you're game, come ahead." So she said, "Sure! It doesn't matter to me." I said, "Nothing will happen. There may be some people who will stare, and others won't even think about it. And none of it will spoil my lunch." So in we went. It spread like wildfire to other board members: "She doesn't have to be fed in her room."

GS: *Wouldn't that make you feel disgusted with that whole bunch, so you would want to quit? Why did you want to continue with your association with these people?*

EO: But you're not looking at the important goal! The important goal was not just my personal comfort or discomfiture, but a concern that basic principles in human relations be established and maintained; that these opportunities and this recognition must come, not just to me, but to any qualified nurse.

Incidentally, when we were pushing on this membership issue, we found some discrimination against quite a few white nurses, in different ways. So it helped them. There are few issues that affect one group in society that don't affect others, if you look at it. I was on the A.N.A. board for four years. And when the I.C.N. was meeting in Stockholm in 1949 and we could have only four delegates from the whole United States, I was one elected by the A.N.A. board.

Leadership

GS: *Do you consider that your greatest leadership role?*

EO: I do. I think in terms of what that embodies: membership, the right to belong, the right to have something to say about the policies of the whole American Nurses' Association, a right to be a part of the international group. That's the only way one can be a member of the I.C.N. through the A.N.A.

GS: *What were the other key issues going on in nursing or in the United States at the time?*

EO: The Structure Study. On the A.N.A. board there was sharp division between those who wanted a new structure and those who didn't. And I happened to be one of those who wanted new structure. Without any caucusing we were finding ourselves voting the same way on certain issues, and there was another bloc voting another way. But the Structure Study was the heart issue at the time. I was on the boards of two organizations. As someone said to me once when I was at N.Y.U., "Estelle, don't you think you get elected to all these committees just so they can say they have a black person there?" I said, "I don't know. I just couldn't tell you what the motivation is. But I can tell you how I act after I get there; I vote for and against just like every other person. I can nominate people, and I nominated some very good people. They weren't black, but they had a philosophy that would carry out good programs for all of us. To be sure, I recommended black nurses."

GS: How, and in what ways, have opportunities for black nurses improved today?

EO: Let's start at the basic thing, and I think that's employment and recognition of qualifications irrespective of color: upgrading. There was a time when black nurses with high preparation couldn't be elevated beyond a certain point. Black nurses were not nominated for important elective, and certainly not to appointive, posts. But they are now. The schools discriminated, not accepting black students. Now fewer and far between are the schools that don't integrate their student bodies and faculties.

GS: You said there's a new association for black nurses. What are your views on this? Isn't this a backward trend?

EO: As far as I'm concerned, it is. I was approached by the leaders of that point of view, that philosophy. I said to them, "You know that, to me, is a backward step." The person asked me to come and speak. I said, "I will come to your meeting because *who am I to say what the right way is in a society as complex as ours is?*" I would question whether or not any tangent group can influence the legislation—which the A.N.A. does influence in regard to all nurses in this country—whether any tangent group can do as much for economic security and status. I've been out when half the nurse population thought an economic security program was awful: the A.N.A. doing that? I think I've mentioned the international situation. And so then you get on to the physical thing. We couldn't support an N.A.C.G.N. financially when we had it. Frances Bolton and the Rosenwald Fund underwrote us, largely. The cost of maintaining a separate organization is a mammoth undertaking. What I've seen of their programs, they're very clearly stated. I'll have to include some of them in my memoirs. But they are some of the same things that other nonnursing organizations are doing.

GS: What do you think will happen to this group?

EO: The needs of the black people and the poor people are so intense and varied that some organization can exist on any program which expresses a desire and a program to improve their lot.

GS: Do you think you're not considered radical and activist enough by some of the black . . .

EO: I'm pretty sure.

GS: . . . that you're too conservative because you seem to stress working through the channels?

EO: They are the recognized channels.

GS: Rather than picketing or violence?

EO: But I do not tie picketing with violence, automatically. I have participated in picket lines about housing without violence.

As I looked at some of their objectives, I said, "If I could see you
taking one objective of the A.N.A. and saying, 'I'm going to work
through this and see, and then let the A.N.A. know what's happening.'
But you go out and work on sickle-cell anemia." For a while it was the
password in lots of black organizations. Now they're finding scientifically that it isn't really a possession of the blacks any more than of some
other groups. But other people are doing that.

I went to one of the meetings of black nurses in Detroit. To me it was
really a backward step. At A.N.A.'s convention, there was a session on
black nurses to which white nurses were not admitted. To me it seemed
the major emphasis was on needed social action which, again, like
the National Association for the Advancement of Colored People
(N.A.A.C.P.), the Urban League, and so forth, work upon and welcome
recommendations and financial contributions from all.

I'm on the N.A.A.C.P. Legal Defense Fund. I not only give time but
also give money to that organization. These are the organizations that
are set up to do this kind of thing; they have the structure. For example,
the Legal Defense Fund has about forty young lawyers on its staff. It's
doing things; it's getting things done because that's their goal. So when
we had N.A.C.G.N., we referred many things to them. We brought them
in on certain specific issues. Then out of that we took recommendations
to A.N.A.; they could do something about them.

I was mentioning the freeze-out. I can understand that there are
blacks who just can't go through the rigors of integration; they want
action here and now! You've got to be strong. Look at Boston: just one
example. Boston has a history of having been the emancipators, the
people who gave so much opportunity, who were in the underground.
Now look, here comes an issue about busing.

*GS: What do you think is going to happen in race relations in the near
future? What direction is it going to take?*

EO: I wonder. I think I see a concern of professional nurses with a
broader perspective. I think the National Student Nurses' Association
(N.S.N.A.) has demonstrated concretely how you involve, how you take
up the issue for, all the people, in terms of not only the participation of
the nurses themselves, but also the kinds of people that they are serving, and what they see needs to be done in relation to that serving.

I'm all for people who talk in terms of newer ways of delivering health service; and that's going to create a lot of changes in nursing across the board. I'm all for the involvement of more community people, in terms of the nursing needs of the people. That was part of my satisfaction in working in the N.L.N. I was so pleased the other day to see a write-up of a program the Arkansas League for Nursing is developing with and for the community. Years ago it moved toward arousing the community to the needs in mental health, and really got some things done. The leadership given through the N.L.N. to state leagues was definitely positive; we had ways to measure it. Arkansas I look at with great pride because, as you know, if you can find the leader who has the possibility of embracing many kinds of people and problems, you're doing something.

National League for Nursing

GS: Would you comment on your work with the N.L.N.?

EO: When I went to the League, it was understood that I was working as a staff person across the board for all. Every state has the right to invite League staff. At first I didn't expect many invitations to come from the South. But pretty soon the southern leaders were inviting me for initial and follow-up visits. When we went to states for initial visits, we endeavored to see people who had some connection or interest in "nursing as a community service," such as Community Chest Chairmen, hospital association executives, some community-minded women's organizations, the public health officials, and volunteer agencies, as well as nurses, professional and practical. Who provides money, and how much for nursing in the total community budget? What are the relationships between nursing groups and some of the health organizations, such as tuberculosis, mental health, and so forth? These were some of the questions to which we sought answers. I got to talk to some people who saw the need for mental health facilities. The Arkansas league took the initiative in working toward establishing facilities. Once they began to see what could happen, enthusiasm for the project increased, and facilities were developed.

The Rosenwald Fund conducted a behavioristic study in the rural South. They put fourteen of us into southern rural communities to live. I came out after a year. The Rosenwald Fund offered to give me more fellowships to study under Dr. Lloyd Warner, the anthropologist; Dr. Park, the sociologist; and Dr. Shrieke of Java, the educator. They wanted to give me a year of exposure to those disciplines—not so much on an academic basis, but on a project basis, where the analysis of experiences could be sustained and incisive. But I got married. Dr. Davis was supposed to have said in the presence of a coworker, "See, you can't develop a woman but so far. She got along with whites; she got along with the blacks; she lost no respect; and she got things done."

There was, in the South, the custom of whites to address black people only by their first names; it was a social custom, and it was rampant. How did I keep whites from calling me by my first name? Just introduced myself using my last name and title, and stated that I was "from the Rosenwald Fund. We're here to do so-and-so. Will you help?" Now I wouldn't say that all of them called me Mrs. Some of them would just start talking. I'd just act as if I didn't notice the omission. But I never called myself "Estelle" to them. This represented dignity and indignity to the black, especially in the South.

GS: Did you ever tell them off, the ones that made you mad?

EO: No, not just in that way.

GS: You mentioned that being a strategist is one of your strengths. Could you elaborate a little on that?

EO: Let's refer to my work with the Rosenwald Fund. We were doing a study, a behaviorist study on rural life. We were supposed to do as much remedial work as we could, or initiate it, but not play God. The important thing was to try to stimulate improvement flow through the organized areas of responsibility. I was stationed in Louisiana, and I had done enough to get people saying, "If we had a public health nurse to continue this kind of thing." We worked through the schools and churches. I then decided to offer to teach the American Red Cross Home Nursing Course as a medium to reach all ages of community women.

The regional director was visiting the local office in Monroe the day I went to ask about teaching the course. She was headquartered in New Orleans, but she was up in Monroe on an official visit. Her home was Boston. She had a much broader concept of things than did the local director. So I told them that I was stationed 20 miles out in the rural Mineral Springs doing a behaviorist study. But you don't just go and pull out pencil and paper: you go in there and do some work; get something that identifies you, that you can identify with. I said, "I was wondering if you would like me to teach one of your Red Cross nursing courses out there for the women." The local person said, "We don't have no money." The supervisor said, "What do you mean? We'll find some. This is Santa Claus. These are the things we should be doing, and we don't have personnel. She's a registered nurse. We'll find the money." So with that they gave me vouchers to go around to the furniture store and the drugstore to select the equipment I would need.

In the furniture store, I didn't know the slats to the bed were separate; so it was going to make a difference in the voucher. I had to call her. I said, "Miss Holstein, this is Mrs. Riddle[10] calling." Every secretary in the store stopped. Who was this black woman saying "Mrs." to Miss Holstein? They knew who Miss Holstein was. "Will you approve?" I asked. "Yes," she replied. One of the secretaries came over to me. One's antenna has to be very sensitive; all the little variations and gestures indicate something.

GS: Did you ever think that sometimes you might be just a little paranoid?

EO: No, but it interests me that you ask the question! Fortunately my own life as a member of a large family was secure and well balanced. When quite small, I was helped to weigh values and to differentiate between those which can harm your development and those which can not. I could read my name, "Estelle," since I was about three years of age; but when I saw it connected with "ugly" on a playmate's book, I was really puzzled, so I waited to ask an older sister what the word meant. When I told her where I saw it, she gave me so many positive interpretations of beauty that I have always striven to be beautiful in my inner sense, so that it has never worried me that some may consider my physical characteristics ugly. I have, however, been in some situations where overt pressures caused me to explode!

---

10 Riddle is the name of Estelle Osborne's first husband.

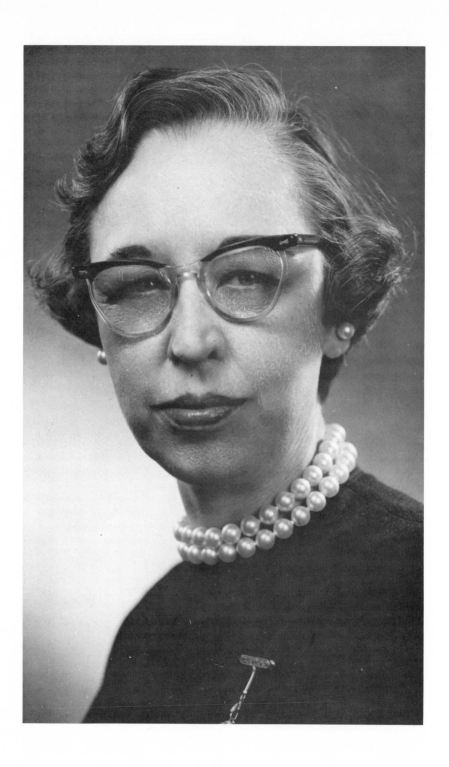

14

One of Nursing's most controversial leaders whose ideas are highly original and who has the personal courage to expound them . . . A quick sense of humor . . .

Martha E. Rogers

EDUCATOR

*M*artha E. Rogers was born in Dallas, Texas, May 12, 1914, the eldest of four children. Her father was in the insurance business. The idea of her going to college was very much a part of both her maternal and paternal backgrounds, and she had many active women suffragists among her relatives. She was doubly fortunate in that she not only lived where there was a state university in the community, she also had a wealthy uncle who provided a trust for his grandnieces and grand-nephews to assist them in going to college.

Dr. Rogers attended the University of Tennessee in Knoxville from 1931 to 1933, and then entered the Knoxville General Hospital School of Nursing, where she received a diploma in nursing in 1936. She received her B.S. degree in public health nursing from George Peabody College, Nashville, Tennessee, in 1937; an M.A. in public health nursing supervision from Teachers College, Columbia University, in 1945; an M.P.H. in 1952 and a Sc.D. in 1954, both from Johns Hopkins University.

She is at present Professor and Head of the Division of Nurse Education at New York University, where she has been since 1954.[1] Her work experience includes: Research Associate, Johns Hopkins University (1953–54); Visiting Lecturer, Catholic University of America, Washington, D.C. (1951–52); Executive Director, Visiting Nurse Service, Phoenix, Arizona (1945–51); successively staff, Assistant Supervisor, Assistant Education Director, Acting Education Director, Visiting Nurse Association, Hartford, Connecticut (1940–45); and rural public health nurse, Children's Fund of Michigan, Clare, Michigan (1937–39).

Dr. Rogers has been active in numerous professional organizations, and served as a consultant to the U.S. Surgeon General, U.S. Air Force, 1969–1973.[2]

Dr. Rogers has received many awards and honors, such as the Award and Citation for "Inspiring Leadership in the Field of Intergroup Relations," Chi Eta Phi Sorority, Omicron Chapter (1960); and the Award and Citation "In recognition of your outstanding contribution to nursing," New York University, Division of Nurse Education, faculty and alumni (1965).

---

[1] Dr. Rogers resigned as head of the Division of Nurse Education in the early part of 1975.

[2] She is a member and has served on various committees of the American Nurses' Association, National League for Nursing, American Association of University Professors, American Public Health Association, School of Education Nurse Alumni, New York University Faculty Women's Club, New York University Faculty Club, Royal Society of Health, American Society for Psychical Research, Museum of Natural History, National Council on Family Relations, Center for the Study of Democratic Institutions, New York State Council of Deans, American Association of Deans.

She is also a member of Sigma Theta Tau (National Honorary Nursing Society) and Kappa Delta Pi (National Honorary Education Society).[3]

She has published extensively in the *American Journal of Public Health, Journal of the New York State Nurses Association, American Journal of Nursing, Nursing Outlook,* and others. She has written three books,[4] and is in the process of writing several more. From 1963 through 1965 she was editor of the journal *Nursing Science.*

Into Nursing

GS: Would you please tell me very briefly why you first went into nursing?

MR: It's always very difficult to look back—reasons are generally quite complex—but I had a great missionary zeal when I was in high school. I wanted to do something that would, hopefully, contribute to the social welfare. I toyed with the ideas of law and of medicine. When I entered college, not being very sure, I tossed a coin and it came out medicine. So I studied science-med for a couple of years. But women in medicine were not particularly desirable animals in those days, not only from the standpoint of the medical school, but also, my parents thought it was rather an inappropriate career for a female. The local hospital had a school of nursing, and a friend of mine had decided she would enter there in September, so I decided I would go along. My parents weren't really any happier over that decision than they had been over the medicine. In considering my career choice, perhaps I should have selected home economics like my two sisters, which would have been quite appropriate, but I never could sew very well anyway.

I had a large social orientation, and I thought it would be nice to be a missionary. That was going to be my goal, but I was going to be different. I wasn't going to be a religious missionary, you know. I don't think I would have made a very good religious missionary anyway.

GS: Did you like nursing?

MR: Yes, I liked the human aspects very, very much. I was a little annoyed with some of the other things; and when I had been in about— I don't know, for about three months—I decided I had really had

---

[3] Dr. Rogers is listed in *Who's Who in America, World's Who's Who in Science,* and other directories and listings of distinguished people.

[4] *Introduction to the Theoretical Basis of Nursing,* F. A. Davis Company, Philadelphia, 1970; *Reveille in Nursing,* F. A. Davis Company, Philadelphia, 1964; and *Educational Revolution in Nursing,* The Macmillan Company, New York, 1961.

enough of it, so I told the director I was leaving and I left. I did a little thinking-over for three days, and decided that I really couldn't come up with anything better so I went back and said did they mind? And they said, no, come on. [*laughter*]

Original Contributions to Nursing

GS: You are considered by your colleagues to be one of the most original thinkers in nursing. What do you think has been your main contribution to nursing?

MR: I would like to think that it has been twofold. One is evolving the conceptual system that provides for a substantive body of knowledge in nursing that will have relevance for all workers concerned with people, but with special relevance for nurses; not because it matters to nurses per se, but because it matters to human beings, and consequently to nurses. I think that health sciences are built pretty much on some false assumptions, and too often serve the workers rather than society. But human beings are quite well put together and have managed to survive this long in spite of it, after a fashion, but I would like to see a little more progress. So I think a body of theoretical knowledge specific to nursing is essential. The other thing that I hope I have contributed is confrontation with reality and an effort to force other people to get their heads out of the sand. I could get into a lot of talk on that. The situation is very critical right now. We have large numbers of nurses who would prefer to leave nursing to be physicians' assistants. We have an amount of antieducationism that sometimes seems almost overwhelming. We have large numbers of nurses who deny that there is anything to know in nursing. We have people who are selling nursing right down the river with such weird euphemisms as "pediatric associate" and "primary care practitioner," and so forth. Nightingale started primary care in modern nursing. Nightingale started the family health practitioner, and every nurse I have ever known, from any kind of beginning program— good, bad, or indifferent—was specifically prepared to practice nursing, to be a nurse-practitioner. How nurses can be so naïve is incredible. So I hope that I have aroused people's awareness. I haven't finished trying, either.

GS: So I gather, then, that these advocates of the so-called expanded role of nursing do not impress you too much.

MR: Well, I think it's a major sellout, and incredibly naïve. Those words are designed to get nurses to be hands and feet to another discipline. As far as an expanded role specific to nurses is concerned, the phrase is empty and misleading. What is expanded role for nursing is equally expanded role for everybody else. And I can find little that these people are talking about as expanded roles that I wasn't taught in a formal classroom setting back in the 1930s, unless one refers to new machinery, which is new for everyone. It's just incredible.

GS: What is unique about nursing from the other health professions, such as medicine and social work and so on?

MR: The difference is in the body of knowledge. As a learned profession the term "nursing" becomes a noun. We've used "nursing" as a verb, and have licensed nurses only for the technical level of practice. We've used the word "nursing" as meaning "to do." A learned profession signifies "to know." It is the body of knowledge that differentiates nursing from other professions, and the body of knowledge then requires an organized conceptual system out of which to derive testable hypotheses. It emerges out of scientific research and logical analysis. Further, the specific phenomenon of concern to nursing is clearly different from that of any other field. Nursing's prescientific concern was with unitary man. Certainly Nightingale wrote a great deal about this. In moving into a scientific frame of reference, it is quite proper that the concept of synergistic man would represent the phenomenon central to nursing's concern. No other field is concerned with synergistic man. Psychologists look at psychological phenomena, and that is not synergistic man. Biological phenomena (medicine is largely physiological pathology) do not deal with synergistic man. This is not a denial of biological or psychological science. Rather, these are different. I would propose for selected conditions that medicine is a very important career. But the scope of medicine is quite narrow. In general it deals with specific areas of physiological pathology. If I break my leg, I would like to have somebody who knows anatomy to set it. Psychologists deal with psychological phenomena; this is fine. But nursing is the only field that both prescientifically and scientifically has concerned itself with unitary man, who is different from the sum of his parts. One can not generalize from parts to a whole. This has been noted in many contexts. It is this particular phenomenon, synergistic man, whom nursing seeks to describe, explain, predict about, and which is unique to nursing, and specifically differentiates nursing from these other fields.

The Martha Rogers Theory of Nursing in a Nutshell

GS: If you could put it into a few words, what is your theory of nursing?

MR: Do you have a couple of months? [*laughter*] I think we get a little confused about what is the theory of nursing because there are multiple theories, and I would hope that there always will be. Rather, there must first be a conceptual system on which one bases a conceptual model. From the system, one derives theories and tests them; and the findings of research are then lodged within the conceptual system. Thus the conceptual system is continually being modified, revised, and altered in the light of new knowledge. Science is never finished. There is no such thing as a single theory of nursing that is then all of nursing. There are multiple theories. There is the theoretical or the abstract conceptual system, but you can't derive principles and theories except as these are preceded by an organized conceptual system. Nurses have worked awfully hard to develop theories in the absence of a conceptual system specific to nursing, with resultant confusion. In fact, I think some of this is perhaps not knowing how or where to begin. One starts with the phenomenon central to nursing. One develops a science which is an elaboration of the particular conceptual model. In this instance, principles of homodynamics, among others, have been derived. The principles of homodynamics, heliocy, and resonance describe, explain, and predict about the nature and direction of synergistic human development, and open wide all sorts of doors. In addition, other theories have been derived from this system subsequent to publication of my book, *Introduction to the Theoretical Basis of Nursing,* and are being discussed in the new book in this area that I am currently writing. It includes such things as a theory of complementarity, a theory of explanation for paranormal events, a theory of accelerating evolution, and so forth. Theories that derive from this system must sooner or later be tested against the real world. Some of these have been tested; some are being tested; and all will in time be tested and retested. After all, Einstein's theory of relativity is still being tested. It's even become a special case for more universal theories. It's been around since 1906, and is by no means fully understood yet.

GS: Would this apply—the way you're using theory—to other than nursing?

MR: I'm using this the way any scientist in any field uses it. It has nothing to do with whether it's nursing or any other field. It's the way one would find the scientist explaining it. If one wants a good reference, I suggest Popper has a very excellent book.[5]

GS: Do you have a title for your new book yet?

[5] Karl Raimund Popper, *The Logic of Scientific Discovery,* Basic Books, Inc., Publishers, New York, 1959.

MR: No. It will be written for general consumption this time. It will not be just an editing. Now there are some books that we need specifically for nursing, but just as we think every educated person ought to know something about the biological world and the psychological world and the social world, so too do people need to know about the synergistic world. A general course in biology or sociology doesn't make a biologist or a sociologist; so too a general course about synergistic man doesn't make a nurse. So, for example, we have a course here that we give every semester that I teach, called the Science of Man, and it's open to everyone with a baccalaureate degree acceptable to N.Y.U. It happens to be a beginning master's course. All graduate students in nursing are required to take it, but it's open to anybody with a baccalaureate degree acceptable to New York University. This semester I have over 220 students enrolled in it.

GS: *Someone said that you stated that no nurse should get a Ph.D. in anything other than nursing. Is that your opinion?*

MR: I think that is not exactly what I stated. The point is that if somebody expects to be an expert in psychology, they get their doctorate in psychology. If somebody expects to be an expert in biology, they get their doctorate in biology. And if this university or any other university is looking for a professor in such fields, it will look at the person's graduate major. The person who aspires to be a professor of psychology, and who has taken his graduate studies in economics, is unlikely to be appointed as a professor of psychology. Now I think there are two reasons why nursing has been very apt to study anything provided it wasn't nursing. One is a low self-concept. The other is a belief that there is nothing to know in nursing. Because they couldn't dream up what there was to know in nursing, they decided to put parts together and think that somehow they would have something in spite of the fact there have been many symposiums, and so forth, dedicated to demonstrating that this does not work. Further, there is a paucity of resources for doctoral study in nursing. Certainly twenty years ago, in order to get off the ground, nurses had to secure almost anything they could. And certainly twenty years ago, this seemed necessary. It was an emergency. In spite of that, we had some people in nursing who decided it was to be all outside of nursing, and worked hard to sell this case. The thing was that while they were running around spending time and money to train so-called nurse-scientists, the doctoral program in nursing at N.Y. U. had more students than all the nurse-scientist programs put together. It did give me a great deal of faith in nurses who believed in nursing.

I believe that if one is to be prepared to teach nursing, then one has to study nursing; and I do not believe that because somebody studies biology or sociology or psychology, it gives them some strange knowledge that is magically transmuted into nursing knowledge. Certainly anything we know is potentially useful, but, just as I say, if anybody's going to teach my child college math, I'd like to know that they were a little more than one page ahead of the student, and I'd like to know that their graduate study was in math. We do not hire anybody here who does not have graduate education in nursing. And we are in a real tight situation when someone gets to this institution where we must employ faculty who hold an earned doctorate. Occasionally we can employ some instructors, providing they are engaged in doctoral study and there is absolutely nothing else on the horizon. Today a majority of this faculty we have, of course, have earned doctorates. But it has been one long, hard haul.

GS: You say doctorates . . .

MR: And they are pretty much in nursing. For many reasons we have explored nurses with doctorates in other fields and have employed them in a few instances, but they are unfamiliar with the philosophy and theoretical base we teach, and are so strongly oriented to their own outside field that to make the transition really requires a period of formal study in the science of man. Otherwise they do not have the nursing content to teach. What we have is a good portion of our faculty with doctorates from N.Y.U. who are familiar with nursing science. We also have a few from Teachers College, Columbia, who have some orientation to this conceptual system. The person coming from someplace else generally needs a great deal of orientation. The other thing is that while it is true the bulk of our doctorates are here, their undergraduate and master's degrees are from many places. We are concerned that we don't become too inbred, so I would guess that about 80 to 85 percent of the faculty have one or more degrees from places other than N.Y.U. We have variety and diversity all over the place. I believe we have a lot of good, healthy discussion. Faculty differ on many things. We have a total faculty. We don't have an undergraduate faculty or a master's faculty, and so forth. Students have opportunity to be exposed to a range of faculty and a range of different ideas. Faculty are quite free to state their own beliefs, to indicate this is the point I take and it differs here, here, and here. The students are free to end up determining their own sets of beliefs. The idea is to give them enough knowledge so that they can work their own way through to rational judgment on their own part and learn to think. Perhaps it's learning to think that is one of the most important things we do for students. We do give them a lot of substantive content in nursing. We do give them exposure to many different ideas. We force them to think, and we do try to get them accustomed to the idea that change is not only rapid and inevitable, but it's accelerating, and they had better learn to be flexible.

GS: What to you, then, is the scientific basis of nursing?

MR: The scientific basis of nursing is an organized body of scientific knowledge arrived at by logical analysis and scientific research. It's an abstract system out of which to derive testable hypotheses. And the phenomenon specific to nursing is synergistic man.

GS: What is your conception of nursing research?

MR: I think it's the same as for any other research. I think the word "research" has been vastly misused. You know, one may hear that third-graders look up words in the dictionary and say they are researchers. The scholars and scientists more often talk about a study or an investigation. But I don't think that the criteria for scholarly research are any different for nursing than for any other science. I think nurses have proposed that some things were research that weren't. Certainly the kinds of questionnaires that get over my desk sometimes . . . I'll never forget the one that asked me to respond to whether there should be round pockets or square ones in a public health nurse's apron!

I think one thing is, we have been so anxious to achieve research that we have forgotten (1) research isn't done in a vacuum; and (2) it requires substantial knowledge and marked sophistication. We expect our undergraduate students to exploit knowledge for the improvement of practice. We expect that they will be able to design and initiate epidemiologic studies and to carry them out with proper use of statistics, and so forth. This is *not* research in the scientific, scholarly sense. We expect our master's graduates will be able to identify more complex problems, that they will possess more sophisticated tools, greater resources in evaluating and carrying out significant investigations than the baccalaureate graduate. When it comes to a doctoral person, this one must carry out the scholarly, knowledgeable, theoretical research. And of course the thing that is needed so desperately in research in nursing is study of the nature and direction of synergistic human growth and development. It is not the study of "how to do it." Whether one calls it pure research or theoretical research or basic research—I don't care what adjective you apply—what is needed is the study of synergistic man. There is also a very real place for applied research. I don't think it's an either/or; they feed each other. But applied research does not contribute to new knowledge. It cannot go beyond the basic research. They are both important, but where we are desperately in need of research is in the study of the science of nursing.

There are research categories that are being used, and studies are listed in *Nursing Research* journal that do not identify research in nursing. And it's unfortunate. Research that is classified under psychological, biological, or what-have-you is not research in nursing. It does not contribute to nursing knowledge. I get equally concerned when I hear someone say that the science of the unitary man that I propose is a physical science or it's a psychological science or a biological science. It is none of these things. It is a basic science. None of these other fields even deal with synergistic man; so that, as far as these research categories are concerned, they are really devoted to how to do it, analogies, and to research in fields other than nursing. Unfortunately this doesn't give substance to nursing practice based on knowledge in nursing.

Some Views

GS: Do you think that theoretical researchers should be involved in policy formulation, that they should use their findings in nursing policy?

MR: Policies for what?

GS: In terms of health education, care, health insurance, and things like that.

MR: Yes. But one doesn't have to be a researcher for this to be important. I think we jolly well have to participate in policy making, and I don't think it takes a doctorate to do that. I think people with different preparations will have different bodies of knowledge to contribute, and I think anything we know ought to be used for all it's worth. I think the public has been had, and I think that nursing has a singular responsibility. Unless nursing picks itself up and really pushes ahead to lead in achieving decent health services for the public, the Dark Ages may, by comparison, look bright.

GS: Do you think that nurses in general have improved their self-image?

MR: I don't think we will get anywhere until we quit pussyfooting around and openly declare what has been in existence for a long time. Specifically, there are different careers in nursing. We do have technical nurses, and it's all we have ever licensed as registered nurses. Hospital school graduates, associate degree nurse graduates, and practical nurses are technically prepared. "Types of programs" is a misnomer. This is how we have covered up antieducationalism. Cer-

tainly no professional person is prepared in less than a full baccalaureate degree program of study. A baccalaureate degree itself isn't a
guarantee. Certainly we have many schools which are giving baccalaureate degrees in the absence of any semblance of a baccalaureate
education in anything, but anything less than a full baccalaureate degree that includes a substantive upper-division major in nursing is not
professional education. Graduates of valid baccalaureate programs
represent a whole new population, a different career in nursing. They
are not an upgrading of hospital schools. Associate degree nurses were
developed to see if they provided a better preparation in an educational
institution than in a service agency. And they do. We are moving in the
direction of beginning to develop legislation for licensing a professional
worker in nursing. There are several groups in different parts of the
country who have already initiated steps toward this. In New York State,
a committee of deans is working on a draft of legislation for professional
licensure. This would supplement the current technical licenses. It
would not throw out the registered nurse. We have a technical license.
Everybody knows this except nurses, but nurses generally use the word
"professional" to mean to work for "hire." Nursing needs a license that
will identify a professional worker in the same sense that lawyers, engi-
neers, M.D.'s, dentists, and so forth are licensed. A baccalaureate degree is the equivalent of the M.D. degree or the dental degree. The
M.D., D.D.S., D.V.M., Pharm.D., and so on, are first undergraduate professional degrees. Certainly the associate degree nurse, hospital
school, and practical nurse group constituted a peer group in the sense
of similarities with the dental hygienist group, with the physician's assistant, the engineering technicians, whatever. These fit into the overall
pattern that we have in society. We need these groups. I think nursing
is extremely fortunate because we do have both professional and technical personnel. There are many jobs that need to be done, and the
ratio of professional to technical personnel in nursing has been going
up over the years.

*GS: Dr. Rogers, you are considered by most of the other nursing
leaders as being the most controversial figure in nursing, and I think
you are aware that not everyone agrees with you.*

MR: Yes, I know.

*GS: What do you have to say to your critics, and how do you feel
about it?*

MR: Well, you know, I think that people either think I'm great or they
think I should have died a long time ago. Ten or fifteen years ago, when
I would give a speech, the first thing I would do would be check how far

the windows were from the ground because, really you know, some people got pretty upset. After a while, I suspect, when people asked me to speak it was partly because at least I wouldn't put people to sleep. They had a better idea of what to expect so they didn't have to get angry, because after I spoke I went away. Today it is different. Many more nurses are comfortable with my ideas.

GS: What do you mean, they were angry with you? What were the ideas you have that upset them?

MR: It has varied from time to time. Certainly differentiation of careers and my attacks on antieducationism in nursing have been particularly sore points. Attacks on current euphemisms and the idea of a nurse is a nurse is a nurse, and so on, have been part of it. These, I think, are the things that have been most upsetting to large numbers. When it comes to nursing science, arguments are becoming less frequent. Certainly people are more and more interested in what we are doing in nursing science as far as synergistic man is concerned, and, as far as I know, there haven't been any big fights over it. I think more because it really isn't that well known or that well understood. I have done a number of papers on it at different places for different-sized groups. I know that many schools are using my book, and also that many students are being oriented to this sort of thinking. But I don't think that it's so much argumentative as it is people deciding whether to do this or that. This would be my guess.

GS: In your long, distinguished career, could you pick out what seem to you to be several of the main, key issues in nursing, and your own particular role in them? We have touched upon this in other ways, but I wanted to have you put it in a different way.

MR: Picking out any one thing, of course, is really never that simple; but if I were going to identify one single thing, then I would say differentiation of professional and technical careers in nursing, legally and openly and honestly, is the most critical point that we have because all of these other things will fall into shape, once careers are openly admitted and lead to honest recruitment, for example. We would begin to be honest and accountable to the public, which we are not. We would quit the head-in-sand cover-up. We would begin to develop a little self-respect. We are so busy apologizing to hospital school graduates that it gets to be pretty bad. I wonder when we are going to start apologizing for what we are doing to baccalaureate graduates. The human waste in terms of knowledge; the misuse of graduates; the human waste in students; and the financial cost to parents who invest money in their children to send them to college and then have them leave nursing because what happens in the real world is "for the birds." What about the public, who are denied not only any guarantee of professional services, but even their existence? And one can go on and on and on. Nursing does have professional and technical careers. This is a fait accompli, nothing to argue about. That American Nurses' Association (A.N.A.) Position Paper on the diploma schools—wow! I will give you a copy of my answer, which was titled "Eulogy to Obsolescence."[6] It was one of the most incredible documents that I have seen in a long time. It was incredible, and the authors were also highly dishonest. So, if I were going to pick out one area that I think is most critical, that is it. The other thing is we needn't talk about fulfilling our responsibilities and accountability to society until we differentiate careers honestly. We have to allow that there is a knowledgeable population in nursing that does possess substantive knowledge. Professional education does start with the baccalaureate degree. I can't imagine any of us wanting a dental hygienist to make decisions for dentistry, or a dental hygiene license as adequate for dentists. But this is precisely what we do. And then we make a whole group of second-class citizens out of hospital and associate degree nurse graduates when we tell them they have to go on, and if they don't go on for a baccalaureate, something is wrong with them. This ladder game is nothing in the world but setting up second-rate citizenship and denying the right to respect and dignity to nursing technicians. It's little wonder that in the last year, in *The New York Times* crossword puzzle on Sunday, there has twice appeared in the list of words "hospital aide," and what do you suppose the synonym was? "R.N." Well, this is the picture we get that includes failure to differentiate careers and continuation of many hospital schools. The public knows the latter are essentially service-centered, apprentice-type modifications. These are not higher education. In fact, a fifth of the faculties who are teaching in hospital schools have had no college education themselves. Now just how are they going to teach anything on a college level?

GS: When you stated your reaction to the A.N.A. position on the diploma, you called it incredible.[7]

MR: I called it some other things too. Incredible is my nice word. It was untrue.

GS: Where do you think nursing is going?

---

[6] Martha Rogers, "Eulogy to Obsolescence: A.N.A. Board Statement on Graduates of Diploma Schools of Nursing."

[7] Dr. Rogers stated that the need for action in opposition to this degrading and incredible document is urgent.

MR: I know where I'm going to try to help it go. Where it will end up, I wouldn't know. I think there are several things that we need to do. One, we need to really differentiate careers, and we need to pass professional licensing laws. Secondly, I think that all these nurses who want to be physicians' assistants, under whatever title, should go be physicians' assistants. Now it's very interesting: The American Medical Association (A.M.A.), the physician's assistant group, and no end of other persons have already pointed out, strongly, in the literature that all of these roles—paramedic, family health practitioner, pediatric associate, and so on—are physicians' assistants, and it's time they are called what they are. Now, I think that's grand. I think the public has the right to know, and I think that nurses who want to practice as physicians' assistants ought to be called what they are. They are no longer practicing in nursing. Society has a right to know what it is getting. And these nurses, if they want to take care of machines and declare dependency to another field, this is all right. I think people have a right to pick what they want to do. Let's get them into what they want to do. Let them get whatever certification or licensure they want, but they are no longer in nursing; they are no longer entitled to the privileges of being a nurse. They should no longer be permitted to claim identity nor lay forth to the public that they are practicing nursing when they are not. So let's help them to be what they want to be. Then we will have left a group of people who are committed to nursing; who want to know what this body of knowledge is, whatever it is; who want to practice nursing; who are committed to social needs and nursing responsibilities, if you like; and then let's get on with the job. That is critical.

GS: What have been some of your biggest disappointments?

MR: Maybe I would count them more as frustrations: the naïveté of nurses; their lack of commitment, either to nursing or to society; their dependency; their antieducationism; their running after anything, providing it's something other than nursing. We make a lot of noise about hospital school graduates. We really ought to be praising them, because they have gone beyond what we had any right to expect. And they have done a very remarkable job many times. But when I look at the people who have been privileged to be exposed to the higher learning, who have had all kinds of experiences of many sorts, and who are also often least committed to knowledgeable nursing, then these are the people who have discouraged me, not the people who haven't been privileged to have all this. For those with limited preparation, I can understand their feelings. I may not agree with them; I may think they are wrong. I do think they are wrong. But I can understand it. But I can't understand those who have gotten the halos and big names and who are selling nursing right down the river.

GS: As an example of that, do you mean the nurse-practitioner?

MR: Yes, that's a good example. Or like somebody else who sets up a national commission to study the expanding role of the nurse and makes the chairman and the cochairman of that both M.D.'s. And then there was another commission that provides a very fascinating example of what might be called medical malpractice. The commission was really committed to medicine, and the areas where nursing came in were those in medicine would belatedly like to claim. In a recent report of a medical-legal commission, one item hit me because there is a recommendation that all students of nursing in the future should have some exposure to anatomy, physiology, psychology, and human relations. Now, there were three nurses on that commission. Three of them! And two of them are on university faculties of schools of nursing. I happen to know who they are, and they wouldn't be employable here; but the point is that they were on it. From Nightingale on, content in the aforementioned areas has been part of every nurse's training. It doesn't even have to be the registered nurse. This really is incredible. And these are only part of the story. Do you see those two piles of papers on the desk over there? I've just run through them, and one after another gives a similar picture of ignorance by nurses. These physicians' assistants that parade under titles like "pediatric associates," and so forth, I just plain don't understand.

GS: Do you think it may be because they are used to the submissive role, and they think they don't know as much as the others do?

MR: I think there's no question that there's been a lot of indoctrination, and certainly nurses have been slow to move on in general. In fact, many nurses have not only been most inactive in this area; they have really been quite on the other side of the fence. There are the dependent individuals in nursing, and we also have some very active, liberationist people; but in general, nurses are not thought of as people who will initiate and actively look for how we can really use ourselves effectively for people. When we talk about women's lib, of course, if you happen to be a male chauvinist, there are ways in which one interprets it. But the concept of people's lib, of really freeing people to use themselves, cannot take place except as this involves a whole complete change in women. But nurses are . . . One of the things we know from earlier studies is that people who selected nursing were predominantly those wanting to take orders.

We have a large group of antieducationists in nursing, and it's tragic when they are in positions of power or strength. Their commitment is often to themselves, so that they'll say, "Yes, ma'am!" But this is people. The way I understand it is, I have some assets and somebody else has some others, so . . .

GS: Did you ever feel the stigma that the nursing profession has had in the past, such as the nurses not being too bright and from mainly the lower social class?

MR: I get mad, but I don't think there is anything remarkable about one person having certain kinds of characteristics and somebody else not. I don't think it makes one person any better or worse than anybody else. I think one thing that we in nursing as well as in our society have not learned is to respect differences; and I think that (for example, nursing technicians) it certainly doesn't take the same kind of interest and abilities to be a top-notch nursing technician as it would to be a theoretical researcher; but it doesn't make the researcher one bit better, or one bit more important, as a matter of fact. We need all of these kinds of people. We need to respect them as equally important in the social milieu. I still think Gardner's book titled *Excellence*[8] is about the best little thing I have ever read. The point is we do need differences. I don't think there is anything worse than having everybody all alike. I don't like all sorts of things, and I like all sorts of people, and I'm no better than or different from anybody else. Well, maybe I have had my name in the paper more often.

GS: Do you think that nurses will become more assertive and become leaders in nursing and in social reforms? Can leadership be taught?

MR: There already are nurses who are active. I think one of the things that we have to get past is acting like a nurse is a nurse is a nurse. We are talking about two different populations. Both are equally important, but one makes the larger judgments. Now I think that in both instances, however, we need social leadership with judgments consistent with the knowledge that each possesses. As for building leaders, at this point I don't even know what a leader is. But in the sense of assuming professional responsibility, we hope we are building this into every student we have here. Now some of them may never set the world on fire, but there are others who will. But we are talking about a professional self-image that is different. But what right have we to expect professional responsibility of a group of people who have had no professional preparation? You see, we are confusing starch with words. And as the starch is wrung out, the words are pretty empty. But in terms of social responsi-

[8] John Gardner, *Excellence,* Harper & Brothers, New York, 1961.

bility and social accountability of a learned profession course, yes, this is part of it. And in moving to be aggressive in this, there will be many different kinds of leadership; but it had better be socially activist. And we tell the students, "You know, some people tell you not to stick your neck out or you will get it chopped off. But that's all right. You just pick it up, screw it back on, and go on." This is expected, and by the time they graduate, at any level, I think they are ready to get their heads chopped off. If they aren't, they sure don't let me know.

GS: *As a summary, then, what is it that you want to make certain will be in the chapter about you that you think is valuable for whoever will be reading this book now and many years from now?*

MR: The things that people might want to read aren't always printable.

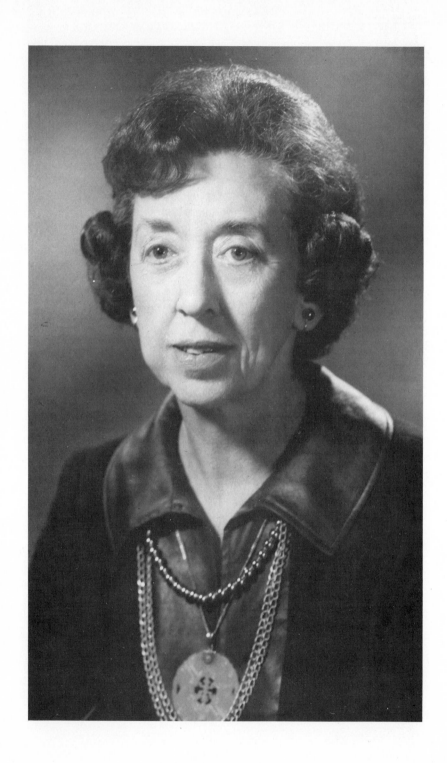

15

An outstanding scholar of nursing . . .

One of nursing's most original thinkers.[1]

. . . an educator with innovative, progressive and sometimes startling concepts of education for nurse practitioners . . . (she) is unafraid of censure, she probes nursing's problems and insists that there are no solutions. She asks for nothing she is not willing to give, but she gives much more than she would ask of others.[2]

Dean Schlotfeldt exemplies the characteristics represented by (this) award—deep concern for people—those who serve—those who learn—those who teach—those who suffer and those who must be helped. She is vigorous, informed, and articulate.[3]

[1]Quotes about Dr. Schlotfeldt from nursing leaders throughout the United States.
[2]From the American Nurses' Association Honorary Recognition Award, May 1969.
[3]From Wayne State University Centennial Celebration Award, April 11, 1968.

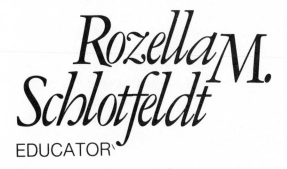

Rozella M. Schlotfeldt

EDUCATOR

*D*r. Schlotfeldt is one of the nation's foremost nursing scholars. She has emphasized the importance of nursing research, the teaching of research and writing, and the importance of exemplary professional practice.

Rozella M. Schlotfeldt was born in the small town of DeWitt, Iowa, in 1914. She was the younger of two girls. Her father, proprietor of his own business, was a regional poultry and dairy products distributor. He died suddenly as a consequence of the influenza epidemic when she was four years old. Her mother, who had almost completed a program of study in preparation to become a registered nurse prior to her marriage, worked as a practical nurse.

Dr. Schlotfeldt was valedictorian of her high school class and, as a consequence, earned a scholarship for study in a liberal arts college. Instead of accepting the scholarship, she decided to enter the University of Iowa's combined liberal arts and nursing program, thereby fulfilling a career goal she had held from the time of her father's death. She worked twenty-one hours weekly in a private home for her room and board while enrolled for full-time study in the university. In 1935 she was awarded the bachelor of science degree in nursing, magna cum laude. She received a master of science degree in nursing education and administration from the University of Chicago in 1947. In 1956, she received a Ph.D. degree in education and curriculum development, also from the University of Chicago. Her dissertation was entitled "The Educational Leadership Role of Nursing School Executives and Faculty Satisfaction."

She has had varied experience: She has been a staff nurse at the State University of Iowa (1935); a staff nurse and later a head nurse in a U.S. Veterans Hospital (1936–1938); an instructor and supervisor in maternity nursing at the State University of Iowa and the University of Iowa Hospitals (1939–1944); and a second and first lieutenant in the U.S. Army Nurse Corps (1944–1946). After World War II, she was a faculty member at the University of Colorado School of Nursing, and in 1948 she joined the faculty of the College of Nursing, Wayne State University. In 1952–1953 she took a one-year educational leave in order to begin a program of doctoral study. In June 1955 she resigned her position as Associate Professor and devoted full time to graduate study. After her Ph.D. degree was awarded in December 1956, she returned to the College of Nursing at Wayne State University as Professor and Associate Dean for Research and Development. In 1960 she was appointed Professor and Dean of the Frances Payne Bolton School of Nursing, Case Western Reserve University, Cleveland, Ohio.

Under her leadership the school of nursing has achieved prominence in nursing education and research. Among the accomplishments have been the revitalization of its faculty, the planning and construction of a new facility in the health sciences complex, the expansion of the school's graduate programs, and a research program that has enabled the school to be one of the first two in the country to be awarded a general research support grant.[4]

As dean, Dr. Schlotfeldt developed the Frances Payne Bolton School of Nursing into the number-one nursing school in the United States.[5] She "developed a significant program of research in the School but had also been an active participant in ongoing study."[6] She resigned from the deanship in 1972, but has remained on the faculty as a professor until the present.

Dr. Schlotfeldt has been active in many professional activities on local, state, and national levels. They are too numerous to list them all here. Her elections and appointments since 1967 include, among others, Chairwoman and later member of the American Nurses' Association (A.N.A.) Commission on Nursing Education; member of the National Advisory Council, Health Services and Mental Health Administration Administration; the first nurse appointed as a member of the Council and Executive Committee of the Institute of Medicine, National Academy of Sciences; and member of the Defense Advisory Committee on Women in the Services, Department of Defense.

She has published over eighty articles in medical, nursing, and education journals.[7] In addition, she has been the keynote speaker or has

[4] *Nursing Outlook*, p. 12, January 1972.
[5] R. Z. Margulies and P. M. Blau, "American's Leading Professional Schools," *Change*, 5 (9): 21–25, November 1973.
[6] Margene O. Faddis, *A School of Nursing Comes of Age: A History of the Frances Payne Bolton School of Nursing*, Case Western Reserve University, Howard Allen, Inc., Oberlin, Ohio, 1973.
[7] Among them are "The Nurses' View of the Changing Nurse-Physician Relationship," *Journal of Medical Education*, 40:442–477, August 1965; "Emerging Patterns of Education and Practice in the Health Professions: Nursing," *Pharmacy, Medicine, Nursing Conference on Health Education*, Richard A. Deno (ed.), University of Michigan, Ann Arbor, 1967, pp. 11–20; "Response: Responsibility of the University for Preparation of Members of the Health Professions," *Response to Change in Health Services*, The Johns Hopkins Hospital, Baltimore, 1967, pp. 36–44; "The Nurse Scientist Program at Case Western Reserve University," *Extending the Boundaries of Nursing Education: The Preparation and Role of the Nurse Scientist*, N.L.N., New York, 1968, pp.35–44; "An Experiment in Nursing: Implementing Planned Change," *American Journal of Nursing*, 69:1247–1251, July 1969; "Nurses and Physicians: Professional Associates and Assistants to Patients," *Ohio Nurses Review*, 45:6–12, March 1970; "Ph.D. in Science," *Future Directions of Doctoral Education for Nurses*, U.S. Government Printing Office, 1971, pp. 120–142; "Nurses, Physicians, and Physicians' Assistants: An Anecdote," *Ohio Nurses Review,* 48:5–7 September 1973; "Research in Nursing and Research Training for Nurses," *Nursing Research*, 24:177–183, May-June 1975.

presented papers at more than one hundred professional meetings throughout the country and abroad.

Dr. Schlotfeldt has received many honors and awards. She was one of the first fifty persons elected to the Institute of Medicine, National Academy of Sciences (1971). She received a doctor of science degree, honoris causa, from Georgetown University in 1972, and the Distinguished Service Award from the University of Iowa in 1973. A Rozella M. Schlotfeldt Scholarship was established in her honor by the Frances Payne Bolton Alumni Association, and a lectureship in her name was endowed at Case Western Reserve University (1972). In 1974 she was elected to fellowship in the American Academy of Nursing and was selected for listing in the 1975 edition of the *Cyclopedia of American Biographies*.[8]

Dissertation and Wayne State University

GS: What did you do your dissertation on; what is the title of it?

RS: The title of the dissertation is "The Educational Leadership Role of Nursing School Executives and Faculty Satisfaction." It's kind of a joke, because I had always vowed that I was not interested in administration, but I became very interested in what they were doing at the Midwest Administration Center in theories relative to administration. I also became quite interested in, and studied extensively about, the newly developing concepts of leadership and role theory. Perhaps the title of the dissertation represented a hidden goal.

It was an interesting study. I designed an instrument whereby I was able to contrast faculty members' expectations for the leader's role as it related to educational planning and their perception of the nature of educational leadership. I then looked to see the extent to which faculty satisfaction was a consequence of their perceptions of whether or not their expectations for educational leadership were fulfilled.

There was the opportunity for me at Wayne to give leadership in the development of a research program when I returned there in 1957. I think we were reasonably successful in getting several projects off the

---

[8] There are many other awards, and the reader is referred to Dr. Schlotfeldt's listing in *Who's Who in America*, *Who's Who in American College and University Administration*, and *Who's Who of American Women*.

ground. In addition to that, several curriculum changes were brought about; and I was privileged to be a part of many new things that were developing during the 1950s. For example, the Kellogg Foundation had given money in order to help support universities (in about 1952, I think) in developing graduate programs in nursing administration. It was recognized that then very few of our nurse leaders were formally prepared in the science and art of administration. So that program had gotten off the ground at Wayne. The Kellogg Foundation had also given financial support to several institutions to help them develop graduate programs in clinical nursing. And those were always in a state of continuous development. Wayne was an exciting place to be. We were developing new programs in education, administration, clinical practice, and research. Ours was a university that neither owned nor operated hospitals; and so it became necessary to try out ways of developing relationships with many types of clinical facilities in the large metropolitan area and in rural areas as well. The Wayne program had contractual arrangements with many different institutions, and was one of the first university nursing programs to develop such agreements. That really was quite an experience, and truly an experiment in developing interinstitutional arrangements. Regrettably, it wasn't looked on as an experiment, and thus was not reported as such.

I used to get very restive when I would hear complaints about the quality of nursing care that was exemplified in some institutions across the country. And I recall very well saying to faculty colleagues, "Well, what can be done about it?" And the answer invariably was, "Well, faculty are not in a position to do much directly because we really are guests in those institutions." And that was a true statement. My concern that faculty should be actively involved in patient care, and be in a position to exercise quality control over nursing care in institutions used as clinical learning environments, led me to consider the possibility of accepting a deanship. I developed the notion that maybe there would be a new way to approach relationships between educational institutions and service agencies—to develop a plan that would effect an exemplary clinical learning environment for students. I envisioned a relationship that would be receptive to faculty members' active involvement in nursing practice and research, and one that would foster collaborative efforts between and among institutional staffs of service agencies, faculty, and students. I was convinced that nursing knowledge would not be advanced without active involvement of faculty and students in clinical practice; and I was convinced also that knowledgeable staff members had much to contribute to nursing education and research.

Dean of Frances Payne Bolton School of Nursing, Case Western Reserve University, 1960–1975[9]

GS: What led you to take the position of dean?

RS: John S. Millis, then President of Western Reserve University, wrote to me and said that they were looking for a dean here (Western Reserve). Originally I gave him my standard answer: "I am interested in graduate study and research and I really don't want to become an administrator." He wrote back to say that if I wouldn't come to Cleveland, he would come to Detroit to talk with me. And then I talked with myself and said, "Look, you're not close-minded; you could go down there and investigate in order to see what might be interesting." So, I came once and I came twice and I came three times; and by then I was thoroughly convinced that I really did want to come here, because it presented a very unusual opportunity to try out some of my ideas about leadership in nursing education. I would say to anybody who is contemplating being a dean, "Pick your president!" John Millis himself is a great intellectual, a scientist, a humanist, a man who has considerable knowledge in the health sciences, and a remarkable administrator. President Millis saw that nursing could become a learned profession, and he was willing to give a dean all the freedom posible in working with faculty in an attempt to contribute to attaining that goal.

In some ways, being a dean is kind of a lonely job; but it's also a job of great opportunity, because a dean has the tremendous privilege of working with people who have great minds. President Millis is a good example: here he was President of the university, and sometimes I just called him up and said, "I need to talk to you." I would go to talk with him, and we'd bat ideas back and forth, and talk about new directions in which we ought to be going. It was really a wonderfully rewarding experience, working with university colleagues, and especially with the nursing school faculty.

I came here in 1960, and by February of 1961 we had developed (we always worked together as a faculty) a paper on the school's future. President Millis had asked all the deans of the university to set forth goals for the next twenty years; and then he asked a central planning committee for the total university to correlate all of those plans.

---

[9] She resigned from the position of Dean in 1972, but remained on the faculty.

We predicted what this school was going to become, because we had quite a clear vision of where we were going. There was no question that this School of Nursing was going to become a research center. It was going to become a center in which we would find a new way to relate the educational institution to the community and to the nursing service staffs. We began working on that immediately, but even before I came, I ascertained that it was going to be possible to do it.

When I came here, the budget for this School of Nursing was something like $600,000; last year it was $2.5 million.

GS: Where did you get all your money?

RS: Well, from many sources. We raised tuition fees first of all; and that was the first really difficult, courageous thing that we did. We said, "Okay, over the next number of years we're going to raise the tuition substantially, so that fees charged are comparable with those assessed by the rest of the university." So that was one source. We developed a fine relationship with our alumni. When I came here, we had something like $2500 annual income from that source; alumni members gave $65,000 to the school during the last year of my service as Dean. We sought grants from the federal government. We went to foundations to enlist their interest in and support of our programs. Grants and gifts could be considered to be "soft" money, but a lot of it was "hard" money too. And we established the principle that all of the efforts of the school had claim on the "hard" money as well as the "soft" money. Thus, if we were committed to seeking grants, we could apply for grants to support innovations in teaching as well as research and patient care.

We developed further the plans for a new interinstitutional relationship, and we tested it initially with the University Hospitals of Cleveland. That magnificent, 1100-bed institution is not just ideally located in the Health Sciences Center on campus. It offers high-quality acute care and, additionally, there's a huge ambulatory care service; and it offers clinical learning opportunities for students of all of the health science schools.

We developed the concept of "joint" rather than "dual" appointments, rationalizing the amount of time available to those persons who were the joint appointees so that they were not expected to do two jobs rather than one. We negotiated practice and research privileges for all faculty. We appointed directors for the clinical programs who were really experts in their field, and never compromised our standards for quality. We waited until we could appoint the real experts for leadership positions, and then we recruited for and prepared specialists for all the clinical fields of nursing. That meant that we started new graduate programs in pediatric nursing and in psychiatric nursing. So then, as we developed new people as well as recruited vigorously, we had a larger pool of qualified candidates from which to appoint. But, more than that, I was committed to the notion that we had to get persons from all over the United States, because only then can students be brought into contact with faculty representing varied points of view. I recall that after my first year in the Dean's position the school made recommendations for appointments of nineteen people, and their advanced preparation was obtained in fourteen different institutions, from all over the country.

Our school was awarded a Faculty Research Development Grant, and that was followed by a Research Development Grant. Both were very helpful to us in supporting a research program. Additionally, individual investigators sought and obtained research grants. In 1963 along came the Nurse-Scientist program, and ours was one of the first two of such awards made. So they all kind of meshed together and allowed us to advance knowledge, provide excellent programs of education, and be actively involved in nursing care in a variety of settings, not just University Hospitals.

GS: Would you say that recruitment of well-qualified faculty was one of your biggest problems in the job?

RS: Absolutely! It was one of the most important responsibilities. Back in 1960 it was not easy to find people who were prepared at the doctoral level and who were really experts in their clinical fields. After our pilot study convinced us that our concept of interinstitutional relationships was a good one, we went to the W. K. Kellogg Foundation and got some support for the experiment so that we could keep the show on the road as well as introduce planned change. You can't ask people to do a double job. You can't ask them to keep on doing what they're doing and then do something else besides.

GS: Did you think that you could begin a doctor of science nursing degree?

RS: No. Actually we began our deliberations about doctoral study solely with the idea of supporting nurses to obtain Ph.D. degrees in relevant disciplines. And, as a matter of fact, my thinking has come 180 degrees, all the way around, for later we decided to develop a Ph.D. in nursing degree, not a D.Sc. in nursing. We started a Nurse-Scientist program, and that was with full sanction of the faculty for we never did anything without discussing it with the faculty and having their full support. For example, when we sought a research development grant, everybody voted for that, so there was some commitment to it before we really got it off the ground. When the Nurse-Scientist program came along, we discussed the kind of Nurse-Scientist program we wanted, and decided that in this university we would like nurses to have opportunities to study in the departments of physiology and biology, sociology, anthropology, and psychology. We envisioned opportunites also for nurses to obtain Ph.D. degrees in history on this campus, hopefully with support from the Nurse-Scientist program. (That did not eventuate.) And then Case has a big name in systems, and we wanted nurses to have the opportunity to study there. Eventually several students studied in systems-operations research and in all of the disciplines I have mentioned. But in the early stages we did not want to develop a program at the doctoral level in nursing. It was our belief that when we could get a large enough cadre of persons who were prepared at the doctoral level in the relevant disciplines, we would then address the question of what kind of doctoral program we wanted. And we did, in fact, do that. In 1971 we took to the Graduate Council of this university a proposal for a Ph.D. in nursing program (a research-oriented program). It was approved, and two students were admitted to it in the fall of 1972.

We built this building with support from our many friends in the community, our generous alumni, some foundations, and several divisions within the federal government. The building was designed by a committee of the school. This is a forward-looking building. There are facilities and space here for every kind of research that investigators will likely design in the near future. I have told you the kinds of things that we wanted to do here, and we developed long-range plans for all of them. And I think we accomplished quite a bit. I felt good about having accomplished what we did accomplish in the period of time that I served. It was a great opportunity and privilege to serve as Dean.

Resigns from the Deanship

GS: Why did you resign from the deanship?

RS: I think one of the marks of a good administrator is having a sense of timing. And I think there is a time to come and there is a time to go. I was growing very tired. I had had twelve years of service without much time off. The dean's role is very demanding. I decided that perhaps it was time for me to think about doing something else. I'm not even real sure what it is I am going to do yet, but I decided that I needed time to think about it, so I took a sabbatical for a year. Actually, I did schoolwork during much of the sabbatical year; because I had been the principal investigator for the research development grant in the school, it was my responsibility to write that report, which I did.[10] Also, during the last year of my deanship, we were preparing for the regular school accreditation visit, which took place in the fall of 1972, during the time that I was on sabbatical. And, since I had appointed all the task forces to do the self-study, it seemed appropriate for me to collate those reports from the task forces and to write the accreditation report. I did that during the summer after my sabbatical began. Actually, there were many things that I was involved in for the school. It is very hard to dissociate oneself from that kind of endeavor summarily. And so I did complete those responsibilities that I felt were mine; and then I did a great deal of writing and I began thinking about the next thing that I would like to do.

GS. In your job, what were some of your frustrations and disappointments?

RS: Well, I suppose there were some. Basically I'm a supreme optimist, but when good and necessary goals seem too remote for their accomplishment, I do get very frustrated. One of my faculty said to me one time toward the end of my tenure as Dean, "You used to always say, 'We will find a way.' Once in a while now you say, 'I'm not sure we can.'" That was undoubtedly an indication of frustration.

Case Institute of Technology and Western Reserve University became a federated institution in July 1967. President Millis became Chancellor, and the President of Case became the President of the federated institution. We immediately began a long, very difficult, but also stimulating, period of combining the two institutions. We had a constitutional assembly to write a constitution for this new university. Some of us went Saturday after Saturday as members of the constitutional assembly in order to hammer out a constitution for a new kind of institution. That was a remarkable experience. President Morse, who was the first presidential appointee of the federated institution, is a delightful, beautiful man. He has written some magnificent things about the nature of higher institutions. It was a privilege to work with him. The federation made visible the financial needs and problems of the new institution, because there were, for example, two departments of physics and two departments of chemistry, both having appointees with tenure, resulting in larger departments than were actually needed, I suspect. So the financial difficulties that are now quite common to higher institutions became visible earlier in this institution than in others. In a certain sense, that was a blessing because we had a bit more lead time for financial planning. But almost immediately after federation, we began to hear budget, budget, budget throughout the year; and we spent so much time in budget planning that there was little time or energy left to devote to educational planning. And I am a person who consistently keeps an eye on the future, and must have some time for

[10] *Creating a Climate for Nursing Research,* Frances Payne Bolton School of Nursing, Case Western Reserve University, Cleveland, 1973.

thinking ahead and for developing new goals and new approaches for meeting them.

I don't know; I think probably the decision I made represented an awareness that there comes a time for new leadership in any enterprise.

Now I must say that I think that I had some part in the great legacy this school has. There was much money brought into the school. The hard money support from tuition income was sound, and we had developed many sources of gifts and grants. Many of the grants are still ongoing, including foundation support. We had had very little help with increasing the school's endowment, although we were beginning to make some progress with that also. The school had established very fine relations with its alumni and with the community. We have a magnificent building and a fine faculty. The curricula were in good shape; there was research ongoing; and we had effected a relationship with service agencies that was productive of excellent programs of nursing care and fine educational and research climates. For all of those reasons I decided that the time had come for the school to have new leadership.

GS: *Is there anything you wish to add about the deanship, then?*

RS: I think the image of nursing was somewhat enhanced in this institution. I often say that the university should also be enhanced by all of its divisions; and I believe that this school has enhanced the image of this university. I believe also that the efforts of this faculty and its students and graduates have helped to move nursing toward its becoming a scholarly discipline. We were able to demonstrate that research does have a legitimate claim on the total resources of the institution, and I know that we have been able to demonstrate a workable, good approach to having faculty involvement in patient care, and to have good practitioner and investigator models. I had many more ideas that I would like to have helped move forward. I shared those, hoping that they would be picked up and carried on.

GS: *Would you say something about when one retires or resigns from the position, the concern she has for the role and what she has left behind for the successor? Or doesn't that concern you too much?*

RS: I think anyone who has invested a great deal of himself or herself in a leadership role must be very eager for assurance that the institution will maintain the level of excellence that it has achieved, and of course I was concerned with that. I would have been devasted if the commitment for faculty's involvement in care of patients would all of a sudden be turned off. That would have concerned me very much indeed. Similarly, my commitments to research and to the climate of inquiry that had been developed in this school were intense. It would worry me very much to have the research commitment deteriorate. On the other hand, I think that everyone has to live on his or her own record. I think it's appropriate for a person who has been a part of the leadership to disengage from that role. Someone else has to take over. The person who leaves is neither responsible for nor involved in the school's leadership. I certainly am not responsible for the direction the school takes under someone else's leadership. Nor do I think I have the right to indicate what that leadership should be. Of course I shall continue to be involved and concerned, but henceforth in the full-time role of professor rather than in the role of leader, or dean.

GS: Is there anything else you'd like to add about the dean's role generally?

RS: I think one thing that is terribly important for an administrator is always to look for opportunities to learn. One learns more from colleagues than one could possibly ever teach them. Imagine the opportunity of being a dean or being a president or any kind of an administrator and of learning from all these bright people that you surround yourself with. The smart thing is always to appoint people who are much smarter than you are, and then learn from them. It is important to let them get together so that the combined wisdom of the group can be brought to bear on ideas emanating from any or all of them. That's one of the strategies I've tried to develop—always to learn and to make it possible for other people to learn and to be supported and helped. Everybody ought to have a chance. I think administrators have to *take* chances too.

GS: You have to be willing to take risks?

RS: Absolutely. But I've always been very fortunate, and have a lot of self-confidence as well as confidence in others. I came from a good home in which learning and effort were valued. I was educated in a good high school. I went to a good university nursing school. I went to a good higher institution to earn master's and Ph.D. degrees. I've always practiced and taught in good institutions. I've had wonderful colleagues; I've had opportunities to work with very bright people. In our home we used to say, "The good Lord gave me a brain—and I am expected to use it." That means proposing some new ways to resolve problems, and taking some risks.

I have never given up my interest in patient care, and I believe that designated leaders have obligations to improve circumstances of practice, whatever the field may be. I probably did as much to help improve patient care by giving leadership in the experiment that we conducted (interinstitutional relationships) as persons do who are giving direct services to patients. In many ways that was a "risky" endeavor, for it meant making planned changes in two highly bureaucratic institu-

tions—the university and the hospital. But we demonstrated that investment in competence is good for patients, for students, for the faculty,
and for nursing. Someone was asked. "What's going to happen when
the experiment is over?" And one of the nurse-director-chairmen said,
"It's not an experiment; it's a concept." Which is a good answer. It was
looked upon as an experiment because it was partially supported by
outside funds. But it truly is a concept. Simply stated, it is having people
who know, do. And the people who know a very great deal, and are
eager to learn more, are those who give leadership in the doing. That's
the concept.

A View on Leadership

GS: Do you think that nurses can be taught to become leaders?

RS: Sure. But I think we have an awful lot of potential leaders—maybe
they're the bumptious kind—who need to have somebody give them a
pat on the head and say, "Yes, you can become a leader." I can give
you an example of a leader who needed to be discovered and encouraged. I had asked to have all alumni questionnaires returned to me if
there were any negative comments on them. I recall one especially on
which there was a very negative comment. So I wrote the young woman
a letter and invited her to come to see me. She was obviously a very
bright young woman, who had a real gripe; but her efforts were not
being directed in a very constructive direction. She was encouraged to
develop her leadership potential by obtaining more education and by
seeking opportunities to give leadership. She now holds a responsible
facuty position, has learned the rewards that inhere in working with and
through others, and is giving fine leadership within the profession. She
has a brilliant future, I am sure. Nursing needs to seek out and develop
its bright, probably rebellious, innovative young people, and cultivate
their leadership potentials. Actually, the women's movement should
help to raise nurses' consciousness about their great leadership potentials.

*GS: Aren't you active in the A.N.A.'s class-action suit against the
Teachers' Insurance Annuity Association (T.I.A.A.)?*

RS: Yes, and I believe that that represents appropriate action on the
part of so-called leaders. I had long been concerned about the low
visibility of women in the university and their relative paucity of opportunities. I had personally hit many resistance points. I realized that women
really were getting a bad shake within all universities, including this one.
And I was always forthright. I would communicate immediately every
time I saw evidence of any kind of adverse discrimination. So when the

A.N.A. came along and said that they were willing to introduce a class-action suit against the T.I.A.A. for discriminatory policies unfavorable to women with regard to retirement annuity, I thought that was right. I think such action makes an important social contribution. And so I thought about it and then communicated with the President. I told him that inasmuch as he had gone on record as saying that he wanted to eliminate all discrimination within the university, I was going to help him. I told him that it was necessary to name the university as well as to name the T.I.A.A. in such action, and that I made the assumption that he would encourage me to be actively involved in the action. His response was that he would encourage faculty to do anything that they thought was right in order to right a wrong; and so it was with his knowledge and with his written sanction that I joined the group. I think such forthright action makes a great contribution. However, it has not been something that has helped me at all; as a matter of fact, I'm sure that I've been criticized greatly. But leaders must be courageous; and those who take stands on issues are often criticized. As a matter of fact, in a social setting, one of the supporters of this university really attacked me for my part in the T.I.A.A. action. I finally told him that I was doing what I thought was right; and that it was done with the full knowledge of the President. That really surprised him when I told him that. And I said, "What is more, I shall communicate with the President about this conversation." And I did, by letter, and I sent a carbon copy to the gentleman who was so critical of my action. That's the way I operate—on top of the table. And I always try to communicate effectively.

I know that I make mistakes; but if I do, it's not because I want to make them, and surely I'm not going to hide my actions under the table.

Leaders surely must take positions on important issues. They must also, I believe, contemplate the future and determine wherein change is needed; and then help to bring it about. They must also, in my view, stimulate inquiry about the need for new types of institutions. I should add that I was one of the prime movers in beginning the inquiry about the wisdom of having an American Association of Colleges of Nursing (A.A.C.N.), which I very strongly believe must be further developed in this country.

I have had the privilege of representing nursing in all kinds of national endeavors: Accreditation Board; National Institute of Mental Health; Policy and Planning Board of the National Institute of Mental Health. I've served on the Nursing Research Study Section. I've been on the Health Services and Mental Health Administration Study Section and on its National Advisory Council. I'm on the Institute of Medicine's Council and its Executive Committee. I've been invited to many national meetings, and have been able to speak for nursing and nurses and for nursing's contributions to the world. It was my privilege to serve as the

Vice Chairwoman of the Steering Committee of the Council, Department of Baccalaureate and Higher Degree Programs, when we were making progress relative to development of a joint National League for Nursing (N.L.N.)–A.N.A. career counseling effort. And I was fortunate to have been a member of the A.N.A.'s Committee on Education (later the Commission of Nursing Education) during the time we issued the first Position Paper on education. That was a historic document that represented forthright action. My tenure on the commission encompassed issuing the papers on continuing education and on graduate education in nursing, and, additionally, preparing the A.N.A.'s Standards for Nursing Education for their first review at the 1974 convention. Those were all marvelous experiences; and I believe they all helped to set directions for the future.

Nursing in the Future

GS: Where do you think nursing's going to be in the future?

RS: I think we're at the crossroads. We've said that for I don't know how many years, but I think now we're at the moment of truth. Actually, in some ways I'm really quite worried about nursing at the present time. Being the optimist that I am, I like to think that we will have a sufficient number of bright people who will act wisely and give the kind of leadership that is needed. However, I see too much of this selling out to the notion that nurses should become physicians' assistants. They don't call themselves that, but some so-called nurse-practitioners are serving as physicians' assistants, hoping thereby to get prestige and rewards and money that they believe are not concomitants of practicing nursing. There's entirely too much of that, and there's entirely too much publicity and sanction being given by persons in leadership positions in nursing. Maybe the action of the American Academy of Pediatrics will wake up a few people. I think nurses have to stand up and be counted. Nursing must control its own destiny. Forthright leadership that's of a good kind recognizes that nurses have a great contribution to make, and such leaders communicate confidence in nurses who are competent.

GS: Why do you think that some of the nursing leaders are selling out?

RS: I don't know. I was at a meeting not long ago in which I spoke quite forcefully about that silly term "nurse-practitioner." And one dean replied, "You might as well give up on that. We have all accepted it." Well, I don't plan to give up. Why deal in tautology? Isn't the nurse a practitioner? And when you say one is a nurse and another is a nurse-practitioner, the implication is that the nurse is not a practitioner. And this is the greatest put-down of nurses by nurses! You know, like Pogo said, "We've met the enemy and the enemy is us." I don't know what the outcome is going to be. I worked very hard while I was Dean of the School of Nursing, to be sure that graduates were competent practitioners of nursing, asking questions such as: Have we delineated the competencies that *should* be expected of persons who are professionals in the field? Can they assess the health status of the people? Can they use nursing strategies appropriately? Can and do they evaluate the outcomes of nursing care?

GS: Do you think the name or term "nursing" will change to something else?

RS: I hope not. There are all kinds of reasons given for wanting to change the name "nurse" or "nursing." It's a feminine profession. Well, what does it say if you change the word "nurse" to something else because "nurse" has a feminine, nurturing, kind, accepting derivation? It says that kindness, nurturance, and femininity aren't worth preserving. I don't believe that.

When teachers were primarily women, and when the teaching profession decided that it wished to have teachers who truly were educators, they didn't change the name. They took forthright action. They said that after a certain date, all persons who were certified were going to have educational preparation, first at the baccalaureate level and then later at the master's level for certain kinds of credentials. To my knowledge they didn't say, "We're going to take this action because we want men to come into teaching." Interestingly enough, men did come into teaching in increasing numbers; and the teaching profession said that young kids need to have models of men teachers as well as models of women teachers. And that forthright action was for appropriate reasons; and in my view it was right. They didn't change the name "teacher" because it once had a feminine connotation.

All of those suggestions to change nursing's name come from people who don't care about nursing, who don't care about women, who think nursing should be put down, and who think women should be put down. Not I. I believe in nurses; I believe in nursing. I think people need nurses and people need nursing, as well as medicine and other helping professions. Nurses don't do their legitimate work just because there aren't enough physicians. That silly rationale for needing competent nurses is reiterated, I don't know how many times. A similar put-down is calling nurses "physician extenders." Do nurses want to be physician extenders? Be two-bit physicians? How will that help the world when people need the services of first-rate nurses! But I was heartened by a conversation that transpired lately. I happened to be attending a meeting in Washington, D.C., of the Institute of Medicine. There was some discussion about health care and the need for more people, and mention was made of the contributions of nurse-practitioners. Subsequently one of the scientists rode out to the airport with me, and I think I can quote almost exactly what he said. It was something like: "I don't know why nurses want to go that practitioner route, and thereby deny their professional contributions and their professional identity in order to become feldshers." I thought that was a tremendous observation on the part of a scientist. People need to hear those kinds of things.

GS: Would you call that consciousness raising?

RS: Yes, I think so. At one of the meetings in this health center, somebody commented about the lack of physicians in certain geographic areas. And in some geographic areas, of course, there is a paucity of physicians and of available medical care. And a physician said, "Well, if I were in general practice, I would get me a couple of nurse-practitioners." That reminded me of an article published in a medical journal in which physicians shamelessly reported that they hired nurse-practitioners—pediatric nurse-practitioners—and enhanced their intake of patients. And they had the gall to quote how much they had to pay their "practitioners" (around $8000 a year), and they even gave a statistical prediction of how frequently they would have to add one in order to obtain particular increments in their own incomes. But of course physicians couldn't do that if nurses weren't fool enough to cooperate. And some of them call themselves "nurse-practitioners."

GS: Do you think, then, that the nurse-practitioner is going to stay?

RS: I have no idea. I don't know what those who use the term mean. When anybody says something to me about a nurse-practitioner, I ask, "Do you mean a nurse?" That's my standard query. And if you ask the question often enough, maybe the question will be addressed. But you asked me to discuss where I think nursing is going. I think if this kind of thinking persists, I'm not at all sure that nursing won't take a real nose dive. Nursing has a real contribution to make, and that contribution is health care. How much better it would be to have a group of nurses who have competence and self-confidence say, "I'm a nurse and I'm proud of it." Everybody knows that competent, knowledgeable nurses make tremendous contributions, including those people who are trying to make them into nurse-practitioners!

The goal of nursing as a field of professional endeavor is to help people attain, retain, and regain health.[11]

[11] Rozella M. Schlotfeldt, "This I Believe: Nursing Is Health Care," *Nursing Outlook*, pp. 245–246, April 1972.

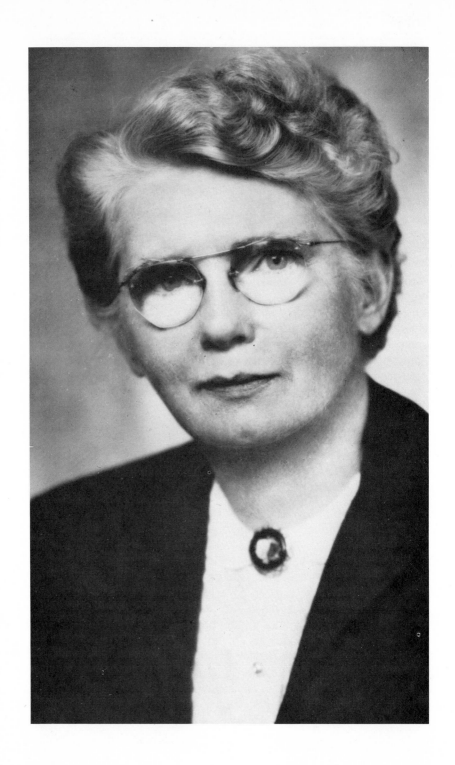

16

For her inspiring leadership, skills, and unswerving devotion to her 'visions of a better world'. . . . Her creative thinking helped to mold plans which enabled nursing to play its proper role throughout World War II in health protection on the home front and mobilization of nursing personnel for the Armed Services. Her comprehensive program of nationwide action in the field of nursing became the blueprint which initiated and will guide progress in nursing for many years to come. As Director of Public Health Nursing in New York she pioneered new methods that set the pattern for her own and many other states.

With ability and courage to reach difficult goals Miss Sheahan has forged a record of superb achievement by her accomplishments.[1]

[1]Citation from the Lasker Award presented to Marion Sheahan Oct. 25, 1949. Marion Sheahan was the first nondoctor to receive a Lasker Award, which consisted of $1000 and a gold replica of the Winged Victory of Samothrace to symbolize victory over death and disease.

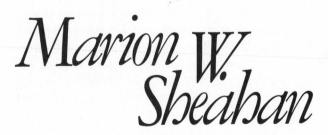

Marion W. Sheahan

PUBLIC HEALTH ADMINISTRATOR

*M*arion Sheahan[2] is described by everyone who knows her as a "wonderful person." She has been one of the nation's outstanding leaders in nursing and public health. In 1913 she received her registered nurse diploma from St. Peter's Hospital, Albany, New York.

She lectured and taught public health administration at Teachers College, Columbia; the University of California at Berkeley (spring 1948); and the University of Minnesota (summer 1948).

Marion Sheahan was the first nurse to be elected President of the American Public Health Association (A.P.H.A.). She has been active in many organizations, including the former National Organization for Public Health Nursing (N.O.P.H.N.), of which she was a president. She was chairman of the committee that studied the Nurse Practice Act in New York State and was instrumental in bringing about helpful revision of the statute requiring the licensing of all classes of nurses in New York. In 1944 she was named Vice President of the A.P.H.A., and was a member of the War Manpower Commission on recruitment of medical personnel during World War II.

She was a member of the 1952 President's Commission on Health Needs of the Nation. She has served on advisory committees to the U.S. Public Health Service (U.S.P.H.S.) and the Veterans Administration; has been a consultant to the Army Nurse Corps (A.N.C.); and has served as a member of the Surgeon General's Consultant Group on Nursing, which issued the report "Toward Quality in Nursing: Needs and Goals." She was a member of the National Commission on Community Health Services, sponsored by the A.P.H.A. and the National Health Council to stimulate community studies of the health services needed by the American people. She was a member of the forum planning committee of the National Health Council and of the New York State Hospital Review and Planning Council. She still serves on the Health Committee of the Public Affairs Committee, publisher of pamphlets on health and welfare matters of public concern.

Along the way she received two honorary degrees: a doctor of laws from Case Western Reserve University and a doctor of humanities from Adelphi College, New York State. Three awards she especially cherishes, because they came from her day-by-day associates, are the Sedgwick Medal from the A.P.H.A., a Medal of Achievement from the New York State Public Health Association, and one from the Board of

[2] Sheahan is her professional name; she was married to Frank W. Bailey in 1937; he died in 1947.

the National League for Nursing (N.L.N.). She also received the Florence Nightingale Award from the International Red Cross.

Early Background

GS: Could you please say something about your early life?

MS: I was born in New York City on September 5, 1892. My father was in the building business. Mother was a housewife. My father's people came from Vermont; Mother's from the Hudson Valley area of New York. Father's father had a business selling building supplies; Mother's father was a farmer. There were four children in our family: I had two sisters and one brother, and I was the second-eldest of the four. My father moved to New York City from Burlington, Vermont. We moved to Albany in 1901.

GS: How would you describe your childhood in general?

MS: We were a close, middle-class family. We enjoyed singing, doing puzzles, and playing games together. As we grew older, one favorite game was poker. Mother kept a fancy tin box into which the pennies went to be used the next time. We were encouraged to express our ideas but with due respect for our elders. We had plenty of books around the house, among them Darwin, Mills, and Newton. I was a good reader with plenty of Jane Austen and the Elsie Dinsmore series type of "growing-up saga" along with more serious reading. My father discussed the social issues of the time with us as though we were sages.

GS: Did you decide at an early age that you would like to be a nurse?

MS: I think so. In fact, my mother hoped I would be a schoolteacher, but both parents encouraged me to go into nursing if I wanted to go. I went to St. Peter's Hospital at the advice of our family doctor.

GS: When you graduated, did you have career plans at that time?

MS: No, I didn't have set plans. While doing private-duty nursing, I volunteered to help in a South End child welfare clinic in Albany for two summers. This sparked my interest in public health.

My career plans really started after I met a friend of my parents who was a supervising nurse at Henry Street. I became enamored with the idea of the Henry Street Settlement from the way our friend described the work. My mother was doubtful, but my father encouraged me. In short order I was accepted, and started the career of my life.

GS: Could you please tell a little bit about your experience at Henry Street, because I think from a historical perspective that would be interesting.

MS: My first day there, Annie Goodrich gave a lecture to the staff. She contrasted the two sides of Fifth Avenue, east and west New York. If I was ever in doubt of my father's social philosophy, I certainly became a crusader for social betterment from that point on.

GS: What did she say?

MS: She contrasted the different living of the two sides of Fifth Avenue, west and east New York, and the growing poverty and the causes of it. I don't remember exactly what she said about correcting the inequities, but my whole concept of my mission changed as I entered the homes of East Side New York. One other thing I remember that helped me grow up: I was a babe in the woods as far as sex problems were concerned; I got disturbed about the tales women would tell me about too many children, and thought I should be doing something about it.

My father had written me about a lecture he had attended where Margaret Sanger was to be the speaker. She had been pulled off the platform by local authorities. Dr. Arthur Elting, the Chief of Surgery when I was in St. Peter's, invited the rather small audience to meet in his home to continue the lecture. This letter prompted my action to do something about my problem. A friend and I dressed in our severest costume and marched down to see Margaret Sanger. You remember, her early training had been nursing. She greeted us as though we were important people. She told us what we could do, the religious taboos that had to be respected, and what we had to be careful of. She gave us literature and set us straight about our limitations to reform the sex lives of people in the district where we worked.

GS: Could you, in a few sentences, describe your impressions of these two very well-known women, Margaret Sanger and Annie Goodrich?

MS: Well, as I remember Margaret Sanger, I thought she was a highly dedicated person. She made us feel important and respected our inexperience without making us feel uninformed or stupid.

Annie Goodrich, of course, was Annie Goodrich. She had the kind of social consciousness that communicated itself. She was an unusual, dynamic person. Her belief in the dignity of people and their right to live above the poverty line, and her belief that we nurses could help, was something that communicated itself for keeps.

There is another experience that lasted me throughout my future work. While at Henry Street I attended a series of lectures at Teachers College, Columbia University, given by Dr. Louis Dublin on "The Drama of Records." I carried this reasoning into my future experience, such as when I was Chairman of the Records Committee of the N.O.P.H.N. This committee developed the Family Health Record and worked on the "cost-per-visit study" basic to the financing of public health nursing costs.

In Public Health and Administration

GS: Why did you leave Henry Street, and where did you go?

MS: The war needed nurses, and I had applied to go overseas with the unit of the Albany Hospital, which was the recruiting unit around Albany. I was disqualified because of some rales in my chest, and I was very much underweight. So then I stayed in Albany working in the City Health Department to relieve a nurse who went with the unit.

Then I went to the New York State Department of Health on a temporary arrangement designed to help local physicians to improve medical care. This was through a series of regional clinics manned by specialists who gave consultation to physicians who elected to bring their patients. My task was to visit physicians and, when requested, to visit patients. Later I gave the same service for tuberculosis control clinics, immunization against diphtheria, and so forth.

After that experience I worked in Cohoes, New York, on a summer assignment. The infant mortality rate was very high. I volunteered for the summer to get the families to bring babies for physical examinations and advice. It was very successful; in fact, there were so many baby carriages around the street near the city hall where the clinic was held that the police complained that they were blocking traffic. I stayed there all summer. That was under the auspices of the TB and Public Health Association.

Then, through that and the interest of the lay president of the TB and Public Health Association, I went for that organization out to Niagara County as a county tuberculosis nurse. I was there a little less than two years, and then returned to the Division of Public Health Nursing, State Department of Health.

GS: How long, approximately, were you there before you became the Director?

MS: Several years. I worked on communicable disease outbreaks during my first years. I worked on getting patients to the clinics for tuberculosis control, orthopedic or child health care, and immunization. A good deal of my life seems to have been getting patients to care of one kind or another. Before I became Assistant Director, I had had a good experience in the staff work required of the divisions of the state department as a whole and in the status of public health in the state. I pay tribute to my predecessor, Mathilde Kuhlman, who taught me much. Her untimely death in 1932 elevated me to the directorship. At Mathilde Kuhlman's death, Dr. Thomas Parran, then the Commissioner, appointed me the Director. I became the Director of the Division of Public Health Nursing in 1932, and was there until 1948, when I retired.

The Lasker Award (1949) and the Presidency of the A.P.H.A. (1961)

GS: What was the Lasker Award?

MS: The Lasker Award was provided by the Lasker Foundation to recognize persons who had contributed significantly in the fields of medicine, science, or administration in public health. My award was for administration in public health.

Social Security came along in 1937, and with it came the need and the opportunity to prepare more public health nurses. The American Red Cross had done a fine job in several communities in New York State through its demonstration program, "Town and Counties Health Nursing." This program emphasized employment of nurses by towns. Several counties employed tuberculosis nurses. Some city health departments employed nurses. As I remember, all told, New York State had around 1500 public health nurses. Many of the city public health nurses were sort of the handmaidens of the health officers. At that time nurses were tacking up signs on doors for measles and scarlet fever and other communicable diseases and delivering birth certificates. In surveying what was going on, and in all the work I did around the state, I got a pretty good idea of what public health nurses, so called, were doing and what they shouldn't be doing. One of the objectives had been to help to get public health nurses prepared, but the advent of Social Security gave the impetus.[3]

In planning for the development of public health, the overall objective

---

[3] "The State Health Department, in which Marion W. Sheahan was Director of Nursing, promptly developed a practical program for the employment of nurses under public health nursing agencies, which seems to have provided a pattern for programs subsequently developed under federal auspices." Mary Roberts, *American Nursing: History and Interpretation,* The Macmillan Company, New York, 1954, p. 226.

was to organize on a unit basis sufficient to develop and maintain a health unit with adequate direction, supervision, and staffing. In New York State, counties were considered the base for adequate support. To that end the nursing plans were made with a *generalized* public health nursing service the goal. We had a very good staff. That's one thing I have always been blessed with: working with really fine medical men and nurses. So again, it's a combination of factors that makes for success. Nursing attitudes and perspectives in the *total* scheme are basic, but nursing leadership cannot think in terms of nursing alone.

Several progressive plans were envisaged to improve currently employed nurses. We started with a correspondence course under the aegis of New York University. I think the university gave, as a bonus or an attraction, two credits to anyone who completed the course. A great many enrolled, but relatively few finished the correspondence course; evidently there weren't enough who were self-motivated to do the work at home, and it was unfamiliar material. We then reorganized the course and selected from the nursing agencies of New York State the best-prepared supervisors. We recruited the supervisors who would undertake leading a group in many communities for three days, once a month, based upon homework given out by the university, and again New York University gave some credit. We had several hundred nurses enrolled before we finished. It became the thing to do. I think the difference between the nonsuccess of the correspondence course and the success of this was that the nurses who enrolled came together every month. It was almost like Alcholics Anonymous. They motivated each other, and the leaders of the group were well prepared.

GS: Peer group stimulation?

MS: Yes, peer group stimulation; that was exactly the reaction. And of those who started, practically everyone finished.

We kept that up for several years with growing sophistication in subject matter. Nurses really began to understand what their jobs were. In the meantime, selected nurses were given scholarships to get the formal preparation to progress. This was a long-range plan, of many years.

GS: Did they have to pay for this correspondence course themselves?

MS: That may have been another important factor, I think. The fee was a nominal sum; I don't remember the amount, but there was an enrollment fee. And I presume the university based that enrollment fee on whatever it cost for two credits. It was a very small motivation, in one way, to finish the course, but it was enough anyway.

One factor in the nurses' response was, I think, that we started where they were. The state had no control to dismiss them, even when we wished to, so we started where they were. Just as the correspondence course failed, then some other method was tried.

After a period, promotion and new appointments depended upon at least four months in an approved public health nursing program as a start, and a commitment for another four months in a year or so. The use of scholarship money helped a great deal.

Some people criticized the course, I'm sure, thinking it wasn't of college level. Well, it wasn't of college level, but it was at the level that most of the nurses who took it were when we started. Many of the employed public health nurses at that time were married women; they had commitments, and the plan allowed them to do some studying to improve themselves and to stay home. And then—it was rather interesting—once they became motivated to get more and more formal preparation, many accepted scholarships. I think it was because they began to get satisfaction out of their jobs. It was amazing how they began to make plans, and it wasn't too hard: we had a list five years ahead of those nurses who were going to take at least four months of college work. If they were going to take supervision, they had to take what was then the standard year of public health nursing.

The program to promote public health nursing on a county basis was a long-range plan, still in progress. Through Social Security funds we employed in the State Health Department a large number of public health nurses, many of whom had received preparation through the federal government nurse scholarship plan. These nurses were assigned to counties on a demonstration basis. Evaluation was carefully planned, based on how many counties actually carried on and supported the program after the terms of demonstration expired. The first plan did not bring results. A second plan was developed. It was successful. Counties did appropriate funds and carried on. I give credit to citizen committees who were part of the plan to bring to bear influence as they were convinced of the value of the service. In most instances the demonstration nurses became permanently employed.

GS: Did you go back to school?

MS: I never received an earned degree. I just took extra courses here and there, including a week-a-month year-long course in public administration given by the School of Public Administration at Syracuse University. At the time I started, in 1918, Minnesota was the only school that had a course.

I think, in retrospect, I was promoted too fast. My predecessor, Mathilde Kuhlman, died suddenly at age fifty-seven in 1932. Had she lived her normal span, I feel certain that with the impetus of the Social Security movement in 1937, I would have been the first recipient of a scholarship and a mandate to get formal preparation. I can say for myself that I was a student without benefit of formal guidance.

GS: Would you please mention what you consider to be your main contributions to nursing?

MS: Remember, I started my public health nursing work, which has been most of my nursing experience, when there were very few prepared people. That was way back before 1918 or 1920, so that my contribution would be entirely different if I were entering nursing even within the last twenty years. I think, as I look back, my contribution was to be absolutely convinced that nursing was an important part of the whole health team. I think I have always tried to establish nursing in that context in relation to the medical men with whom I have worked. Maybe all my life my major idea was to start where we were at any given point. At the time I entered nursing, for instance, there were very few—in fact there were no—"prepared" nurses in the formal sense. The most important thing was to get nurses prepared so that they could make their contribution and really be accepted as coequal with the medical men of the time and with the other people in the field of public health. As I say, on a coequal basis; but in order to be coequal they had to be prepared.

An important objective of the New York State Department of Health, to which the nursing division gave leadership, was a long-range plan to promote county health departments of comprehensive health service to serve all of New York State. The nursing division did its full share while directing its special responsibility in nursing.[4]

GS: Could you comment on your becoming the President of the American Public Health Association in 1961?

MS: Yes. It was, of course, a great satisfaction and an honor to be nominated to become the President of the A.P.H.A., for two reasons. I had great respect for that association, and worked very closely with its committees and with its executive director, and I thought it was an honor for nursing, too, to have a nurse selected.

The time had come when others in the health profession had to be

---

[4] During her career, Marion Sheahan was active in the study of the nursing organizations; she was on the National Nursing Council for War Service, which highlighted the clumsiness that resulted—in terms of effective, concerted action—when six national nursing organizations were involved in a critical period nationally. She became the Director of the National Committee for the Improvement of Nursing Services, which was, in essence, a mini-national league for nursing. Nurses and nonnurses worked together to solve some of the crucial problems. This committee organized and conducted the study of schools of nursing that led to the accreditation program of the N.L.N. An interim Joint Committee for the Accreditation of Schools of Nursing was a step along the way, with Helen Nahm as its able Director. After the N.L.N. was organized, Marion Sheahan became the Deputy Director, serving until her retirement from active nursing.

recognized by an association like the A.P.H.A. It represented all of the disciplines in the public health field. I think timing is a factor in many events. The time was ripe and I was there, and I was nominated. Again I repeat, if the timing is right and you happen to be in the spot and you seem to be the right person at the right time, some surprising things happen. I'm not saying that I hadn't earned a reputation of having a head on my shoulders, or of ever hesitating to speak up when I thought speaking up was appropriate, so that I'm sure I wasn't nominated because I would be a silent president. Anyone who knew me knew that that wasn't the case. I think I knew my full role in nursing and as a member of a broader team—health professionals.

GS: *How long is the presidency term?*

MS: One year is the pattern.

On President Truman's Health Commission⁵

I'm now reading *Plain Speaking,* Merle Miller's book on President Truman, and I would agree, as I read it, on President Truman's integrity. I recall some of his conversations with us in the White House rose garden and around the table, when we would report our progress to him. I remember very clearly his commitment to us not to make this a political commission; he wanted a good report. I remember at one of the meetings he said, "Of course I would like to have this report published before I leave office. But," he said, "I don't want it published prematurely at the expense of a good report that will stand the test of time." The report wasn't published before he left office, and it really never made its impact for political reasons. I believe it was a very good report. It was called "The Truman Health Commission Report." It was published when Dwight Eisenhower became President. I have been told that it was taken off the governmental shelves. In other words, it was assumed that since it was President Truman's Commission, it didn't represent President Eisenhower's philosophy. I believe the report is as sound today as it was when it was published.

GS: *What were the findings?*

⁵ In 1952 President Truman appointed a commission of fifteen persons to investigate the health requirements of the United States and to report within the year. Marion W. Sheahan was the only nurse on the commission.

MS: It was largely the reorganization of medical and group practice, and with more emphasis on preventive medicine. There was one chapter on nursing. My role there was as a member of the commission in general and in particular representing nursing in the total. I wrote the material that had to do with nursing, presented the facts, and so on.

GS: Could you please tell me what you thought of President Truman, since you had the opportunity to meet him?

MS: I thought he was a very down-to-earth kind of a man, and I particularly admired his statement to us at the meetings about our commitment. He was unpretentious and easy to meet, and gave me confidence in his national leadership ability.

GS: What was the next Commission that you served on?

MS: It was the National Commission on the Health Care of the Nation, and that was foundation-supported. (The Truman Commission was government-supported.) The National Commission on the Health Care of the Nation was quite a few years after the Truman report. This Commission was financed from nongovernmental sources.

GS: How did you get on the commission? Who appointed you?

MS: I don't know.

GS: Did you get a letter asking you to become a member?

MS: A letter came from the chairman; he was Marion Folsom of Eastman Kodak Company. The members were representative of professional, business, and lay interests. I was instrumental in getting a social worker added as the work got under way. I have great regard for social workers if they know their jobs, just as I have for public health nurses if they know their jobs.

The modus operandi was interesting. The group was divided into committees to work on initial presentations to come up at the next meetings. Let me tell you how we worked. The work committees could invite consultants as they saw fit. We could be sent off to various places to work for about two days to thrash out concepts, and so on. I think there were about eight or ten work committees of that kind. And then in the final analysis, when the final discussions were over, we were divided into work groups to review the material that would be included in the final report. We had very good staff workers at the committee's disposal.

In the interim the separate reports would go to the expert in the area under review, and he or she would write a critique. For instance, Dr.

Crosby was the hospital specialist, and everything that pertained to that went to Dr. Crosby. He sent in his critique. Everything that had to do with nursing came to me, and I sent in my critique. Also, all members got all reports.

The subcommittees to review the whole worked separately for about three days. Then the whole group got together to agree or disagree on the content that went into the final report. The result was truly a "committee report."

GS: Is there anything that you want to add about your work on this or any other commission?

MS: No, except to comment that the National Commission on the Health Care of the Nation was organized in such a way that every single member of that Commission singly worked in all subcommittees and as a whole group in an interesting organizational pattern. If there was ever a report that expressed the thinking of a group, it was this particular commission's report.

GS: Of all the committees and commissions you've been active on, which one did you enjoy the most?

MS: I enjoyed the Truman committee, maybe because I admired President Truman and it was my first such experience, and I was proud of the report. I was glad I was a part of it. I endorsed it, and still do. I enjoyed the real workouts of the National Commission on the Health Care of the Nation because I liked the method. The recommendations in both commission reports are supportive of each other. They both deserve study. It will be many years before their recommendations are implemented.

I came to the National Committee for the Improvement of Nursing Services (N.C.I.N.S.) with only a year's commitment. I had recruited Anna Fillmore when I was President of the N.O.P.H.N., to become the director. She wrote me at the School of Public Health in Berkeley: "You recruited me for the directorship of N.O.P.H.N.; now I'm recruiting you to become the Director of the N.C.I.N.S." It was an interprofessional committee with nonnurses and other professionals who were interested in nursing as a whole. We worked for three years before the N.L.N. was organized and the N.O.P.H.N. was abolished. If something appeals to what you have in your mind and there's an opportunity to help, I guess I feel the urge to keep on. I stayed on the job.

When the N.L.N. came into being, Anna Fillmore became the Director. I became her assistant. I was with the N.L.N. until I retired in 1962. I went for one year but stayed on and on and on. (In fact, I never joined the pension system of the League because I never expected to be there that long.)

I think that what the League has accomplished nationally is good. It has not been successful in developing dynamic local links. There are reasons for it, but I think that nationally it certainly has done a good job. I don't think the American Nurses' Association (A.N.A.) could have established the comprehensive accreditation of schools which the League has accomplished. I don't think the A.N.A. would have sought the number and variety of nonnurses who have really become influential in helping to improve nursing. I think the professional nursing organization now is broader in respect to its interprofessional relationships and in its interpretations of aims in terms of society's needs.

GS: *Is there anything else you care to add about your work with the League?*

MS: Nothing, except that it was a very gratifying experience. We had very understanding nonnurses who, from their own points of view, contributed a great deal. If one looked over the roster of the committee members who were nonnurses, as well as members of the board of directors, the evidence would speak for itself. When anyone who thinks that outstanding nonnurses aren't interested in nursing, they should note the roster of the N.L.N., the N.C.I.N.S., or the commissions I served on. Nursing was never slighted. After all, each of us has two major competences: we are first of all citizens with social concepts in general; and then there is our special competence as a nurse or a physician or whatnot. Our citizen's role is as broad and effective as each of us makes it; our nurse's role is a more circumscribed, single part in a corps of related health professionals.

Major Issues in Nursing

GS: *What do you see as major issues today that nursing has to take a certain leadership in?*

MS: I think that nurses should recognize the imminence of an entire change in the organization for health care. Nurses have to be prepared to take their part in the change that's coming, organizationwise and socially. There are too few of our group who really have a concept of where we are going and how we are moving. In my early days we moved relatively slowly toward any social change, but in the last, well, say fifteen or twenty years, there has been an enormous change in people's concept of what is due to them. We are not a passive society. We no longer have a complacent labor group. We no longer have a complacent group of patients. The population is beginning to demand what relatively few of us are willing to face up to. Not every young nurse will have a college education, but that doesn't stop them from keeping abreast of the times and trying to see their role in terms of social development as well as patient care.

GS: Do you think that leadership, as it relates to nursing, can be taught?

MS: I think that there are personalities that lend themselves to being willing to take responsibility, and that's the essence of leadership—not only deciding what to do and having commitments to certain objectives. Sometimes the leadership is in the wrong cause. We have a good many illustrations of that. But I think all leadership is the willingness to be committed and take responsibility for the mistakes you make as well as the successes you have. It is good that a substantial amount of health leadership is for the good. Important, too, is the ability to interpret your concepts and goals to the end nursing leadership is accepted on a coequal basis with other components in agency and community affairs.

GS: How would you describe your own personality?

MS: I don't know. I have ideas. I think I have always been willing to listen to other people even though I don't agree with them or have very little respect for what they have to say. And I think I always did face up to any responsibility I had. I was willing to face up to my mistakes. I always read a great deal of socially oriented material, and material from other professional fields.

GS: Would you say, then, that you were thrust into your leadership positions and roles, rather than actively seeking them?

MS: Yes, I am certain of that. I was thrust into becoming the Director of Public Health Nursing of the State Health Department because of the early death of Mathilde Kuhlman. Dr. Parran sent me a wire to say I was being appointed provisional director. We were under civil service in New York State. I feel certain I would have taken the time off and I would have gone to school to receive formal preparation. But I was thrust into a position of responsibility, first as assistant and then as Director, and I took it. Dr. Parran expected me to take the job, and he was a convincing man.

GS: You obviously succeeded in your job.

MS: I think so. With all modesty I have to say that. The program was never static, and I made friends over the years. Nursing was considered coequal in planning, in general, with the other divisions.

GS: *What would you say you considered to have been some of your biggest decisions that you had to make?*

MS: I think the decisions were to decide to take whatever opportunity presented itself that interested me.

GS: *What would you say was your biggest frustration?*

MS: Not moving fast enough.

GS: *For nursing or for yourself?*

MS: No, not for myself. I never had any feeling that I should go beyond where I was, but one of my regrets was that I didn't follow the orthodox pattern of getting professionally prepared. That probably was a frustation of my own making. With all due respect to myself, I feel I am reasonably well educated with degrees to document it.

GS: *What is your opinion of the advocates of the concepts of physician's assistant and nurse-practitioner?*

MS: Well, as I understand the physician's assistants, they are helpers to physicians in more or less the type of activities that interns have done in the years gone by. They would be employees of physicians. In other words, they would be obligated to follow the rules and regulations and the kind of medical practice that their employer follows. Now nurses, by and large, will be employed by agencies. I have been interested in the—I don't think it's a movement yet—but in the experiments that a few, certainly brave, nurses have started in developing their own practice in nursing, which I think is a very interesting concept. But even in back of their practice there must be a physician who has the broader knowledge of diagnosis. But I can see the role of the nurse in doing a lot of screening, particularly in the home, and in certain clinic services, and in making what Ruth Freeman calls "null diagnoses"—just as we did during the war when so much screening was done by nurses. Then I visited all day long, seeing families that reported flu; took their temperatures; used my judgment as to whether to give the usual prescription or whether to decide to refer them to a physician. Well, I can see the newer role of more independent nurses—but I still do not dissociate nursing from the broader aspects of medical diagnosis and medical prescription. I am rather intrigued, too, by what is happening in professional nursing: What a basic education for nursing with a modern college course can give, as compared with the average diploma program. I can see the reason for a growing group of nurses with that kind of background becoming specialists. I think, with medicine going as it is, and with the short hospital stay of even seriously ill patients, that the specialist nurse is going, in the future, to be a very important part of health care. Public health nurses for many years have carried a major role in "null diagnoses," to quote Ruth Freeman.

GS: Do you see that as the major trend now?

MS: Yes. Louise McManus first suggested a change of title of the professionally trained nurse to nurse-therapist. I believe what she was thinking of is the nurse-specialist, well prepared for her role. She was really trying to differentiate the nurse who was going to be well prepared for responsibility, independent judgment, and so forth.

GS: What is your opinion of those who advocate that the word "nurse" is obsolete?

MS: Well, I don't think a change in name is going to do any good. "Doctor" means a great many things. People doctor themselves. There are all kinds of doctorates floating around. So I see nothing wrong in keeping the word that has meant so much through the centuries. Because nursing means "care," and I see nothing wrong in the nurse who is the prepared, caring type of person, versus the amateur. If nurses really live up to their obligations as a professional group of people who have preparation for general or special care of patients, I do not reject the word "nurse."

GS: If you had to name the biggest one issue in nursing today, what would you say that it is now?

MS: I think it is the failure to speed up the preparation of nurses so that they can take their place in the emerging new concept of medical care in the country, which is certainly based on maintenance of health. A speedup in the nurse-specialist group is surely indicated.

GS: Now when you say "speedup," just what exactly do you mean?

MS: I mean having enough nurses who are prepared to take their part in the emerging pattern of health organization.

GS: Do you see nursing education, then, as being in the junior colleges or the colleges?

MS: I think in both, because there is a place for a level of nursing to work in relation to professional nursing, comparable with physicians' assistants to physicians. And I don't think it makes any difference whether the nursing profession as it is now continues to call itself "nurse" or not. The skills will be needed. Someone is going to be needed who is going to take the role, as I see it, of the nurse today who is the prepared nurse, capable of growing as society moves along. Specialization means supervision and administration and education, as well as nurse specializing in hospital, office, or the community.

GS: How has public health nursing changed over the years since you first started in it?

MS: Well, way back at Henry Street, it started with the kind of nursing that was important at that time. Many, many children with pneumonia had mustard paste to the chest, hot mustard foot baths, and pneumonia jackets, and were desperately ill. Antibiotics changed the character of treatment. Now community nursing, as it is called, has really developed to care of family needs. Prevention is the keynote. The public health nursing agencies are community nursing services now, with health teaching a service. Visiting nursing agencies are becoming home health care agencies. They are beginning truly to meet family needs, and I believe will still further expand service beyond nursing. Some former visiting nurse agencies have changed their title to Home Care, employing physical therapists to round out nursing care. Now most of these agencies have nursing direction because nursing has the experience, and I think it's to the credit of the nurse directors that they have seen the necessity for branching out and perhaps losing their identity as a nursing agency only.

GS: What are your ingredients, or what advice would give on how to be a successful administrator? What skills, talents, training, or whatever?

MS: A good basic education for nursing is needed and that, before too long, will be a college-oriented program. Specialization of any kind, I believe, will be at a master's level. For certain positions, such as in educational institutions, a doctoral degree is already the requirement. The direction is already charted.

Leadership positions above all must accept responsibility. Persons holding them must be abreast of not only the agency but also the general societal changes. They must be positive enough to spearhead action and to take responsibility for failures as well as successes. They must be able to attract qualified staff. They must be able interpreters of their plans and developmental needs. They must be able to follow as well as lead.

GS: Well, in addition to the so-called orthodox, formal educational preparation, what other talents or skills do you view as necessary for a successful administrator?

MS: I don't know how anyone can teach personal relationships as such. I think you get that from the time you are born and through experiences in life, but there are some concepts of human behavior, sociological and anthropological concepts, that are important to understanding human development and in understanding the different cultures we deal with in today's society.

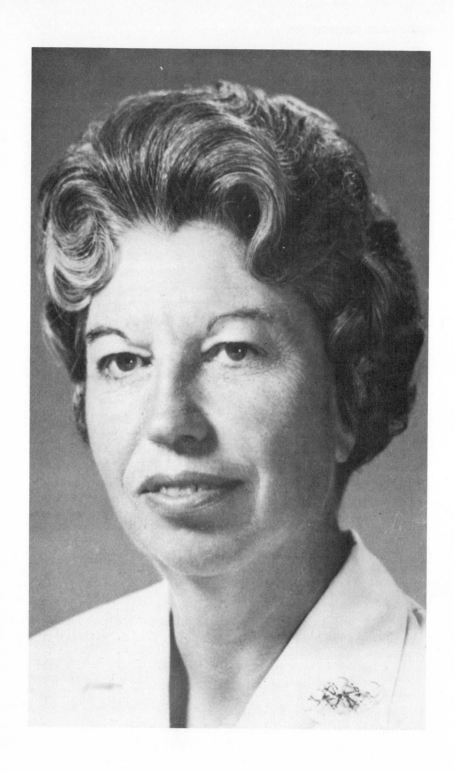

17

After my name I think I just like to be recognized as "nurse" because really in many ways that's what I've been. My whole life I've felt that it was a privilege and an honor to be a nurse, and the fact that I was a nurse brought me all the goodies and the advantages and satisfactions that work could bring. When I say "nurse," I mean it in the fullest sense of the word, with patients. That's what I think makes me a little different than a lot of other people in nursing, that I found plenty in nursing to satisfy and stimulate my intellect because I think there are still so many unanswered questions. So I just like nurse. Not R.N. (registered nurse) necessarily, but *nurse*.[1]

[1] Interview with Dorothy Smith, Gainesville, Fla., May 5, 1974.

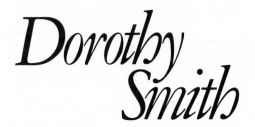

Dorothy Smith

NURSE

*D*orothy Smith has vigorously emphasized the necessity of combining nursing education and nursing practice. She was one of the first nurse educators to say that the faculty, even the Dean herself, should be involved in nursing service.

Dorothy Smith was born in Bangor, Maine, in 1913, the oldest of three children. Her parents had little money, and growing up during the Depression was a struggle.

When I graduated from high school in February, I still didn't know what I was going to do, but my best friend went into nursing, and I thought, well, why not? You could make a living at it, and that's why I was really interested in it at that time, since I didn't know what else I could do.

She received her registered nurse diploma from Quincy City Hospital School of Nursing in 1936. "I enjoyed nurses' training," she says, "and never felt exploited."

She earned a B.S. degree in nursing education in 1941 from Teachers College, Columbia, where "I had a fantastic experience with a host of fantastic women (Isabel Stewart, Maude Muse, Virginia Henderson) who really killed themselves to get good courses for nurses." In 1947 she received a master's degree in personnel and guidance from Harvard University, where she had gone initially to study student organization.

Among her many positions,[2] two serve as examples of her leadership: Assistant Dean at Duke University (1947–1952) and Dean and Professor of Nursing at the College of Nursing, University of Florida, Gainesville (1956–1971), until she retired.

Dorothy Smith has published extensively. Her articles, particularly from 1963 to 1971,[3] discuss a clinical process that she felt was missing from nursing practice: collecting data, establishing of objectives based on some kind of a diagnosis, and then carefully monitoring whatever treatment is devised to handle the problem.

She has been active in professional organizations and committees and has received various honors and awards.[4]

---

[2] Staff nurse (1936–1937) and head nurse (1937–1939), Quincy City Hospital; science instructor and Assistant Educational Director (1942–1945) and Educational Director and Science Instructor (1945–1947), Quincy City Hospital School of Nursing; consultant (1952–1954), National League for Nursing, Division of Nursing Education, New York City.

[3] "From Student to Nurse," *Nursing Outlook*, 11(10): 735–736, October 1963; "Myth and Method in Nursing Practice," *American Journal of Nursing*, 64(2): 68–72, February 1964; "A Clinical Nursing Tool," *American Journal of Nursing*, 68(11): 2384–2388, November 1968; "Is It Too Late?" *Nursing Clinics of North America*, June 1971.

[4] Nursing Leadership Award, Florida Nurses' Association, 1970; honorary doctor of science degree, University of Rochester, 1972; Teacher of the Year Award, University of Florida, 1973.

Duke University

GS: When and why did you go to Duke?

DS: I went to Duke in 1948. I was thirty-five. I decided I had to leave home—literally—Quincy Hospital as well as my own home. So I went to Duke. Up to that time I really didn't have any . . . well, I had some ideas about teaching. One of the things that bothered me was that nursing courses pretty much consisted of medicine plus a few lectures on watering and feeding and diapering the patients. The doctors were giving all the lectures or it was mostly medical textbook stuff. I felt that if there was anything to nursing, we better find out what it was. If there was something to nursing that was different from medicine, that we really ought to find out what it was. I also realized that my training wasn't too bad, but during World War II and the advent of the Cadet Corps I saw the diploma program—I'm not saying it was good from an educational standpoint, but my own personal training wasn't all that bad—I saw the diploma program deteriorate to nothing, literally nothing. My teachers were working with patients. After World War II nobody seemed to want to work with patients. The people who came back from the Army wanted to go to school because of social and economic rewards. Nursing was hard and paid poorly.

GS: What was the reason you went to Duke rather than somewhere else?

DS: I guess it was because I wanted to get into a university program. I felt by this time that diploma programs were wrong and that nurses should be educated like everybody else in educational institutions. At Duke I met Helen Nahm, and she encouraged me a lot.

I almost didn't take the job at Duke when I saw two water fountains side by side, one for whites and one for blacks. The whole thing was absolutely repulsive to me, and I had my problems at Duke because they wouldn't let me call any black person by their last name. You couldn't say Miss or Mr. or Mrs. anything. I said, "Okay, I'm going to do it; you can fire me," and they didn't fire me. It was an educational experience. The other thing I found out at Duke was that here was this big university, well known, good, and a nursing school plunk in the middle of it, and there was absolutely no control of the nursing school by the university. There seemed to be no relationship between the university and the School of Nursing. The School of Nursing was in the Medical Center and it went its own way, and uneducational things went on in that nursing school.

GS: Such as?

DS: Such as students working in the operating room for months on end because they needed them. It was even worse than my diploma program. And it was called a university program. And then Helen Nahm and I really worked hard trying to get it to be a real university school, and I found out then that many people didn't believe that nurses needed education. It was a real rough time. Eventually it did become an honest-to-goodness university program and it was probably due to the work that Helen Nahm and I did; although we both left before it happened. I also learned the necessity of deans of nursing schools and medical schools to communicate with one another. I had some great students at Duke. I probably had some of the best students I have seen in my whole life. And it really bothered me to see these bright women come there and get such a water-bed kind of programming; because really all that many people wanted them for was to run Duke Hospital. That's exploitation. That was really pretty bad, and actually it was pretty much the same situation all over the country, as portrayed in Esther Lucile Brown's book.[5] That book and Dr. Brown had much influence on me.

I deliberately went to Duke as an Assistant Dean of Nursing Education, and I stayed there to definitely take leadership in trying to make an honest-to-goodness university program. I didn't think of myself as a leader. But I knew the job had some authority, and I thought it was high time I moved on to a place where I had some authority to do anything about it. I think I've always been a leader, in a way. Either chosen or, you know, because I stood out in some ways, in height and partly brains.

I resented leadership sometimes because I've got big holes in me from never having been a child or an adolescent; I have big gaps. So I said, "Why can't they get somebody else?" But that's the way it was. Anyway, at Duke I thought it was high time we did something about nursing. Now you have to remember that all this time, no matter what job I had, I was always on my own, working with patients.

GS: For what reason?

DS: Because of my curiosity. Because I couldn't understand why it was that we couldn't teach nursing students what was real, and the only way I could think of to do this was to keep getting more data myself. Now I do have a thing in me that will always be for underdogs— rejected, sad, miserable, lonely people—because I have had those ex-

---

[5] Esther Lucile Brown, *Nursing for the Future,* The Russell Sage Foundation, New York, 1948.

periences myself. But over and beyond the emotional factor there was a big intellectual factor because I got tired of people answering a question with, "Oh, we can't help you; you'll have to find that out from experience." I thought there ought to be a better way than just from trial and error and from experience. There ought to be some data somehow so you could tell students that if this and this occurs, the probability is that this will occur. But all I ever got was, "Well, I really don't know. I do it this way; you just have to learn it from experience," which I thought was pretty wasteful. So then I went to Duke, and I saw that a nursing school could be in a university and it could still be lacking in data for nursing care.

GS: That must have been a disillusionment to you.

DS: Well, it was a shock. I don't know if it was disillusionment. It was a challenge. [*laughter*] And Helen Nahm was there, and we had great students, and, as I said, I learned. I talked to all the people in the science departments on campus and all the people in the medical school, and I could see how little respect was given to nursing. I guess I had my first conscious evidence of male chauvinism. Now I'm sure I'd experienced it before, but this was the first time I'd been aware of it, and it was really an experience! But I also learned that nurses had power too—to do or not do for patients—and that nursing without data and records was intuitive and not scientific.

GS: Did you ever at all consider during this period of time that you might have more power, and ultimately were bright enough to go to medical school and become a physician?

DS: I didn't want to be a doctor. No way! I didn't want to make the decisions they did. I really thought that nursing had something creative and required intelligence and the use of everything you had if there could be a place for us to use it, and if . . . you see, my greatest difficulties have not been with doctors but with nurses.

GS: Why is that?

DS: I don't know why. I don't have any idea why, but most people who go into nursing, unless they're bright—in which case they to into education or administration—seem to be people who want the routine, technical side of nursing. And so they don't want anybody like me coming along and saying, "Look, I want you to interview patients and make a problem list and write this on the chart."

GS: Why did you leave Duke?

DS: I was in an intense situation at Duke, trying to push a real university program with a degree, and hassling with almost everybody because I was too impatient; and Helen Nahm left, and things just closed in about 1951.[6]

In Florida: Dean of College of Nursing, University of Florida, Gainesville, 1956–1971

GS: What took you to Florida—to become a dean?

DS: Somebody had given my name to the University of Florida. They were opening up a new nursing program, a new medical school, and a new health center, and so they wrote me and asked me if I would be interested in the dean's job. I wrote back, "No, thank you very much." And they wrote and said, "Please come and let us try to persuade you." And so I wrote back and said, "No, I don't want your job, but I am interested in getting to Miami and I have no money, so if you want to take your chances and pay my way down I'll stop in Gainesville." So I did, and I was very intrigued. There was a very small group there because, you see, we didn't take in our first students, medical or nursing, until 1956. This was in October of 1955. And there was nothing except Quonset huts; there were no buildings, although one was under construction.

GS: Why did you take the job, as you evidently did?

DS: The more I thought about it, the more I realized that I had some very definite ideas that I had gotten from being at Duke and from being at Hartford and from being at the National Nursing Accrediting Service (N.N.A.S.). I thought things were terribly wrong and that I could go along the rest of my life saying how wrong everybody was and nobody would let me try things, and so forth, and so on, or I could put my hat in the ring and become the authority figure, and try these ideas in a brand-new setting where they probably had more hope of succeeding if they were ever going to succeed anyway. And so I thought about it, and I talked with a good friend, and he thought I could do anything I wanted to do anyway. He was kind of disappointed I wasn't coming to Miami, but he agreed with me that it was probably time for me to become the boss and see what I could do. Sort of growing-up phase. But he agreed

---

[6] Dorothy Smith became a consultant, National League for Nursing, 1952–1954; and Assistant Director in Nursing, Hartford Hospital, Hartford, Connecticut, 1954–1956.

with me also that I would hate the protocol and the fuss that go with it, which I did. Also, the group who would be working with me seemed to want a health center, not a medical center. The Provost (or Vice President for Health Affairs) was a nonmedical man, which also influenced me.

One of the things that we sort of said before I took the job was that I would have some say in the kind of nursing that went on in the hospital, because I didn't think it was right to teach our students something they never saw in a hospital; I thought that was just a waste of time. There were one or two things that I really fought for. One was that I wanted practice privileges for the faculty. I didn't know if the faculty would take great advantage of those privileges, but I wanted that. The only way I could get practice privileges for faculty was to organize us as medicine was organized. That was that the Dean of Medicine was in charge of medical practice in that hospital. And so, if I were to get faculty practice privileges, I had to become Chief of Nursing Service, as George was Chief of Medical Service. Now that didn't bother me, because I knew that I could handle it; but what bothered me was that throughout the country, people were very critical. I wanted faculty practice privileges, and if you want privileges you have to take on accountability and responsibility. This got to be a big thing across the country—which I tried to explain, but nobody really listened. The other thing was that I had gone around enough to see that the highest-paid people in nursing service rarely did anything with patients. There were all kinds of head nurses and supervisors and assistant supervisors. This wasn't true in physical therapy or medicine; it wasn't true in anything but nursing and in hospital administration, of which nursing was sort of a part. So we did a study of what some of these people did, and gradually they could see what I was talking about.

We met about our hospital as soon as I came in—the dean of the medical school, a pharmacist, a microbiologist (who was here already), a photographer, a hospital administrator, a secretary, and maybe about ten other people who were there early. And we set down everything patients ought to have in our hospital. I maintained, and medicine maintained, that unless you have the kind of practice in the hospital that you want students to emulate, the whole business is a farce. So they agreed about that with medicine, but they never thought about it in nursing. I was there to make them think about it. So we set down everything we wanted patients to have, from clean floors to warm, loving handshakes, and then we said: Okay, who should do these things? Well, there was a long list of stuff that everybody said nursing should do, and I said, "No way. That's not nursing; that's secretarial or dietary or something." "Well, why isn't it nursing?" I said, "Because I'm not going to teach the students how to do those things.'' Well, that was the only thing that made sense to them. They didn't agree with me, but if I wasn't going to teach the students how to do it, then I got away with it on an education-al principle. That was what started the whole business of unit manag-ers, which we really started, although it had been tried about ten years previously; but it had failed, and it had failed in my opinion because it had been put under nursing service instead of under the hospital. So we started unit managers and put it under hospital administration. I believe in decentralization, so we tried to set up a decentralized hospital with the nurse on a unit having the authority as well as the responsibil-ity, together with the medical resident; but hospital administration was never willing to give up authority to the unit manager. The other thing was that some wanted the hospital administrator *not* to be on the Health Center Council. And I insisted that the hospital administrator had to have the same status on the Health Center Council as the deans, be-cause I didn't want him to be under medicine or under anybody; it just wouldn't work that way. We had students who had been waiting two years or three years to get this thing opened, so we had no trouble getting students. And I was very lucky with faculty because I was able to get, right off the bat, some of the best. We started out with a group of people who all—not that we agreed about everything—pretty much had the same goals in mind: to try to orgainze in such a way that nursing service and nursing education wouldn't be hassling; to be pa-tient-centered, rather than curriculum-centered; to work cooperatively with other disciplines and not go off into the wild blue yonder, you know, trying to do something that we couldn't possibly do.

GS: *What do you consider your biggest contribution?*

DS: At Florida, we did devise a tool for collecting data from the pa-tient, which is a very practical tool and which does give us data from which we can make a problem list and devise methods of solving the problems, the writing of progress notes, and so forth. This is probably our biggest contribution. The book describing this process was pub-lished in 1975.[7] However, it does, if one accepts this, call for an entirely different kind of teaching; and it does mean that the students need to see somebody doing it, either faculty or nursing staff, and of course preferably nursing staff. One of the problems of nursing is that we teach these things, but students see nurses using skills on work that the nurs-es are overtrained for, or actually overeducated for. I had a call from a former student the other day, and she said she was working as a night

---

[7] Eileen Pearlman Becknell and Dorothy M. Smith, *A System of Nursing Practice*, F. A. Davis Company, Philadelphia, 1975.

nurse on a surgical floor, and she left her brains at the door when she went on duty because all she really was, was a technician. That's all she had time to be, and that's all that was expected of her. She is staying in that job because there are other values outside of her job that are important to her. But you multiply this very intelligent woman by the thousands, and you can see perhaps why nursing is, to me, in a bad way. As I say, we did develop the process; we did teach the process to our students; we tried to teach more around patients. We didn't neglect the sciences because you can't even diagnose the problems, or certainly devise ways of solving the problems, unless you have some scientific basis.

We also pushed very strongly that baccalaureate education needed to be different in terms of knowledge and skill from diploma or junior college education—not better or worse, but different.

GS: What has been a big decision for you?

DS: One of the things that I think that I should make clear is that most of my decisions, in terms of jobs, have been made on the basis of my own learning. Almost by accident I found myself at Florida as Dean, with the opportunity to test out these ideas that I'd had for some time. The reason we spent so much time in the early days on establishing practice privileges in the hospital was because I felt that in order to find out what skills were necessary that patients were not then getting, one needed to work with patients. Practice privileges for nursing faculty had never been established in as clear-cut a way as they have for medical practitioners, so that my decision to take on the hospital nursing service had nothing to do with the fact that I thought I could run it better than nursing service directors. It was to enable us to get to patients in a way that we could never have done otherwise. For some time at Florida, because of that decision, nursing service personnel and nursing education personnel were working very closely together. The students did not see the usual hassle. Frankly, it was most difficult to find nursing service directors who approved of this way of operating. It almost seemed that they wanted the separation. Physicians approved until we became short of staff. Hospital administration did not approve. So one of the things we found out was that although everybody had been talking for years about nursing faculty being more involved with patients and patient care, when we provided this, hospital administration and nursing service administration, and, eventually, physicians weren't so sure that it was a good idea. You see, my notion of patient care was that there were different kinds of skills and patient techniques that were needed to give a patient total nursing care, and that one should provide for these different skills and techniques. Hospital administration, nursing service directors, and physicians felt that one was only patient-oriented when one carried out essentially the medical orders in an efficient way and kept the place neat and tidy; so that, although I am very patient-oriented, sometimes I had the reputation of not being patient-oriented because, for example, I would not allow the students to be exploited for nursing assistants' work, except in a great emergency.

GS: What changes did you introduce?

DS: The change we tried to implement was to introduce a clinical role in nursing service that would carry out the process I talked about earlier. That is, getting data from the patient, getting a problem list, getting methods to solve the problem, writing progress notes, and so forth, and evaluating. We also tried to have unit managers do most of the non-nursing, clerical work so that nurses would be free to nurse. I would say that for a period of four or five years we were fairly successful, although we hadn't developed the process to the extent that it's been developed today. I would say that between the years 1958 and 1964 we were pretty successful; we were really making progress. But then the whole thing began to deteriorate because of shortages of nurses in our area due to the opening of the Veterans Administration Hospital and due to our very low salaries. When the shortages began to occur, then hospital administration and physicians wanted to go back to the old bureaucratic system with floats and all the horrendous things that seemed not to work, although on the surface they work for the organization but they don't really work for the patient. So in the long run I would say that we probably were not successful in creating any significant change that was lasting. In the faculty group we tried to have faculty who were scholarly or who had a scholarly attitude, but had the scholarly attitude toward problems in nursing, which necessitated their working with patients, rather than a scholarly attitude toward some other discipline or toward administration. Again, I think we were very successful for about seven or eight years, but we were a small group and it was easy to keep all the channels of communication open. I think our students were turned on at that time but then, as we got larger, with more students and more faculty, and more problems in the hospital, and more problems in the County Health Department, again there was deterioration. I think that some of the students we graduated would never be happy teaching nursing if they weren't working with patients, and I think that's true of some of our faculty, so we did make some changes in individual people. I think also, because of the fact that I wrote a good bit and went around making speeches and did workshops, that probably we've had some effect on some schools and some agencies, and probably a good many individuals.

GS: What was a big conflict you faced as an administrator? And how did you resolve it?

DS: Probably one of the biggest conflicts that existed at Florida was between hospital administration and the College of Nursing. Hospital administration wanted the bureaucratic kind of nursing service, and of course we didn't. It got pretty nasty at times, but I tried to deal with issues rather than with personalities. If it was a conflict between other people—that is, students and faculty or faculty and faculty—then I would generally try to get both groups together or both people together. I tried not to get trapped by acting only on what one person said or what one group said, although sometimes it was difficult. I don't particularly like conflict for reasons, again, that I'm not going into; it goes back to my childhood, but because of my years of psychotherapy I learned to deal with it fairly well.

GS: Where, in your opinion, is nursing going?

DS: I can't make predictions without really being in the situation. If enough people can be found who are career-oriented, and they can be really motivated toward patients rather than something outside nursing, then I think great things could happen in nursing in ways that I can't even perhaps imagine now. I would say this, that to me patients, sick people, are not getting good care. I believe in prevention; I think a lot of things could happen in a community in the way of prevention. I think there will always be sick people, and, to me, if one gets good nursing care in the hospital today, it's accidental rather than planned. This saddens me. Of course this was what my whole work life has been about. The forces that operate against good nursing care are tremendously strong, and they include not only hospital administration and doctors; they include a tremendous number of nurses, who really don't want things to change. I think I underestimated the resistance; in fact, I know I did. And of course as we got larger, it was more difficult to get faculty who would really be involved with clinical studies or patients or whatever.

GS: What have you been doing since you retired?

DS: I left the dean's job because, again, I had learned all I could from being a Dean, or all that I wanted to. The job was becoming more politically oriented. People were fighting for money, and these were matters that I didn't really want to deal with. I decided to stay on for two years because I had a place to practice on a medical unit while at the same time teaching students, and I wanted some more patient data, frankly; so again it was for my own learning. At the end of two years, even though I was only sixty, I decided to retire early, again for my own learning, because I was in a rut. The hospital wasn't being subsidized properly; we didn't have equipment; there wasn't enough staff; there were too many students; everything was at sixes and sevens; the nursing service was becoming more bureaucratic by the minute; and there seemed to be very little evidence that anything would change in the near future. And so I decided to leave to study my own data that I had collected through the years and to see what I could come up with in terms of writing a book or writing articles. I also wanted to learn to play the piano. I wanted to learn more about the community because I had been pretty hospital-oriented, and so I wanted to learn about being a volunteer. And I've done all those things. We have one book to the publisher already, and we're assembling data now on the thousands of nursing histories that we have.

I think it's important, again, that every step I've taken has really been a selfish one in a sense, in that I have done it for my own learning, for my own intellectual stimulation. Once I have exploited a job so that it is no longer fun and a challenge, then I move on, regardless of whether it means moving to a different part of the country or taking a cut in salary or whatever. As far as what's going to happen to nursing, I don't really know. It may sound odd, but I'm not sure that I care to the extent that I used to. I intend to do something with my own data; I intend to see what can be done in the community. I will make a few speeches and perhaps act as a consultant on the basis of the data I have, but I have a trait of "letting go," and I can't make predictions without really being more involved. One of the things that I wish we had done when I first came to Florida was to build our program on top of a baccalaureate program. In other words, use the old Yale and Western Reserve models and give a master of nursing. The students would come in with a baccalaureate degree in something. Then I think that we might have turned out people who had enough career orientation as well as preparation to really change some things. I found that in the undergraduate program most of the students we had, by career orientation, belonged in technical programs. They really weren't career-motivated. You get a few. I think this is the most crucial thing in nursing: whether or not there are enough career-motivated people who, regardless of marriage or family or whatever, intend to keep on growing in nursing, not in something else but in nursing.

I'm not sure I belong in your book. I probably should say that I have done my duty in terms of nursing organizations and committee work; I was on every program committee for every organization in Massachusetts and North Carolina. When I came to Florida, I let most of that go because I just didn't have the time, and I thought it was only fair that younger people take over; and I never really did enjoy it. I was pretty good at it, but I didn't enjoy it. I did allow myself to be put on the board of the Florida Nurses' Association for a two-year period because it was very important that I be on it, but I didn't enjoy it. I've been on several national committees, but I don't feel that my contributions have been along those lines.

GS: *What then do you consider to be your greatest satisfactions in your nursing career?*

DS: This is a pretty hard question to answer. I think—and I'm not sure if these are in the order of priority, and I'm not sure there is any priority—certainly the students I've had, seeing how they developed intellectually and emotionally; and I got great satisfaction out of seeing them achieve. The same thing is true for faculty members that I worked with, particularly here at the University of Florida. Another great satisfaction has been the patients with whom I have worked. In some ways maybe that's been my greatest satisfaction in nursing, because I learned so much from them; and most of the questions that I've tried to find answers to came from the patients with whom I worked, so that I was stimulated intellectually by the patients. I also got a good bit of satisfaction out of working with the physicians, and caring for patients. Again, I got a good bit of intellectual stimulation from them. I think the development of the nursing history, and then the development of the entire process, which was mainly problem-centered, was also a source of great satisfaction to me. It was something that I worked on for about twenty years, and it's finally culminated in the book *A System of Nursing Practice.*

    I think nursing has been very good to me because, the way I pursued it at least, I was able to get both emotional and intellectual stimulation and satisfaction, which I very badly needed. As far as the satisfactions in my personal life are concerned, I think that being essentially a career woman, the fact that I was so happy with my chosen profession, certainly was a satisfaction in my personal life also. I always feel sorry for people who don't seem to like what they're doing.

18

Summary and Conclusions

This book has presented seventeen nursing leaders.[1] As of January 1976, all seventeen of the leaders were living; fourteen of the seventeen were retired, and three of the seventeen were close to retirement. The method of selection, the tool of oral history, and the boundaries and limitations of this book were discussed in the Introduction.

Background

With two exceptions, the women's fathers were not professional men; that is, they had not completed college and were not in professions such as medicine or law. The mothers had not been to college, and if the mothers worked outside the home, it was because they were widowed and had to work out of economic necessity. The women and their parents were all born in the United States. With the exception of one black,[2] Estelle Massey Osborne, no minorities are represented.

Choosing Nursing

The women entered nursing essentially for one of three dominant reasons: altruistic-humanistic—they wanted to help people; economic—nursing was a poor woman's way to get an education, and they could always find a job; and "rerouting"—that is, the women may have wanted to go into medicine or science, but were actively discouraged and

[1] Some of this chapter appeared in Gwendolyn Safier, "I Sensed the Challenges: Leaders among Contemporary U.S. Nurses," *The Oral History Review*, pp. 30–58, 1975. This article is a revision of a paper delivered at the Ninth Annual Colloquium of the Oral History Association held at Jackson Hole, Wyo., Sept. 14, 1974.
[2] Mabel Keaton Staupers, a black nurse, had been included on the original list of leaders to be interviewed, but she was too ill to participate in this work.

385

rerouted into a socially accepted, for the times, occupation for women. Nursing was frequently looked upon as a "stopgap" until marriage, which was the socially approved ultimate goal.

A phenomenon, although slight, that bears mentioning is that today's women and men who are entering nursing come from a different socioeconomic background; that is, many have fathers and mothers who are physicians, lawyers, or college professors. They enter nursing for essentially the same altruistic-humanistic and economic reasons. Incidentally, an increasing number of people who are entering nursing have degrees, even doctoral degrees in other disciplines. They want to now pursue a career which will enable them to find a job when finished with their schooling.

Going into nursing is not, however, looked upon as a stopgap until marriage. Today's nurse has multiple roles available—marriage, family, and a career.

Marriage

Nine of the seventeen married. Of the nine, five married for the first time after age thirty. These five were active in their careers, and most stressed that they were too busy to get married before they did. Generally, they all reported "very happy" marriages. Four of the women married early in life, before age thirty, and they combined marriage and a career. Of the four, only one had children. They all emphasized that it was essential to have a supportive, helping husband. Of the five who married after age thirty, only one had children.

There were eight who never married, and the general response was that they were too busy with their careers. They all stressed that they had rich and satisfying lives, and they did not indicate any regret at not ever having married.

The Times and Types of Leaders

The *times* dictated the type of nursing leader which was needed. For example, the accreditation of nursing schools was gaining momentum as a movement. Nursing education was gradually moving into colleges and universities. There was a need for qualified faculty, curriculum revisions, and implementation. This may be one reason why about half of the seventeen leaders were deans or directors of nursing schools at one time.[3]

World War II demanded additional administrators and educators in nursing. Creative leadership, too, was necessary in research and clinical specialization because of the advances that had been made in science and technology. The nursing leaders were *thrust* into leadership positions, whereas today's leader would probably choose a leadership role.

Style

The women used different strategies to obtain their goals. Most of the leaders thought in advance quite carefully about possible strategies. In terms of decision making, they had to be willing to take risks. Some of the leaders were quite forceful and outspoken in trying to get their ideas across. Some of the leaders had creative ideas, but they had others develop them; so that in some cases the person who had the original ideas did not gain subsequent recognition.

In terms of *stature,* the leaders presented here are not even in their accomplishments and contributions. Some achieved more than others. These women were pioneers. They had a difficult time in getting their ideas accepted. Their work was not easy in that at times it provoked much controversy, and it took considerable courage and determination on their part to forge ahead. They worked tremendously hard, at times at very low salaries, and faced much resistance and many obstacles along the way; but they had strong convictions for which they fought. One dominant characteristic of the leaders was that they all liked *challenges.* When a job, though difficult, was finished, they moved on to a new challenge. The words which describe the leaders are courage, vision, and humility.

Issues

The two outstanding issues as expressed by the leaders revolved around education and the expanded role of the nurse.

---

[3] There are at present reportedly over forty deanships in nursing vacant in the United States.

Retirement

All the women who are retired are still extremely *active* in nursing as consultants, writers, and guest lecturers. In addition, they are very active in community affairs.

Oral History and Feminist Studies

In a recent article, Betty E. Mitson concludes that "oral history brings rewards beyond mere historical documentation—it yields understanding. And that, of course, is one of the fundamental purposes beyond all historical inquiry."[4] While engaged in this project, the author has been increasingly struck by the relevance of Betty Mitson's observation. Although the project was not orginally undertaken to make an explicit contribution to feminist studies, the accumulated testimony from leaders about their experiences within the nursing profession assuredly yields understanding about the plight of women in American society. Since the obstacles nursing leaders confronted and the strategies they used to cope with overt and covert discrimination parallel those of women in other professions, a brief overview of their situation in this respect might well serve as a suggestive model for oral history forays into feminist studies.

It may be recollected that one of the questions which the interviewer posed to each nursing leader was: "Why did you enter nursing?" The answers to this question have proved quite revealing because of their sexist implications. Some leaders, for example, claim that one of the determining reasons for their career choice was that they received active discouragement for aiming at something like medicine or science. This pattern is apparent in quintessential fashion in the case of Pearl Parvin Coulter, a woman who had received both a B.A. and M.S. degree in biological sciences and had taught several years in elementary school before going into nursing. Asked why, in spite of her training, she turned to nursing, she explained:

I married my professor, who was a botany teacher, but he was killed in an automobile accident. We had only been married two years. I was pretty upset over that. I then went on to medical school and took some bacteriology. I

---

[4] Betty E. Mitson, "Oral History and Japanese-American Evacuation," *The Oral History Review,* p. 51, 1974.

talked to Professor H. of the University of Colorado, and he told me he wouldn't do it if he were me. He said that women have a hard time in science, and even though he thought I had the capability, I'd have to be a whole lot better than the men, and it would be a struggle to get anywhere in that department. I'd been around the medical school and hospital so I thought I'd try nursing.[5]

Two other examples also illustrate this point. Martha E. Rogers recalls that she "toyed with the idea of law and medicine." And, while certainly not forbidden by law from entering medical school, she refrained from enrolling because "women in medicine were not particularly desirable animals in those days."[6] Another interviewee, Estelle Massey Osborne, had a brother who was a dentist. After working in his office for a while, she decided that she too wanted to be a dentist. She, too, was retarded by male chauvinism: "My brother told me very emphatically that's [dentistry] *not* a profession for women. No, nothing like that for you!"[7]

Once having entered the nursing profession, the various leaders encountered new varieties of discrimination. Sometimes the prejudice was of a racial nature and emanated both from within and outside the profession. Estelle Osborne, a black who sought leadership positions, had to fight overt racial discrimination so frequently that she seriously contemplated leaving nursing altogether. Nonetheless, she did not back off from the challenge and through struggle eventually reached a position of eminence within the profession.[8]

How would you obtain your goals?

Well, I would get mad—angry—but I always told myself, "You don't gain anything by just exploding. You think through what's the best strategy."

We had to fight for black nurses to have memberships. There would be a freeze-out. I would go to a membership meeting. See, it's one thing to say, "Yes, you can come. You can join." But when you get there, nobody sits beside you, nobody says hello. I've been in meetings where, when I have spoken,

---

[5] Pearl Parvin Coulter, Nov. 12, 1974. For a good example of how a brilliant woman faced discrimination in science, see Margaret Mead, *Ruth Benedict,* Columbia University Press, New York, 1975.

[6] Martha E. Rogers, Oct. 11, 1974.

[7] Estelle Massey Osborne, Oct. 9, 1974.

[8] For a brief biographical overview of Estelle Osborne's professional career, see Sylvia G. L. Dannett (ed.), *Profiles of Negro Womanhood,* vol. 2, Educational Heritage, Inc., Yonkers, N.Y., 1966.

they would look at me with the amazement that you would get if you bought a dog and he suddenly spoke. They would look at you with such an amazement, and no follow-up on what you said; just let it hang. So the freeze-out is a very difficult thing to take.[9]

Other times the discrimination involved inequitable salary. One interviewee, Ruth Freeman, has recounted such an episode. It takes on added significance because she, unlike many others facing similar situations, did not allow herself to be supinely victimized. For strategic reasons she turned down the opportunity to develop a nursing program at Johns Hopkins University and chose instead to become the nurse in that institution's department of public health—at a salary commensurate with her responsibilities.

I never accepted a salary less than what physicians got. I got the same salary at Johns Hopkins that they got, and more than physicians in lesser positions. At a previous job, when they started to talk to me about salary and they had placed my salary at the same level as that of the head of the nursing service, which they assumed to be satisfactory, I told them, "No, it's not satisfactory until I know what you're paying to physicians who have equivalent responsibility." I knew they were getting more and quite a substantial difference. I ended up getting it too; otherwise I would never have taken the job.[10]

Still, at other times it was necessary for the leaders to struggle against discrimination in educational opportunity. One nurse, Mary Kelly Mullane, was in a leadership position on the faculty of a midwestern university. In spite of her conviction that it was necessary for her to gain more advanced education, she met with stiff institutional resistance. .

I'd decided that I'd go and start my doctorate, but President H [of the university] wasn't happy about it. Finally, I said, "Well, I'm just going to go anyway," and he said, "That's nonsense." This was in 1949. Finally he said to me, "Well, Mary, all right. If you think that this is necessary, I'll agree with you if you'll bring me the names of a half-dozen women in your profession who think the way you do." But at that time I really had to dig to get them; but from my going to national professional meetings, I personally found six nurses with earned doctorates. I put the names on a piece of paper and put it on his [President H.'s] desk, and he looked up at me and said, "Well, in this case you're right and I'm wrong."[11]

[9] Estelle Osborne, Oct. 9, 1974.
[10] Ruth Freeman, Oct. 31, 1974.
[11] Mary Kelly Mullane, Dec. 4, 1974.

Another barrier was an attitudinal one. In relations with male colleagues within the medical or academic world, the nursing leaders encountered both those who were "people-minded" (that is, regarded them first as people and as women secondarily) and those who were "stereotype-minded" (that is, regarded them first as women and as people secondarily). More often than not they found themselves confronting the latter. At times, as in the case of Mary Kelly Mullane, this stereotypical thinking manifested itself in the form of a backhanded compliment:

You know, for most of the years of my life, at least the last fifteen years anyway, when I've been a dean, I've been the only woman in many meetings. The men would tell me, "Mary, you look like a woman, but you think like a man." Well, why should I argue with them over this? I don't think that I think like a man at all. I think that I think like an intelligent human being. I think like a scholar, that's what I think like.[12]

An unfortunate by-product of a male-dominated professional milieu was that it transformed female members into staunch upholders of sexism. Instead of finding solidarity among women in the profession, nursing leaders—as the comments which follow indicate—met with vicious competition from female colleagues.

Do you think that women help other women?

No, they most certainly do not; in fact, they block opportunities for you many times because they're jealous of you.

Many nurses have had to work very hard and things didn't come easily for them; so they figure that they don't want anyone else to get anything either—especially easier than they did.

No! No! They don't help. I never got any help from a woman—all of my support came from men.

Well, in terms of academics women have not, perhaps, helped other women because some have generally not been secure in universities, such as in getting appointed, promoted, and so on.[13]

In addition to these specific examples, there are some general conclusions which emerge from interviewing this designated nursing elite that have implications for feminist studies. First, most of them were not prepared for specific leadership, but instead had leadership roles thrust

---

[12] Ibid.

[13] The final observation is by Helen Nahm, Feb. 11, 1975. The identities of the three previous respondents have been withheld by request.

upon them as a result of circumstances. Secondly, most of the leaders were forced to choose between marriage and a career. Questionnaire responses reveal that of the seventeen, eight never married, and five married for the first time after the age of thirty.

These conclusions raise questions which can profitably be pursued by others researching women in leadership positions outside the field of nursing. For example, how does the social climate differ today in creating opportunities for women? How and why do women enter the fields they do? What is their career trajectory? What are the social costs involved for those achieving leadership roles? What are the comparative opportunities for men and women who choose the same vocation?

Although answers may further expose the sexist basis of American life, the accompanying consciousness that such knowledge brings can serve as a starting point between bridging the gap between the "is" and the "ought" of American ideals and practices. Viewed in this sense, oral history can be seen as a tool of social reorientation, an instrument in forging a truly free and open American culture.